Thieme

# Surgical Techniques in Moyamoya Vasculopathy

## Tricks of the Trade

**Peter Vajkoczy, MD**
Professor
Chairman, Department of Neurosurgery and Pediatric Neurosurgery
Charité Universitätsmedizin Berlin
Berlin, Germany

471 illustrations

Thieme
Stuttgart • New York • Delhi • Rio de Janeiro

**Library of Congress Cataloging-in-Publication Data** is available from the publisher

Illustrator: Lucius Fekonja, Berlin, Germany



Georg Thieme Verlag KG
Rüdigerstrasse 14, 70469 Stuttgart, Germany
+49 [0]711 8931 421, customerservice@thieme.de

Thieme Publishers New York
333 Seventh Avenue, New York, NY 10001 USA
+1 800 782 3488, customerservice@thieme.com

Thieme Publishers Delhi
A-12, Second Floor, Sector-2, Noida-201301
Uttar Pradesh, India
+91 120 45 566 00, customerservice@thieme.in

Thieme Publishers Rio de Janeiro,
Thieme Publicações Ltda.
Edifício Rodolpho de Paoli, 25º andar
Av. Nilo Peçanha, 50 – Sala 2508
Rio de Janeiro 20020-906 Brasil
+55 21 3172 2297

Cover design: Thieme Publishing Group
Cover illustration: Lucius Fekonja, Berlin, Germany
Typesetting by Thomson Digital, India

Printed in Germany by CPI Books 5 4 3 2 1

ISBN 978-3-13-145061-6

Also available as an e-book:
eISBN 978-3-13-147081-2



MIX
Papier aus verantwortungsvollen Quellen
FSC www.fsc.org FSC® C083411

# Contents

## Part 2 Indirect Revascularization

# Foreword

I have to admit that during the course of my professional career, I have not encountered anything as fascinating as moyamoya disease (MMD). I can still remember those days when MMD was considered a rare disease, mostly seen in patients from Japan, where it was originally described more than 50 years ago. It was fascinating to see the unusual cerebral angiograms of these patients, showing steno-occlusive changes to the brain-supplying arteries in combination with numerous newly formed small collateral channels at the base of the brain. These changes were difficult to comprehend, particularly when compared with vascular changes noticed in common cerebral ischemia. When it came to treating these patients, we had the option of choosing from a variety of procedures, again mostly introduced by our colleagues from Japan. These procedures were later on summarized under the broad category of "indirect cerebral revascularization." Moreover, it was found more difficult from a technical point of view to perform an extraintracranial arterial bypass using the superficial temporal artery as the donor vessel. This was, however, not because the epicerebral recipient vessels were smaller in diameter in comparison to the situation in chronic cerebral ischemia. It was discovered later on that the cortical arteries in patients with MMD have a different morphologic design, with a thinner structure of the arterial wall, which in turn requires increased attention and a greater amount of skills when performing a direct end-to-side anastomosis.

Initially, we came across these patients only rarely, maybe two or three cases per year. But this has changed drastically over the years. At the end of my career, the number of patients with MMD had increased to about 30 to 40 per year, and it was no longer a local phenomenon. Meanwhile, sizable clinical series of patients with MMD have been published from centers all over the world.

So, what do we know now about MMD that we did not know 25 years ago? The lessons from clinical experience and related research data have further substantiated that MMD is a particular form of ischemic cerebral disease that can be differentiated from more common entities of cerebrovascular occlusive disease beyond characteristic angiographic findings. Based on functional studies, we now know that MMD is representative of hemodynamic cerebrovascular insufficiency. A further distinctive feature of MMD is the unique capability of the brain to create new collateral inflow channels to compensate for the impaired blood flow due to the underlying steno-occlusive process within the basal arteries. This is clearly illustrated in patients with advanced MMD, where angiographic findings demonstrate arterial collaterals from meningeal and even extracranial arteries, which is never observed in common cerebrovascular diseases. Considering this observation, surgical revascularization is the logical treatment of choice in patients with MMD.

In fact, it can be viewed as an enhancement of an underlying and ongoing natural process. Even in the absence of randomized clinical trials, it is now generally accepted that surgical revascularization is the only effective treatment for patients with MMD. This is further supported by clinical information derived from large postoperative follow-up studies.

It should be mentioned that this is good news for the field of vascular neurosurgery in general. It was not long ago that in the larger context of vascular neurosurgery, MMD was only mentioned under the heading "miscellaneous." The situation is significantly different now; with extraintracranial bypass surgery for cerebral ischemia becoming obsolete, patients with cerebral aneurysms are increasingly being treated by interventional means, and patients with cerebral AV malformations are being referred to stereotactic radiosurgery. In view of these developments, it is difficult to provide a young colleague with an interest in vascular neurosurgery with good advice on what to do in the future, and I am happy that I do not have to answer this question for myself. However, I'm convinced that the management of patients with MMD will become more important in the future, especially in view of the fact that this disease is still underdiagnosed. It is also good to know that each patient with MMD is usually a candidate for two surgical procedures. There is obviously great potential for further research activities in relation to MMD.

This would not only include research on epidemiology and genetics of MMD but also on its pathophysiology, based on contemporary techniques of molecular biology and other techniques that have become available more recently. We require further information on questions such as what is the optimal surgical technique, if there is one, and if we should use different surgical approaches for pediatric and adult patients with MMD.

We also need more long-term follow-up studies involving our operated patients, and I am quite sure that there will be more surprises.

Finally, coming back to my personal fascination with MMD that I mentioned in the beginning, let me give you another example for purposes of illustration.

I found it most intriguing to study postoperative angiograms in patients who underwent a combined revascularization procedure 1 or 2 years earlier.

It was amazing to see the number and size of the muscular arterial branches that had ingrown and found connection with the cortical arterial network!

Sometimes, it is difficult to differentiate these newly formed muscular branches from the original extraintracranial arterial bypass. This is another unique feature of MMD, and one wonders if the identification of this mechanism or the isolation of the factor that enables this ingrowth of vessels into the brain could be used for the treatment of other ischemic brain conditions as well.

I am grateful that my long-term coworker Peter Vajkoczy has obviously inherited this interest in MMD, and I will follow his future work with great interest.

*Peter Schmiedek, MD*
*Emeritus Professor of Neurosurgery*
*Mannheim, Germany*

# Preface

Moyamoya vasculopathy (MMV) is a rare cerebrovascular disease that is characterized by bilateral progressive steno-occlusion of basal cerebral arteries, with the emergence of coexisting abnormal net-like vessels. In moyamoya disease, MMV is the single manifestation, whereas in moyamoya syndrome or quasi-moyamoya, MMV is associated with a potentially underlying disease such as a genetic disorder or other coexisting pathology. Although MMV is most frequent in Asian countries, it is ranked among the most frequent causes of stroke in children and adults across the world. The incidence of MMV is on the rise due to increasing awareness of the disease.

The relevance of surgical treatment of moyamoya disease by way of bypass revascularization is undisputed, which is in contrast to the surgical treatment of atherosclerotic carotid artery occlusion. The main aims of revascularization are to restore the blood supply to stabilize cerebrovascular hemodynamics and to regress the fragile moyamoya vessels in order to prevent bleeding. A successful improvement or normalization of cerebral hemodynamics will then result in secondary stroke prevention and improved neurological or neurocognitive outcome. Consequently, bypass surgery for MMV has become an integral part of the clinical practice of many microvascular neurosurgeons around the world. While the role of bypass surgery is well accepted, a versatile range of surgical techniques and strategies exists in the field, which makes it difficult to determine and appreciate the subtle nuances of the varied surgical strategies.

Therefore, it seemed logical to create an instructive manual for neurosurgeons with a step-by-step guide to the surgical techniques. The focus of this book is on introducing neurosurgeons (and other physicians involved in the treatment of these patients) to the different surgical techniques, to the inherent strengths and weaknesses of each technique, and to the surgical considerations that need to be kept in mind. We are grateful to the contributing authors, who are all authorities in their respective fields, for sharing their unique knowledge and expertise with the readers. The descriptions provided by each of them are characterized by an expert assessment of the distinct surgical techniques and their variations, as well as by a standardized illustration of the surgical steps. This book will thus serve as the key manual for everyone interested in the treatment of these complexities and for those who find it a rewarding experience to treat these patients.

*Peter Vajkoczy, MD*

# Contributors

**Sepideh Amin-Hanjani, MD**
Department of Neurosurgery
University of Illinois at Chicago
Chicago, Illinois, USA

**Gregory D. Arnone, MD**
Department of Neurosurgery
Penn State College of Medicine
Hershey, Pennsylvania, USA

**Thomas Blauwblomme, MD**
Department of Pediatric Neurosurgery
Hospital Necker
Assistance Publique Hôpitaux de Paris (APHP)
Université René Descartes, PRES Sorbonne Paris Cité
Paris, France

**Kees P.J. Braun, MD**
Department of Neurology and Neurosurgery
UMC Utrecht Brain Center
Utrecht, The Netherlands

**Fady T. Charbel, MD, FAANS, FACS**
Professor and Head, Department of Neurosurgery
Richard L. and Gertrude W. Fruin Professor
University of Illinois at Chicago
Chicago, Illinois, USA

**Marcus Czabanka, MD**
Professor and Vice Chairman
Department of Neurosurgery
Charité Universitätsmedizin Berlin
Berlin, Germany

**Giuseppe Esposito, MD, PhD**
Neurosurgeon, Senior Physician
Department of Neurosurgery
Clinical Neurocenter
University Hospital Zurich
University of Zurich
Zurich, Switzerland

**Jorn Fierstra, MD, PhD**
Department of Neurosurgery
Clinical Neurocenter
University Hospital Zurich
University of Zurich
Zurich, Switzerland

**Bettina Föhre, MD**
Consultant of Anesthesiology
Department of Anesthesiology and Operative Intensive Care Medicine (CCM/CVK)
Charité Universitätsmedizin Berlin
Berlin, Germany

**Menno R. Germans, MD**
Neurosurgeon
Department of Neurosurgery
University Hospital Zurich
Zurich, Switzerland

**Nestor R. Gonzalez, MD, MSCR, FAANS, FAHA**
Professor of Neurosurgery
Director, Neurovascular Laboratory
Neuroendovascular Fellowship Program Director
Cedars-Sinai Medical Center
Advanced Health Sciences Pavilion (AHSP)
Los Angeles, California, USA

**Ziad A. Hage, MD, FAANS**
Novant Health Presbyterian Medical Center
Adjunct Associate Professor
Campbell University
School of Osteopathic Medicine
Charlotte, North Carolina, USA

**Nils Hecht, MD**
Department of Neurosurgery
Charité Universitätsmedizin Berlin
Berlin, Germany

**Satoshi Hori, MD, PhD**
Department of Neurosurgery
Graduate School of Medicine and Pharmacological Science
University of Toyama
Toyama, Japan

**Kiyohiro Houkin, MD**
Department of Neurosurgery
Faculty of Medicine
Hokkaido University
Sapporo, Japan

**Hao Jiang, MD**
Department of Neurosurgery
The First Affiliated Hospital
Zhejiang University School of Medicine
Hangzhou, China

**Jeremiah N. Johnson, MD, FAANS**
Assistant Professor
Department of Neurosurgery
Baylor College of Medicine
Houston, Texas USA

**Akitsugu Kawashima, MD, PhD**
Chief, Department of Neurosurgery
Tokyo Women's Medical University Yachiyo Medical Center
Chiba, Japan

**Ken Kazumata, MD, PhD**
Department of Neurosurgery
Hokkaido University Graduate School of Medicine
Sapporo, Japan

**Catharina J.M. Klijn, MD**
Department of Neurology and Neurosurgery
UMC Utrecht Brain Center
Utrecht, The Netherlands
Department of Neurology
Donders Institute for Brain, Cognition and Behavior
Center for Neuroscience
Radboud University Medical Center
Nijmegen, The Netherlands

**Susanne König, MD, DESA**
Consultant of Anesthesiology
Department of Anesthesiology and Operative Intensive Care Medicine (CCM/CVK)
Charité Universitätsmedizin Berlin
Berlin, Germany

**Annick Kronenburg, MD**
Department of Neurology and Neurosurgery
UMC Utrecht Brain Center
Utrecht, The Netherlands

**Satoshi Kuroda, MD, PhD**
Professor and Chairman
Department of Neurosurgery
Graduate School of Medicine and Pharmaceutical Science
University of Toyama
Toyama, Japan

**David J. Langer, MD**
Department of Neurosurgery
Hofstra North Shore–Long Island Jewish School of Medicine
Lenox Hill Hospital
New York, New York, USA

**Philippe Meyer, MD**
Department of Pediatric Anesthesiology
Hospital Necker
Assistance Publique Hôpitaux de Paris (APHP)
Paris, France

**Alessandro Narducci, MD**
Division of Neurosurgery
San Giovanni Bosco Hospital
Turin, Italy

**Erez Nossek, MD**
Division of Neurosurgery
Maimonides Medical Center
Brooklyn, New York, USA

**Luca Regli, MD**
Professor and Chairman
Department of Neurosurgery
Clinical Neurocenter
University Hospital Zurich
University of Zurich
Zurich, Switzerland

**Christian Sainte-Rose, MD**
Department of Pediatric Neurosurgery
Hospital Necker
Assistance Publique Hôpitaux de Paris (APHP)
Université René Descartes, PRES Sorbonne Paris Cité
Paris, France

**Michael Schiraldi, MD, PhD**
Neurosurgeon
Institute of Clinical Orthopedics & Neurosciences
Desert Regional Medical Center
Palm Springs, California, USA

**Edward Smith, MD**
Department of Neurosurgery
Boston Children's Hospital
Harvard Medical School
Boston, Massachusetts, USA

**Robert F. Spetzler, MD**
Department of Neurosurgery
Barrow Neurological Institute
St. Joseph's Hospital and Medical Center
Phoenix, Arizona, USA

**Gary K. Steinberg, MD, PhD**
Bernard and Ronni Lacroute-William Randolph Hearst Professor of Neurosurgery and the Neurosciences
Chair, Department of Neurosurgery
Stanford University School of Medicine
Stanford, California, USA

**Mario Teo, MBChB(Hons), FRCS(SN)**
Consultant Neurosurgeon
Department of Neurosurgery
Bristol Institute of Clinical Neuroscience
North Bristol University Hospital
Bristol, UK

**Peter Vajkoczy, MD**
Professor
Chairman, Department of Neurosurgery and Pediatric Neurosurgery
Charité Universitätsmedizin Berlin
Berlin, Germany

**John E. Wanebo, MD**
Department of Neurosurgery
Barrow Neurological Institute
St. Joseph's Hospital and Medical Center
Phoenix, Arizona, USA

**Bin Xu, MD, PhD**
Department of Neurosurgery, Huashan Hospital
Shanghai Medical School, Fudan University
Shanghai, China

**Albert van der Zwan, MD**
Department of Neurology and Neurosurgery
UMC Utrecht Brain Center
Utrecht, The Netherlands

# Part 1

## General Concepts

# 1 Perioperative Management and Considerations

*Bettina Föhre and Susanne König*

**Abstract**

Typically in patients with moyamoya disease (MMD), the cerebrovascular reactivity and the cerebral hemodynamic reserve capacity are impaired, causing transient ischemic attack (TIA) or stroke. Therefore the superior aim of anesthetic management for revascularization procedures is to ensure the adequate perfusion and oxygenation of the brain to avoid ischemic episodes.

Special attention is paid to maintain the systolic blood pressure between 120 and 140 mm Hg perioperatively, to avoid hypo- and hypertension and to ensure normoxemia, normocapnia, and normovolemia with crystalloids.

The two concepts of a propofol-based anesthesia and an inhalational anesthesia, either in combination with a short-acting analgesic agent, are both established for surgery in moyamoya patients. The authors favor the total intravenous anesthesia, because of the lower rate of postoperative nausea and vomiting and the better preservation of the regional cortical blood flow in the frontal lobe.

Postoperatively early extubation for an immediate neurological assessment is usually attempted. It demands adequate analgesia and often the use of alpha- or beta-blocking agents to ensure a smooth, stressless, and hemodynamically controlled awakening.

*Keywords:* impaired hemodynamic reserve capacity, ischemic episodes, normotension, normocapnia, total intravenous anesthesia, early neurological assessment

## 1.1 Physiology

### 1.1.1 Basic Physiology of Cerebral Blood Flow

The normal cerebral blood flow (CBF) of 50 mL/100 g/min$^{-1}$ is dependent on cerebral perfusion pressure (CPP), i.e., the difference between mean arterial pressure and intracranial pressure (MAP – ICP).

Three main principles regulate CBF: (1) flow-metabolism coupling, (2) autoregulation, and (3) carbon dioxide ($CO_2$) reactivity. In regions of increased metabolic activity the local CBF is increased by vasodilation of arterioles to deliver more oxygen and glucose, whereas vasoconstriction is encountered in phases of diminished activity.

In healthy adults, cerebral autoregulation keeps CBF constant within blood pressure ranges between 50 and 150 mm Hg, thus preventing cerebral ischemia. Cerebral vessels react to arterial partial pressure of carbon dioxide ($PaCO_2$) by responding to hypercapnia with vasodilation and vice versa.

As described in the Monro-Kellie doctrine, the intracranial volume is the sum of brain tissue, intracranial blood volume, and cerebrospinal fluid and is limited by the non-expandable skull.

The ICP-volume curve is nonlinear and shows the relationship between intracranial volume and ICP. When the initial intracranial volume is low and compensatory mechanisms are not exhausted, an increase in intracranial volume produces a small change in ICP. On the steep part of the curve a similar increase of intracranial volume results in a large increase of ICP, resulting in a decrease of CPP, respectively CBF (▶ Fig. 1.1).

### 1.1.2 What Is Different in Patients with Moyamoya Disease?

Moyamoya is characterized by chronic progressive stenotic to occlusive changes in the terminal parts of the intracranial internal carotid arteries including the proximal parts of anterior and middle cerebral arteries. A compensatory fine vascular network is developed. Classically, moyamoya disease (MMD) is present bilaterally, but may also develop unilaterally. In these compromised areas, the cerebrovascular reactivity and the cerebral hemodynamic reserve capacity are impaired, causing transient ischemic attacks (TIAs) or strokes.[1] The risk of impaired autoregulation may be even higher in pediatric patients.[2]

Furthermore, the fragile moyamoya vessels are prone to hemorrhage. Typically, CBF shows a paradoxic reactivity to a vasodilatory stimulus in the altered areas. The altered moyamoya vessels are already maximally dilated to provide adequate oxygen supply and perfusion to the brain tissue. These vessels cannot react to a stimulus like hypercapnia the way normal vessels do. Thus, in a hypercapnic state flow will increase in brain areas of preserved normal vasculature and decrease in moyamoya affected vessels, leading to insufficient perfusion. This regional redistribution of blood flow to healthy areas is called "steal phenomenon"[3] and might clinically present as a neurologic deficit.

## 1.2 Anesthesia

### 1.2.1 Choice of Anesthesia Technique

The superior aim of anesthesia for revascularization procedures is to ensure adequate perfusion and oxygenation of the brain and to avoid ischemic episodes. The ideal anesthetic agent should deliver smooth and hemodynamically stable anesthesia, good operating conditions ("slack brain"), and a smooth and rapid emergence to allow early neurological assessment. Cerebral perfusion pressure should be maintained, autoregulation and $CO_2$ reactivity should be preserved.

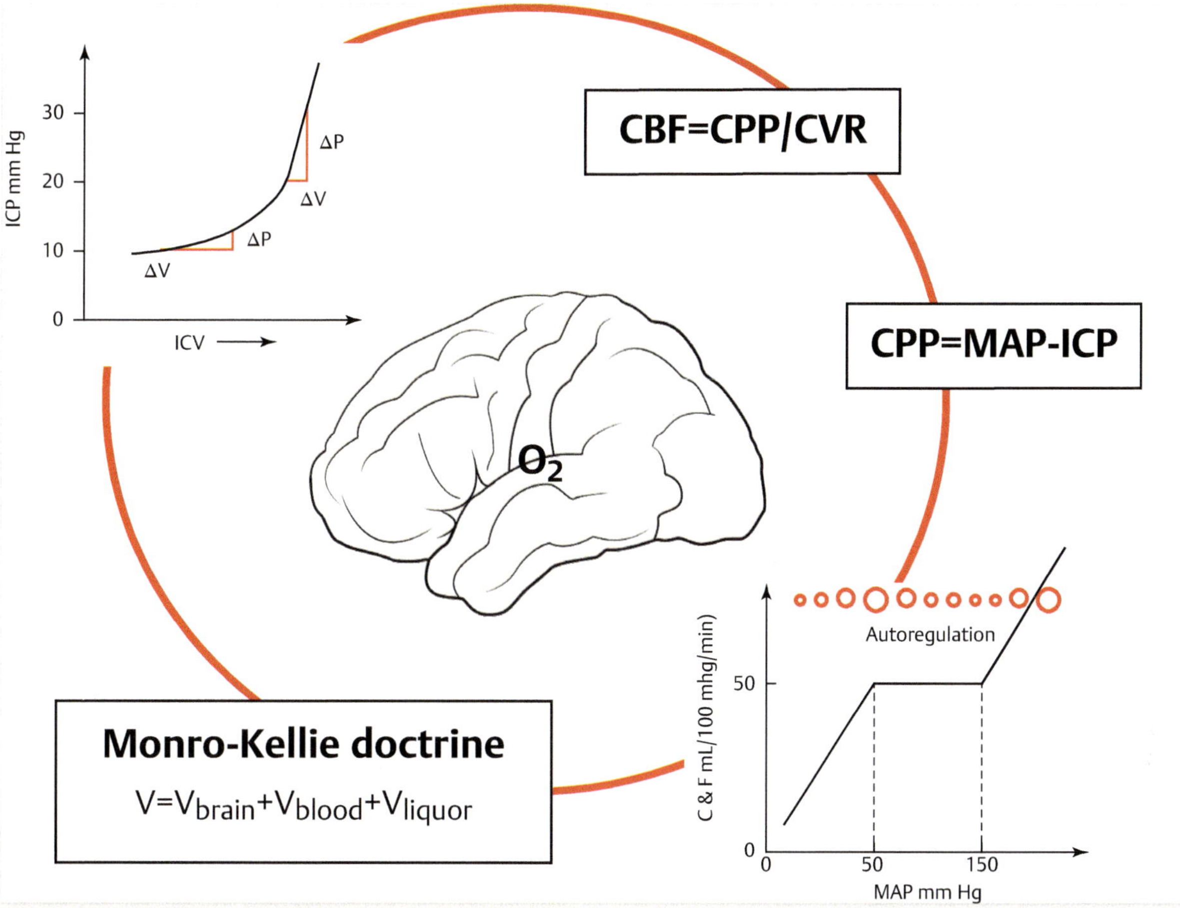


**Fig. 1.1** Basic physiology of cerebral blood flow.

There are some studies that have investigated propofol-maintained versus inhalational-maintained anesthesia in adult patients undergoing elective craniotomy. Both strategies were associated with similar brain relaxation, although mean ICP values were lower and CPP values higher with propofol-maintained anesthesia. The recovery profiles, e.g., eye opening, tracheal extubation, obeying verbal commands, and orientation varied only in the range of minutes without clinical significance. Also the incidence of postoperative pain, seizures, and agitation were similar with both techniques. Nevertheless, the incidence of postoperative nausea and vomiting (PONV) was significantly lower during propofol-maintained anesthesia.[4]

Concerning moyamoya patients, both anesthetic concepts are established and no significant differences in patient outcome were noted. Rather the carefully titrated induction drugs and good control of blood pressure, oxygenation, and stability of $CO_2$ level are determinative.[5]

In authors' opinion, there are some important arguments in favor of total intravenous anesthesia: the lower rate of PONV,[6] the better preservation of the regional cortical blood flow in the frontal lobe in comparison to sevoflurane,[7] the occurrence of steal phenomenon with inhalational anesthesia,[8] and finally, a positive practical experience with this technique for intracranial surgery over the past 20 years in their center.

## 1.2.2 Preoperative Evaluation and Premedication

Patients with MMD often present with many other medical conditions, which may impact anesthetic management. Therefore, a profound preoperative anesthetic assessment is necessary and special attention should be paid to the preexisting neurologic deficits and the neurologic physical status. Motor deficits or epilepsy are signals of chronic ischemia. A history of frequent TIAs, prolonged intermittent neurologic deficits, or stroke should draw attention to an already impaired cerebral blood supply in these patients, and has been identified as a significant risk factor for perioperative complications.[9] Preoperative evaluation must also include the determination of the individual baseline blood pressure, which involves several measurements before the day of surgery. A comparative blood pressure measurement on both arms is recommended to exclude falsely low blood pressure measurement intraoperatively due to, for example, subclavian artery stenosis.

Hypertension is found in some patients as a compensatory mechanism for cerebral vascular insufficiency. Caution is necessary when attempting to treat an elevated blood pressure in these patients.

Special attention has to be paid to the patient's chronic medication. Anticonvulsive and antihypertensive medication should be continued until the day of surgery.

Regarding the antiplatelet-medication in MMD patients, the practice of continuing the medication varies among centers. The perioperative application of aspirin and the postoperative antiplatelet therapy have become controversial. Some centers are giving antiplatelet-medication while others have abandoned them. In our center we determine the effectiveness of aspirin in each patient through a platelet-function test. Thereby detected aspirin nonresponders receive alternative antiplatelet agents.[10]

Premedication should be prescribed carefully. Anxiolysis may be necessary and beneficial in children with MMD, as crying should be strictly avoided, because the resultant hyperventilation may lead to hypocapnia and consecutively to cerebral vasoconstriction, resulting in cerebral ischemia. Vice versa oversedation followed by hypoventilation should also be avoided.

Midazolam is most often used for premedication, but other drugs can also be used.[11]

## 1.2.3 Monitoring

The American Society of Anesthesiologists (ASA) standard monitoring should be extended to invasive arterial blood pressure monitoring and urine output measurement. Anesthesiologists should consider placing the arterial line prior to induction, especially if preexisting medical conditions prompt it, and if the procedure is not considered too stressful for the patient.

Continuous arterial blood pressure monitoring intra- and postoperatively is the key for keeping the blood pressure within a predefined range (see Chapter 1.2.4).

Adequate venous access is essential and can be established by two "well-running" intravenous lines. A central venous catheter is not mandatory but should be considered in patients with very poor venous access or severe coexisting medical conditions.

Cerebral function can be monitored in various ways. Most reliable techniques are the combined transcranial motor-evoked potentials (MEP) and sensory-evoked potentials (SEP) monitoring. Cerebral function monitoring is of crucial importance especially in pediatric patients and in unstable adult patients, because they may experience strokes even after short-term blood pressure drops. Electroencephalography can help identify focal slowing, indicating a compromise CBF. Although near-infrared spectroscopy (NIRS) is only validated for measurement of cerebral oxygen saturation on the forehead, it has been shown that a sustained drop in regional oxygen saturation is closely related to the occurrence of neurological events following surgery,[12] and thus NIRS may provide useful information intraoperatively.

## 1.2.4 Targets of Anesthesia

### Hemodynamics: What Is the Optimal Blood Pressure?

It is very important to have appropriate hemodynamic conditions throughout the perioperative period. Reduction in CBF is poorly tolerated, especially in children because they have a diminished autoregulatory response and a higher cerebral metabolic rate.[5]

Hypotension may cause ischemia or threaten the graft patency because of developing thrombosis. Hypertension may lead to bleeding or cause a hyperperfusion syndrome with clinical symptoms such as an ischemic attack (see also Chapter 1.4.2).

There is not the one optimal blood pressure for all MMD patients. Generally it is recommended to maintain the blood pressure normotensive or to keep it within 10 to 20% of the preoperatively established baseline.[11,13] Some MMD patients induce hypertension and are dependent on higher systolic blood pressure levels. Therefore, the systolic blood pressure target should be determined for the individual MMD patient between the surgeon and the anesthesiologist. It is of tremendous importance to maintain the blood pressure stable perioperatively within the defined limits. According to our experience, in case of hypertensive adult MMD patients, we suggest to keep the systolic blood pressure 20% above the individual baseline systolic blood pressure. For normotensive adult patients, we suggest to keep the systolic blood pressure at 140 mm Hg. The individual baseline systolic blood pressure can function as the lower threshold for the systolic blood pressure.

Careful and smooth titration of anesthetic drugs for induction, maintenance of anesthesia as well as anticipating cardiovascular responses to surgical stimuli is very important for blood pressure control. Episodes of hypotension should be treated immediately with vasoactive drugs, e.g., norepinephrine or phenylephedrine.

The postoperative goal for blood pressure maintenance should be consented with the surgeon. The target blood pressure depends on the quality and diameter (which determines also the flow) of the bypass. It is also to be taken into consideration if additional indirect techniques have been performed, for example, encephalo-myo-synangiosis. Hyperperfusion of the brain has to be strictly avoided as well as insufficient flow and hypoperfusion. Thus, no general rule can be given.[5] An appropriate analgesic management has to be established before emergence from anesthesia and during the postoperative period to prevent hypertensive episodes. Vasodilating drugs such as urapidil or labetalol should be kept handy.

### How to Ventilate the Patient?

Normocapnia should be the target of ventilation, regardless of the ventilator mode chosen. The arterial $pCO_2$ should range between 39 and 43 mm Hg, because the cortical blood flow is maximal in this range.[14,15] A retrospective analysis of 124 children undergoing surgery for MMD showed that those patients who suffered from postoperative ischemic complications had intraoperatively $PaCO_2$ levels significantly above 45 mm Hg. If additional risk factors (preoperative TIA) were present, the incidence of postoperative ischemic complications was even higher.[9] This is consistent with a recent investigation of adult MMD patients. It has been demonstrated that hemodynamically unstable Berlin Moyamoya Grade 3 patients (severe MMD) have the highest risk for perioperative ischemia.[16]

The collateral network of vessels in patients with MMD is in a state of maximal vasodilation. When healthy vessels dilate in response to hypercapnia, they steal the blood from the hemodynamically compromised areas (of maximal vasodilation).[5,8] See Chapter 1.1.2.

## 1.2.5 Induction and Maintenance

### Induction

The major aim of anesthesia induction in MMD patients is to perform a smooth induction, not to allow blood pressure to swing between hypertension and hypotension, as well as to avoid hyperventilation, hypoventilation, and hypoxemia.

In children, it is recommended to carefully guide the separation from the parents before anesthesia to prevent crying and thus an increase of ICP or hyperventilation. Intubation should be performed in a deeply anesthetized patient to avoid any hemodynamic effect.

For intravenous induction the choice of agents includes propofol, thiopental, or etomidate.

Also in children, intravenous induction has some advantage over inhalational induction. For the latter, sevoflurane is the agent of choice. Intravenous opioids are recommended to attenuate the response to laryngoscopy and tracheal intubation. The authors prefer the short-acting remifentanil. Administration may be started at a low dose before the induction agent is applied (e.g., remifentanil 0.1 µg/kg BW/min for 5 minutes) and then continued and increased in dosage (e.g., 0.2–0.3 µg/kg BW/min) throughout the procedure as part of the total intravenous anesthesia (TIVA). Bolus administration of fentanyl (e.g., 3–3.5 µg/kg BW) for induction and repetitive doses throughout surgery is another option.

The ideal choice for muscle relaxation is a nondepolarizing agent, unlikely to cause hemodynamic changes or histamine release.[11,13,17]

### Temperature

Body temperature should be monitored throughout the procedure and measures should be taken to maintain normal body temperature. The proposed beneficial effect of mild hypothermia reduces the cerebral metabolic rate and thus protects the brain against hypoxia and ischemia to some degree. However, as to date, no randomized controlled trial has been conducted to show the benefit of hypothermia for vascular patients in neurosurgery.

Moreover, hypothermia bears the risk of increased bleeding by compromising coagulation and may further precipitate postoperative shivering, and thus increase cerebral metabolic rate.

### Indocyanine Green

Anesthesiologists might be asked to administer an intravenous bolus of indocyanine green (ICG) during bypass surgery. ICG video-angiography visualizes the patency of a bypass graft. Technically the angiography requires a microscope with an integrated ICG camera that applies near-infrared light on the surgical field.

ICG is delivered as a powder (25 mg) that has to be diluted in 5 cc of distilled water. Usually the applied dose ranges between 5 and 25 mg. Following the intravenous ICG injection, a short period of "falsely low" pulse oximetry values has to be anticipated due to the dye. ICG is administered in close communication with the surgeon either through a well running intravenous line or a central line, which is immediately flushed with a bolus of 20 cc sodium chloride.

ICG is generally a safe drug, nevertheless, cases have been reported of patients who showed adverse reaction to the ICG injection, especially hypotension.[18]

### Volume Management

Perioperative fluid management should aim at maintaining normovolemia.

The holding of packed red blood cells or fresh frozen plasma for the surgical procedure should be agreed upon with the surgeon in each institution, depending on the average need for transfusion for the procedure. Intraoperatively, it is crucial to check hemoglobin and hematocrit values regularly. Severe anemia should be treated. There is no ideal hematocrit or hemoglobin level for all MMD patients, but polycythemia should be avoided as much as pronounced hemodilution, because both can lead to cerebral ischemia, the latter by reducing the oxygen-carrying capacity of the blood.[5,13]

## 1.2.6 Emergence

The major target at emergence is a smooth and hemodynamically controlled awakening. Extubation may be performed in the operating room (OR) if feasible, to allow for immediate neurological assessment. At the end of surgery an individual blood pressure range should be agreed upon between surgeon and anesthesiologist individualized for each patient, and any deviations should be treated immediately. Usually, the range for systolic blood pressure in adult patients will be set between 120 and 140 mm Hg. Blood pressure increases may occur during patient awakening and should be carefully treated with a well-controllable antihypertensive agent, e.g., with a beta-blocking agent (e.g., esmolol) or alpha-blocking agent urapidil (the latter is not available in United States and Canada). It is also crucial to prevent coughing or shivering and to administer sufficient pain relief.

Sufficient spontaneous ventilation will aid to maintain normocapnia, which should be regularly controlled via $PaCO_2$ measurement through blood gas analysis. Adequate oxygen supply may be assured through oxygen insufflation via a nasal line. An oxygen mask should be avoided, since the straps put direct pressure on the side of the head where bypass surgery had just been performed.

**Key Points**

**Pathophysiologic considerations**

Impaired autoregulation
Reduced cerebral hemodynamic reserve capacity
Steal phenomenon

**Preoperative evaluation**

Attention to previous transient ischemic attacks (TIAs), preexisting neurologic deficits
Stage of hemodynamic failure (see Chapter 1.2.2)
Concomitant disease
Antiplatelet and anticoagulation management of your center

**Anesthetic goals**

Adequate cerebral perfusion
Normotension, within 10–20% of baseline blood pressure
Normoxia, elevate fraction of inspired oxygen ($FiO_2$) to 1.0 during temporary occlusion
Normocapnia
Normothermia
Normovolemia
Prefer propofol and a short-acting opioid
Sufficient analgesia intra- and postoperatively
Prevent hypo- and hypertension, hypo- and hypercapnia

**Monitoring**

Electrocardiogram, pulse oximetry, noninvasive blood pressure (BP)
Arterial line for invasive BP
Intravenous lines
Central venous catheter if required by concomitant disease
Urine output, body temperature
Near-infrared spectroscopy (NIRS)

**Postoperative care**

Transfer to intensive care unit
BP control within set limits
Ensure graft perfusion (antiplatelet or anticoagulation)

# 1.3 Postoperative Care for Moyamoya Disease Patients

## 1.3.1 Where?

Patients are transferred under continuous monitoring and care from the OR to an intensive care or postanesthesia care unit, where they are monitored overnight. Discharge to the normal ward should be decided the next morning, after neurologic examination and depending on the patient's well-being.

Blood pressure, oxygen saturation, hematocrit, volume status, and urine output should be closely monitored in the postoperative period. Maintaining normovolemia and avoiding blood pressure exaggeration is crucial. Neurologic examination has to be performed frequently to identify ischemia at an early state.[13]

## 1.3.2 Pain Control

Good analgesia is an important factor in reducing the risk of postoperative cerebral ischemia or infarction. In children, pain relief can also help avoid crying and associated negative effects of hyperventilation and hypocapnia. Pain management can be performed according to the institution's standards. Early after surgery, opioids will usually be part of the regimen. There are several options, e.g., piritramid (which is not approved in the United States), morphine, or fentanyl, which can be applied by titrating intravenous doses or by continuous infusion, the latter only if the patient is permanently monitored for signs of ventilatory suppression. Of note, when anesthesia was performed with a short-acting agent such as remifentanil, adequate additional analgesia, e.g., with an opioid such as morphine, has to be applied before emergence.

Additionally a peripherally acting analgesic should be applied before emergence, such as paracetamol or metamizol.

Placement of a skull block may be a useful addition to anesthesia in MMD patients. It has been shown to be helpful in children during encephalo-duro-arterio-myo synagiosis (EDAMS) surgery, providing calm awakening and lower analgesic requirements postoperatively.[19]

# 1.4 Threats of Anesthesia for Moyamoya Disease Surgery

Prevention of any deterioration of cerebral perfusion is pivotal in the care of MMD patients.

## 1.4.1 Ischemic Stroke and Transient Ischemic Attacks

Transitory ischemic attacks can occur as a result of inappropriate cerebral perfusion and cannot be reliably detected while the patient is under anesthesia. Alternatively, a graft thrombosis may be the cause. As pointed out previously, hypotension or suboptimal blood pressure control has to be strictly avoided intra- and postoperatively. Generally, the controlled mild hypertension is of greatest relevance to prevent ischemic events in MMD patients. Clinicians should keep in mind the increased risk for ischemic complications in patients with a history of TIAs (see also Chapter 1.2.2). Patients undergoing indirect revascularization procedures will have a persistent risk for cerebral ischemia until the neovascularization has been completed, which may require months.

Intraoperatively bypass patency should be assessed directly and/or with ICG spectroscopy by the surgeon. Postoperatively, transcranial Doppler evaluation or perfusion CT/MRI are valuable diagnostic tools.

## 1.4.2 Cerebral Hyperperfusion Syndrome

Typically in moyamoya patients the diseased vessels are already maximally vasodilated and show little autoregulatory capacity. The low-flow superficial temporal artery to middle cerebral artery (STA–MCA) bypass might lead to cerebral hyperperfusion in a previously poorly perfused cerebral vascular bed, often presenting as a transient neurological deterioration or an ischemic attack.

Furthermore, cerebral hyperperfusion may lead to intracranial hemorrhage with potentially fatal outcome, thus underlining the emphasis which has to be put onto a strict blood pressure control.

# References


[1] Kuwabara Y, Ichiya Y, Sasaki M, et al. Response to hypercapnia in moyamoya disease. Cerebrovascular response to hypercapnia in pediatric and adult patients with moyamoya disease. Stroke. 1997; 28(4):701–707

[2] Lee JK, Williams M, Jennings JM, et al. Cerebrovascular autoregulation in pediatric moyamoya disease. Paediatr Anaesth. 2013; 23(6):547–556

[3] Han JS, Abou-Hamden A, Mandell DM, et al. Impact of extracranial-intracranial bypass on cerebrovascular reactivity and clinical outcome in patients with symptomatic moyamoya vasculopathy. Stroke. 2011; 42(11):3047–3054

[4] Chui J, Mariappan R, Mehta J, Manninen P, Venkatraghavan L. Comparison of propofol and volatile agents for maintenance of anesthesia during elective craniotomy procedures: systematic review and meta-analysis. Can J Anaesth. 2014; 61(4):347–356

[5] Chui J, Manninen P, Sacho RH, Venkatraghavan L. Anesthetic management of patients undergoing intracranial bypass procedures. Anesth Analg. 2015; 120(1):193–203

[6] Sneyd JR, Andrews CJ, Tsubokawa T. Comparison of propofol/remifentanil and sevoflurane/remifentanil for maintenance of anaesthesia for elective intracranial surgery. Br J Anaesth. 2005; 94(6):778–783

[7] Kikuta K, Takagi Y, Nozaki K, et al. Effects of intravenous anesthesia with propofol on regional cortical blood flow and intracranial pressure in surgery for moyamoya disease. Surg Neurol. 2007; 68(4): 421–424

[8] Sato K, Shirane R, Kato M, Yoshimoto T. Effect of inhalational anesthesia on cerebral circulation in Moyamoya disease. J Neurosurg Anesthesiol. 1999; 11(1):25–30

[9] Iwama T, Hashimoto N, Yonekawa Y. The relevance of hemodynamic factors to perioperative ischemic complications in childhood moyamoya disease. Neurosurgery. 1996; 38(6):1120–1125, discussion 1125–1126

[10] Smith ER, Scott RM. Surgical management of moyamoya syndrome. Skull Base. 2005; 15(1):15–26

[11] Baykan N, Ozgen S, Ustalar ZS, Dagçinar A, Ozek MM. Moyamoya disease and anesthesia. Paediatr Anaesth. 2005; 15(12):1111–1115

[12] Orihashi K, Sueda T, Okada K, Imai K. Near-infrared spectroscopy for monitoring cerebral ischemia during selective cerebral perfusion. Eur J Cardiothorac Surg. 2004; 26(5):907–911

[13] Parray T, Martin TW, Siddiqui S. Moyamoya disease: a review of the disease and anesthetic management. J Neurosurg Anesthesiol. 2011; 23(2):100–109

[14] Kurehara K, Ohnishi H, Touho H, Furuya H, Okuda T. Cortical blood flow response to hypercapnia during anaesthesia in Moyamoya disease. Can J Anaesth. 1993; 40(8):709–713

[15] Yusa T, Yamashiro K. Local cortical cerebral blood flow and response to carbon dioxide during anesthesia in patients with moyamoya disease. J Anesth. 1999; 13(3):131–135

[16] Czabanka M, Boschi A, Acker G, et al. Grading of moyamoya disease allows stratification for postoperative ischemia in bilateral revascularization surgery. Acta Neurochir. 2016; 158:1895–1900

[17] Brown SC, Lam AM. Moyamoya disease–a review of clinical experience and anaesthetic management. Can J Anaesth. 1987; 34(1):71–75

[18] Bjerregaard J, Pandia MP, Jaffe RA. Occurrence of severe hypotension after indocyanine green injection during the intraoperative period. A A Case Rep. 2013; 1(1):26–30

[19] Ahn HJ, Kim JA, Lee JJ, et al. Effect of preoperative skull block on pediatric moyamoya disease. J Neurosurg Pediatr. 2008; 2(1):37–41


# Suggested Readings


Chui J, Manninen P, Sacho RH, Venkatraghavan L. Anesthetic management of patients undergoing intracranial bypass procedures. Anesth Analg. 2015; 120(1):193–203

Parray T, Martin TW, Siddiqui S. Moyamoya disease: a review of the disease and anesthetic management. J Neurosurg Anesthesiol. 2011; 23(2):100–109

# 2 General Principles of Direct Bypass Surgery

*Marcus Czabanka and Peter Vajkoczy*

**Abstract**

Bypass surgery for treating moyamoya vasculopathy (MMV) is often regarded as treatment of choice. In contrast to extraintracranial bypass surgery in atherosclerotic disease, different revascularization techniques are proposed for the treatment of MMV which may be differentiated into direct, indirect, and combined bypass procedures. The superiority of direct bypass surgery in comparison to indirect strategies includes immediate additional blood flow to the ischemic brain leading to reduction of stroke risk in these patients. The following chapter focuses on the general principles of bypass surgery for the treatment of MMV, focusing on general ideas and surgical concepts which are important for indication and planning of the surgical strategy.

*Keywords:* chronic hemodynamic impairment, indirect revascularization, direct revascularization, indication and management of cerebral revascularization in Moyamoya patients

## 2.1 History and Initial Description

After the first description of an arterial end-to-end anastomosis using suture by the French surgeon Alexis Carrel in 1902 it took another 70 years until Yasargil described the most influential direct revascularization technique with the introduction of the superficial temporal artery to middle cerebral artery (STA–MCA) bypass for internal carotid artery occlusion and moyamoya vasculopathy (MMV).[1] In contrast, indirect revascularization techniques had been performed already in the 1940s representing the first attempts to revascularize the ischemic brain. Since the introduction of both revascularization strategies there remains significant debate about the superiority of indirect versus direct revascularization techniques in MMV.[2] Current treatment protocols recommend direct revascularization techniques aiming at immediate supply of additional blood flow to the brain for adult patients as the anatomic difficulties encountered especially in MMV (small and fragile donor and recipient vessels that impose difficulties for the microsurgical anastomosis) are less pronounced in adult patients compared to pediatric MMV patients.[3–5] Consequently, in pediatric MMV patients indirect revascularization techniques have been described to be very effective for treating ischemic symptoms and restoring cerebrovascular reserve capacity.[3,6] Therefore, in adult MMV patients, direct STA–MCA bypass has become the workhorse for revascularizing the ischemic brain, in pediatric patients indirect procedures are regarded as equivalent revascularization strategy often resulting in a combination of both procedures.[7]

## 2.2 Analysis of Hemodynamic Compromise for Direct Bypass Surgery

The most important aim of direct bypass surgery represents correction of hemodynamic compromise and reduction of stroke risk. Hemodynamic compromise is assessed using PET measurements of cerebral blood flow with/without acetacolamide stimulation analyzing cerebrovascular reserve capacity and calculating oxygen extraction fraction (OEF). There are currently different tracers used including $C^{15}O$ PET for cerebral blood volume assessment, $H_2{}^{15}O$ for cerebral blood flow, and $^{15}O_2$ to measure OEF and cerebral metabolic rate of oxygen.[8] Using positron emission tomography (PET) analysis MMV patients have been characterized as patients with high cerebral blood volume due to maximal vasodilation and reduced OEF as a sign of hemodynamic compromise. Single-photon emission computed tomography (SPECT) analysis allows detection of hemodynamic compromise using nonquantitative, relative measurements comparing the healthy hemisphere with the diseased one, which imposes methodological limitations to a bilateral disease as MMV. Even though it remains to be determined whether PET analysis is superior to other imaging modalities analyzing cerebrovascular reserve capacity, our experience comparing SPECT and $H_2{}^{15}O$ PET for detecting hemodynamic compromise indicate improved sensitivity and specificity for PET techniques in this regard[9] (▸ Fig. 2.1).

Another highly reliable tool is Xenon-CT measurement of cerebrovascular reserve capacity. Xenon-enhanced CT has been shown to correlate with increased risk of ischemic stroke in the presence of reduced cerebrovascular reserve capacity and therefore represents a gold standard for detecting hemodynamic compromise.[10,11] Correspondingly, direct bypass surgery significantly improves cerebrovascular reserve capacity in MMV patients.[12] However, significantly reduced availability of this technique due to approval restrictions avoid a broad application of Xenon-CT for detecting hemodynamic compromise in MMV patients. Novel MRI techniques may contribute to the hemodynamic assessment preoperatively. Dynamic susceptibility contrast-weighted bolus-tracking MRI, arterial spin labeling MRI, and blood oxygen

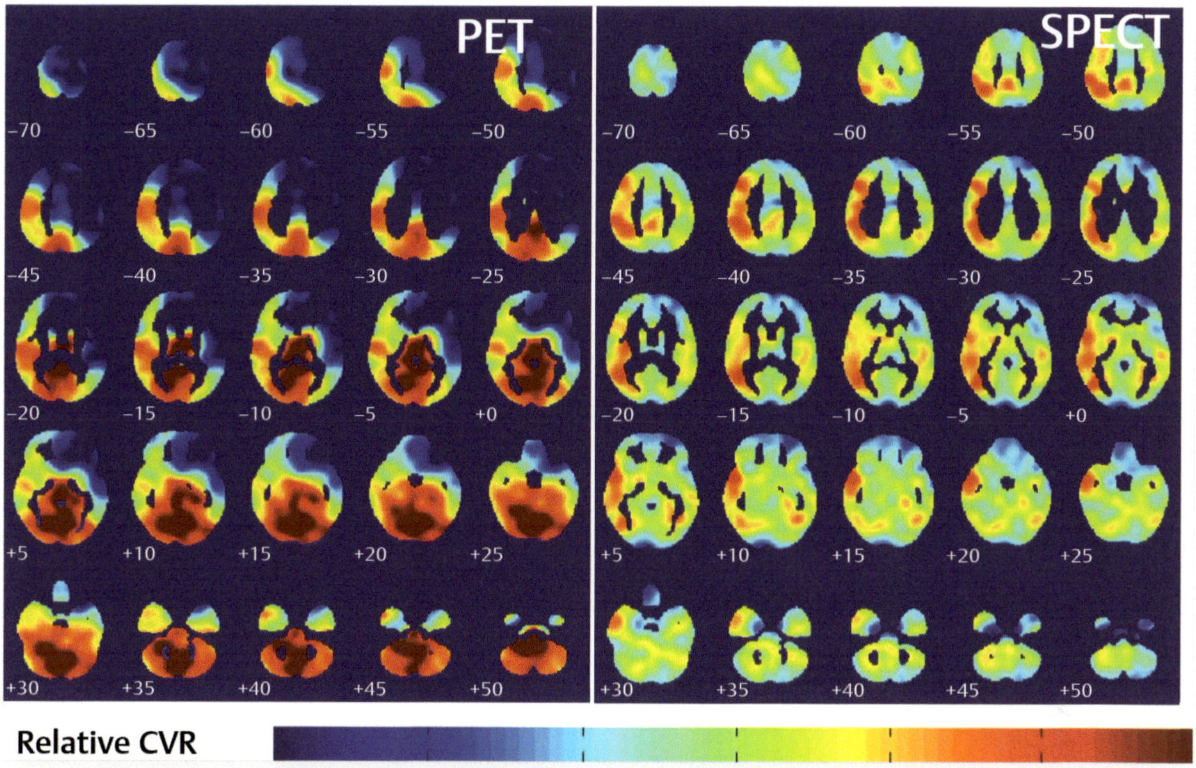


**Fig. 2.1** Analysis of cerebrovascular reserve capacity after acetazolamide stimulation demonstrating highly significant reduced cerebrovascular reserve capacity in $H_2{}^{15}O$ positron emission tomography imaging (left) compared to single-photon emission computed tomography (right) in the left hemisphere of a moyamoya patient.

level-dependent MRI have been shown to potentially identify tissue at risk for cerebral ischemia, hemodynamic compromise, and restoration of hemodynamic compromise after direct revascularization.[13]

Moreover, novel data imply that quantitative analysis of cerebral blood flow or OEF may not yet represent the only decisive indicator for future stroke in MMV as Zipfel et al demonstrate a 10% stroke risk for MMV patients with normal OEF in PET studies.[14] Therefore, other factors must be included in the surgical decision-making process. These include the potential progressive character of MMV and the extraordinarily high risk of ischemic stroke if both hemispheres are affected by the disease (> 80% stroke risk in 5 years).[15] Following the Berlin moyamoya grading system, MMV may be graded according to angiography, presence of ischemic lesions in MRI, and the associated hemodynamic compromised into three different grades that correlate with the presence of ischemic symptoms and the associated risk for cerebral revascularization[16,17] (▶ Fig. 2.2).

Especially, high-grade MMV patients impose a higher ischemia risk during cerebral revascularization than low-grade MMV patients, indicating that early revascularization may be reasonable in these patients avoiding a high complication profile while resulting in a significant reduction of stroke risk[16]. Moreover, the risk for cerebral hemorrhage must be included as STA–MCA bypass significantly reduces the risk for cerebral hemorrhage.[18] The ethnic background of the patient and the risk for cerebral hemorrhage, that varies among MMV populations with a higher incidence of hemorrhagic MMV in Asia as compared to the predominantly ischemic populations in North America and Europe,[2,19–21] in combination with the presence of fragile collateral vessels and microaneurysms further factors that should be considered in the surgical decision-making process for direct revascularization surgery.

## 2.3 Key Principles of Direct Revascularization Surgery

### 2.3.1 Graft Choice

In MMV, the STA is usually used as a donor vessel because standard STA–MCA bypass is regarded as the treatment of choice for direct revascularization procedures. High-flow bypass procedures are associated with a high-risk profile for hyperperfusion syndrome and therefore represent only rescue strategies in cases of failed low-flow anastomosis and/or failed indirect procedures.[22] In this regard, bypass flow in STA–MCA bypass has been described to

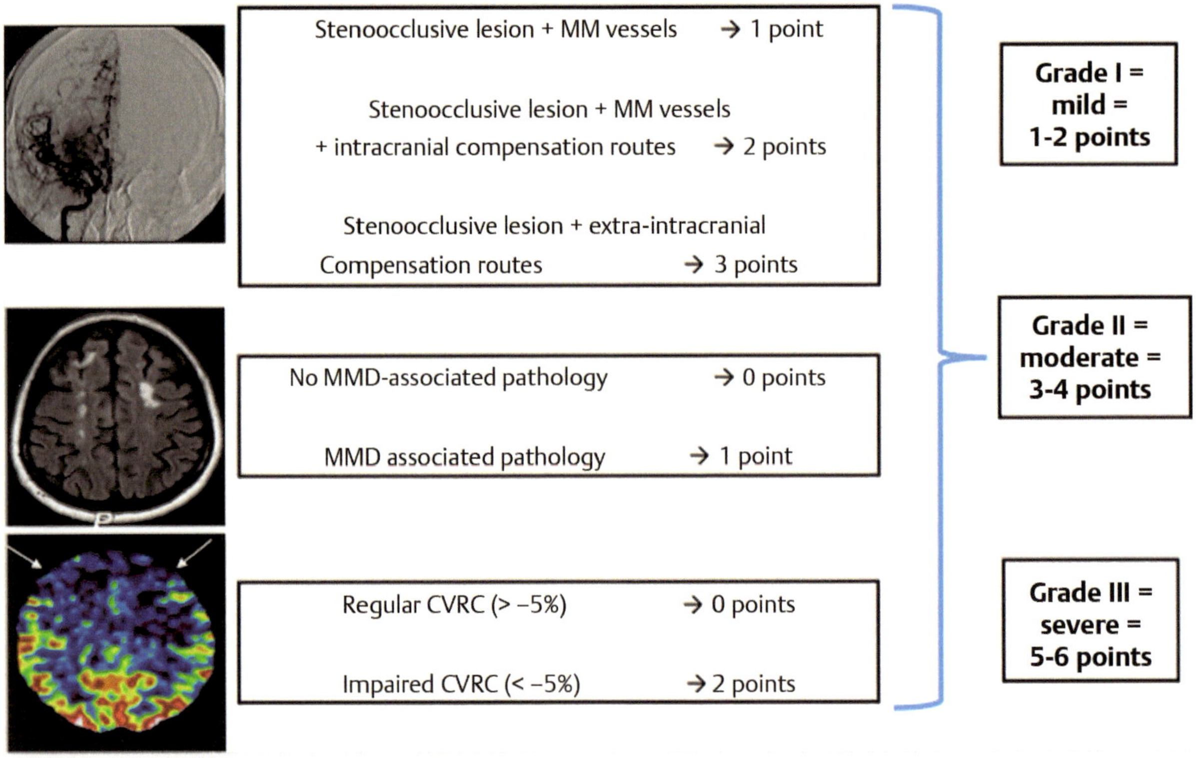


**Fig. 2.2** Description of the Berlin moyamoya grading system.

range between 10 and 60 mL/min while flows above 30 mL/min are associated with increased risk for hemorrhage and stroke.[23] Other direct anastomosis techniques including STA–ACA bypass, occipital artery-posterior cerebral artery (OA–PCA) anastomosis, multiple insertion procedures, and the use of the auricular artery as donor vessel have been described by different bypass-experienced groups, yet all of these procedures do not display superiority to regular STA–MCA anastomosis and they are often associated with distinct disadvantages. Therefore, they play a minor role in direct revascularization of MMV patients and predominantly serve as rescue strategies in cases for failed primary revascularization procedures.

## 2.3.2 Recipient Artery

For direct STA–MCA anastomosis, an M4 segment of the MCA is usually selected as the recipient vessel. In cases of a missing suitable recipient, the sylvian fissure may be opened to select an M3 or M2 segment as recipient. However, in these cases microanastomosis may be technically more demanding and the risk of ischemia during temporary occlusion is unknown. In order to reduce the risk of a nonsuitable recipient vessel craniotomy may be placed above the "target point" at the end of the sylvian fissure.[24] In this area, the risk for a nonsuitable recipient vessel is extremely low as the end of the sylvian fissure is characterized by numerous vessels entering the cerebral cortex.

## 2.3.3 Standardized Strategies versus Targeted Bypass Procedures

There remain debates about the use of a standardized surgical approach (e.g., using the target point as general localization for microanastomosis) versus performing targeted bypass procedures (e.g., using STA–ACA anstomosis in cases of predominantly hemodynamic compromise in the ACA vascular territory). Direct STA–MCA bypass at the target point has been shown to restore cerebrovascular reserve capacity independent from the most prominently compromised vascular territory, which is probably the result of suitable intracerebral collateralization pathways.[12] Especially, MMV patients are characterized by intensive leptomeningeal anastomosis, pericallosal anastomosis, and increased cortical microvascularization supporting the benefits of a standardized surgical approach in order to restore cerebrovascular reserve capacity.[25] Moreover, temporary occlusion of an M4 segment may be performed without the risk of occlusion-induced cerebral ischemia, which may not be the case for more proximal anastomosis.[26] Targeted bypass procedures have been described by different groups,[27] yet targeted bypass procedures rely on definite localization of tissue at risk for ischemia, which still presents a major challenge for imaging modalities. Moreover, surgical techniques are more difficult as multiple insertion strategies with longer donor vessels and larger as well as diverse craniotomies are often required, leading to prolonged surgical time and a higher risk for intraoperative ischemia. Despite these difficulties, several moyamoya groups have reported good surgical outcomes for targeted bypass procedures especially in pediatric patients.[27] For lack of a randomized clinical trial, it depends on the surgeons' expertise and experience which direct revascularization strategy is performed without additional guidelines from the current body of literature.

### 2.3.4 Peri- and Intraoperative Management and Neuroprotection

General anesthesia is recommended for direct revascularization surgery. The most important goal during the peri- and intraoperative period is to maintain conditions that optimize cerebral blood flow and minimize the risk of ischemic or hyperemic injury.[2] During preoperative preparation normocarbia should be achieved especially in the induction of general anesthesia while maintaining blood pressure baseline values. Baseline blood pressure is assessed in the days before surgery with the patient in a normal state of activity. Intraoperative blood pressure management in our institution aims at the patients' baseline blood pressure level plus additional 10% in order to maintain high cerebral perfusion pressure. Maintaining oxygenation, normocarbia, stable arterial blood pressure, and an adequate depth of anesthesia is critical during the intraoperative period. In the case of hypertonic medications avoidance of hypotension after diuresis is another important aspect. During the time period of anastomosis, which requires temporary occlusion of a cortical vessel, oxygenation fraction is increased to 100% in order to further minimize the risk of occlusion-induced ischemia. Moreover, intraoperative monitoring of somatosensory-evoked potentials, motor-evoked potentials, and EEG monitoring may be used to detect phases of critical hypo- or hypertension.[8] Early postoperative extubation is the goal in order to enable early and serial neurologic examinations after direct revascularization surgery. During the postoperative phase, maintenance of blood pressure is achieved aiming at the patients' baseline blood pressure values in addition to adequate pain control and sufficient antiplatelet therapy.

### 2.3.5 Intraoperative Flow Assessment

Intraoperative application of indocyanine green (ICG) videoangiography nowadays allows immediate assessment of bypass patency, which should be performed routinely after microanastomosis.[28] Yet ICG videoangiography does not provide quantitative information regarding bypass flow due to limitations of flow assessment using fluorescence probes.[29] Only intraoperative assessment of bypass flow using microflow probes allow quantitative assessment of flow characteristics before and after anastomosis and may therefore provide information about bypass capacity and bypass efficiency after anastomosis by assessing the cut flow index.[23] Usually a cut flow index of above 0.5 is regarded as sufficient bypass function and indicates good bypass efficiency. In cases of a cut flow index below 0.5, analysis of potential confounders inflicting with bypass function should be performed focusing on problems with the microanastomosis or the recipient artery.[23] In these cases bypass revision or even selection of another recipient may be performed to improve bypass function. Therefore, direct intraoperative flow assessment strategies provide information about potential drawbacks during bypass surgery and may help in the decision-making process in the case of bypass failure or poor bypass function. Additionally, massively increased flow in the MCA after direct anastomosis has been described to predict perioperative ischemia and hemorrhage.[30] Intraoperative detection of this risk factor allows fine adjustment of postoperative management regarding blood pressure control and may therefore help in the complex perioperative management of MMV patients.

In order to monitor bypass induced changes to cortical perfusion, intraoperative laser speckle imaging allows pseudoquantitative assessment of cortical perfusion before and after STA–MCA microanastomosis and may therefore allow conclusions about immediate global effects of bypass surgery on brain perfusion and distribution of additional blood flow in cerebral cortex.[31] Other strategies have been applied including a thermal diffusion flow probe to analyze regional cerebral blood flow before and after anastomosis, a light spectroscopy system for detection of oxygen saturation as well as infrared brain surface blood flow monitoring. All of the above named procedures share the fact that they are applied exclusively in an academic setting without a broad generalized application of these systems.

Intraoperative digital subtraction angiography provides detailed information about bypass flow and filling of cortical arteries via the bypass; however, intraoperative digital subtraction angiography is rarely available and is associated with prolonged surgical time.

## 2.4 General Complications and Risk Stratification

Rates of postoperative ischemia for direct revascularization in the treatment of MMV have been described to range between 3 and 8%, depending on the applied surgical strategy.[2,21] Accepting this risk profile for perioperative ischemia the 5-year stroke risk is reduced to 5.5% with more than 90% of MMV patients being free of recurrent transient ischemic attacks in the case of successful revascularization.[2,21]

A major confounding problem in perioperative management of MMV patients is the phenomenon of hyperperfusion syndrome. This has been reported to occur in up to 38% of MMV patients after direct revascularization even though the exact risk profile remains unknown as surgical series in North America and Europe demonstrate significantly lower risk profiles for hyperperfusion syndrome.[32,33] Hyperperfusion may be associated with significant clinical neurological deficits as dysarthria, paresis, aphasia, and sensorimotor loss. These patients do not present signs of cerebral ischemia in postoperative MRI but rather demonstrate hyperperfusion aspects in postoperative perfusion studies as SPECT or MR/CT perfusion. The most important clinical aspect is to recognize this phenomenon as it requires a totally different treatment decision as postoperative ischemia (which requires an increase or at least maintenance in blood pressure). In hyperperfusion syndrome lowering of blood pressure is mandatory to treat neurological deficits. Especially patients presenting with highly frequent transient ischemic attacks are significantly associated with postoperative hyperperfusion syndrome.

In order to predict risk profiles of MMV patients, a novel grading scale of MMV allows differentiation between three MMV patient profiles.[16] Applying this grading protocol demonstrates that MMV patient with a mild form are characterized by extremely low-risk profile for perioperative ischemia (0%) whereas patients with a severe form of MMV may face a risk profile of up to 16% in the case of one-staged bilateral revascularization.[17] As this risk profile has been confirmed by other surgical groups with different surgical strategies, it becomes clear that revascularization surgery should be performed during an early phase of the disease. Not only to treat ischemic symptoms as early as possible and to avoid manifest cerebral infarctions, but also because the perioperative risk profile is lower during an early phase of the disease when hemodynamic compromise is less severe.

In this regard, many postoperative ischemic events do not occur in the hemisphere that underwent revascularization surgery. Competing flow between native collaterals and the bypass, distinct features of peri-, intra-, and postoperative blood pressure management and the associated hemodynamic fragility of MMV may be responsible for these ischemic events highlighting the importance of an experienced and sensitive interdisciplinary environment during the surgical treatment of patients.

# References


[1] Yasargil MG, Yonekawa Y. Results of microsurgical extra-intracranial arterial bypass in the treatment of cerebral ischemia. Neurosurgery. 1977; 1(1):22–24

[2] Scott RM, Smith ER. Moyamoya disease and moyamoya syndrome. N Engl J Med. 2009; 360(12):1226–1237

[3] Smith ER, Scott RM. Spontaneous occlusion of the circle of Willis in children: pediatric moyamoya summary with proposed evidence-based practice guidelines. A review. J Neurosurg Pediatr. 2012; 9(4): 353–360

[4] Kuroda S. Strategy and tactics of bypass surgery for moyamoya disease. Acta Neurochir (Wien). 2017; 159(8):1495–1496

[5] Deng X, Gao F, Zhang D, et al. Direct versus indirect bypasses for adult ischemic-type moyamoya disease: a propensity score-matched analysis. J Neurosurg. 201 8; 128(6):1785–1791

[6] Czabanka M, Vajkoczy P, Schmiedek P, Horn P. Age-dependent revascularization patterns in the treatment of moyamoya disease in a European patient population. Neurosurg Focus. 2009; 26(4):E9

[7] Liu JJ, Steinberg GK. Direct versus indirect bypass for moyamoya disease. Neurosurg Clin N Am. 2017; 28(3):361–374

[8] Lee M, Zaharchuk G, Guzman R, Achrol A, Bell-Stephens T, Steinberg GK. Quantitative hemodynamic studies in moyamoya disease: a review. Neurosurg Focus. 2009; 26(4):E5

[9] Acker G, et al. Brain perfusion imaging under acetazolamide challenge for detection of impaired cerebrovascular reserve capacity: positive findings with O-15-water PET in patients with negative Tc-99m-HMPAO SPECT. J Nucl Med. 2017; 117:195818

[10] Yonas H, Smith HA, Durham SR, Pentheny SL, Johnson DW. Increased stroke risk predicted by compromised cerebral blood flow reactivity. J Neurosurg. 1993; 79(4):483–489

[11] Yonas H, Jungreis C. Xenon CT cerebral blood flow: past, present, and future. AJNR Am J Neuroradiol. 1995; 16(1):219–220

[12] Czabanka M, Peña-Tapia P, Scharf J, et al. Characterization of direct and indirect cerebral revascularization for the treatment of European patients with moyamoya disease. Cerebrovasc Dis. 2011; 32(4):361–369

[13] Zaharchuk G, Do HM, Marks MP, Rosenberg J, Moseley ME, Steinberg GK. Arterial spin-labeling MRI can identify the presence and intensity of collateral perfusion in patients with moyamoya disease. Stroke. 2011; 42(9):2485–2491

[14] Derdeyn CP, Zipfel GJ, Zazulia AR, et al. Baseline hemodynamic impairment and future stroke risk in adult idiopathic moyamoya phenomenon: results of a prospective natural history study. Stroke. 2017; 48(4):894–899

[15] Kraemer M, Heienbrok W, Berlit P. Moyamoya disease in Europeans. Stroke. 2008; 39(12):3193–3200

[16] Czabanka M, Peña-Tapia P, Schubert GA, et al. Proposal for a new grading of moyamoya disease in adult patients. Cerebrovasc Dis. 2011; 32(1):41–50

[17] Czabanka M, Boschi A, Acker G, et al. Grading of moyamoya disease allows stratification for postoperative ischemia in bilateral revascularization surgery. Acta Neurochir (Wien). 2016; 158(10):1895–1900

[18] Miyamoto S, Yoshimoto T, Hashimoto N, et al. JAM Trial Investigators. Effects of extracranial-intracranial bypass for patients with hemorrhagic moyamoya disease: results of the Japan Adult Moyamoya Trial. Stroke. 2014; 45(5):1415–1421

[19] Acker G, Goerdes S, Schneider UC, Schmiedek P, Czabanka M, Vajkoczy P. Distinct clinical and radiographic characteristics of moyamoya disease amongst European Caucasians. Eur J Neurol. 2015; 22(6):1012–1017

[20] Acker G, Goerdes S, Schmiedek P, Czabanka M, Vajkoczy P. Characterization of clinical and radiological features of quasi-moyamoya disease among European Caucasians including surgical treatment and outcome. Cerebrovasc Dis. 2016; 42(5–6):464–475

[21] Kuroda S, Houkin K. Moyamoya disease: current concepts and future perspectives. Lancet Neurol. 2008; 7(11):1056–1066

[22] Hori S, Acker G, Vajkoczy P. Radial artery grafts as rescue strategy for patients with moyamoya disease for whom conventional revascularization failed. World Neurosurg. 2016; 85:77–84

[23] Amin-Hanjani S, Du X, Mlinarevich N, Meglio G, Zhao M, Charbel FT. The cut flow index: an intraoperative predictor of the success of extracranial-intracranial bypass for occlusive cerebrovascular disease. Neurosurgery. 2005; 56(1) Suppl:75–85, discussion 75–85

[24] Peña-Tapia PG, Kemmling A, Czabanka M, Vajkoczy P, Schmiedek P. Identification of the optimal cortical target point for extracranial-intracranial bypass surgery in patients with hemodynamic cerebrovascular insufficiency. J Neurosurg. 2008; 108(4):655–661

[25] Czabanka M, Acker G, Jussen D, et al. Collateralization and ischemia in hemodynamic cerebrovascular insufficiency. Acta Neurochir (Wien). 2014; 156(11):2051–2058, discussion 2058

[26] Horn P, Scharf J, Peña-Tapia P, Vajkoczy P. Risk of intraoperative ischemia due to temporary vessel occlusion during standard extracranial-intracranial arterial bypass surgery. J Neurosurg. 2008; 108(3): 464–469

[27] Ishikawa T, Kamiyama H, Kuroda S, Yasuda H, Nakayama N, Takizawa K. Simultaneous superficial temporal artery to middle cerebral or anterior cerebral artery bypass with pan-synangiosis for Moyamoya disease covering both anterior and middle cerebral artery territories. Neurol Med Chir (Tokyo). 2006; 46(9):462–468

[28] Woitzik J, Horn P, Vajkoczy P, Schmiedek P. Intraoperative control of extracranial-intracranial bypass patency by near-infrared indocyanine green videoangiography. J Neurosurg. 2005; 102(4):692–698

[29] Prinz V, Hecht N, Kato N, Vajkoczy P. FLOW 800 allows visualization of hemodynamic changes after extracranial-to-intracranial bypass surgery but not assessment of quantitative perfusion or flow. Neurosurgery. 2014; 10 Suppl 2:231–238, discussion 238–239

[30] Lee M, Guzman R, Bell-Stephens T, Steinberg GK. Intraoperative blood flow analysis of direct revascularization procedures in patients with moyamoya disease. J Cereb Blood Flow Metab. 2011; 31(1):262–274

[31] Hecht N, Woitzik J, König S, Horn P, Vajkoczy P. Laser speckle imaging allows real-time intraoperative blood flow assessment during neurosurgical procedures. J Cereb Blood Flow Metab. 2013; 33(7):1000–1007

[32] Hayashi K, Horie N, Suyama K, Nagata I. Incidence and clinical features of symptomatic cerebral hyperperfusion syndrome after vascular reconstruction. World Neurosurg. 2012; 78(5):447–454

[33] Uchino H, Kuroda S, Hirata K, Shiga T, Houkin K, Tamaki N. Predictors and clinical features of postoperative hyperperfusion after surgical revascularization for moyamoya disease: a serial single photon emission CT/positron emission tomography study. Stroke. 2012; 43(10): 2610–2616

# 3 General Principles of Indirect Bypass Surgery

*Satoshi Kuroda*

**Abstract**

General principles of indirect bypass surgery are very unique and specific for moyamoya disease. Previous studies have suggested that the elevated levels of angiogenic factors in the cerebrospinal fluid (CSF) may play an important role in aggressive neovascularization between the brain surface and vascularized donor tissues in moyamoya disease. Previously reported donor tissues include the dura mater, temporal muscle, galea aponeurotica, pericranium, and omentum. Surgical procedures are not difficult for well-trained neurosurgeons. However, the neurosurgeons should be aware of several important issues about indirect revascularization for moyamoya disease. First, indirect revascularization functions as effective collaterals in a majority of pediatric patients, but in only 50 to 70% of adult patients. Therefore, direct revascularization such as superficial temporal artery to middle cerebral artery (STA–MCA) anastomosis should simultaneously be indicated, especially in adult patients. Second, indirect revascularization requires 3 to 4 months to complete the development of effective collaterals, and thus carries the risk for ischemic stroke during and just after surgery, especially in patients with dense cerebral ischemia. Third, the extent of craniotomy and dural opening largely determines the extent of surgical collaterals development, which means that surgical design should be determined according to the extent of cerebral ischemia on blood flow measurements in each patient.

*Keywords:* moyamoya disease, indirect bypass, angiogenic factors, cerebrospinal fluid, craniotomy

## 3.1 Introduction

General principles of indirect bypass surgery are very unique and specific for moyamoya disease. This surgical procedure only requires the attachment of the vascularized donor tissue onto the surface of brain. Gradual, but steady neovascularization occurs between these tissues in moyamoya disease. Nowadays, indirect bypass procedure is indicated almost only for moyamoya disease, although there are a small number of reports demonstrating that indirect bypass is also effective for other disorders, including atherosclerotic cerebrovascular diseases and spinal cord injury. In this chapter, the author describes history, pathophysiology, and concept of surgery of indirect bypass for moyamoya disease.

## 3.2 History and Initial Description

▶ Fig. 3.1 demonstrates the history of main surgical procedures for indirect bypass. For these 40 years, various methods for indirect bypass have been reported for patients with moyamoya disease, including encephalo-duro-arterio-synangiosis (EDAS),[1] encephalo-myo-synangiosis (EMS),[2] encephalo-myo-arterio-synangiosis (EMAS),[3] encephalo-duro-arterio-myo-synangiosis (EDAMS),[4] encephalo-galeo-synangiosis (EGS),[5] and dural inversion.[6] These procedures have been developed to provide collateral blood flow mainly to the territory of the middle cerebral artery (MCA) and useful to reduce or resolve ischemic attacks. However, it is well known that a certain subgroup of patients with moyamoya disease does not respond to these surgery and experiences ischemic attacks of the bilateral legs and/or cognitive dysfunction probably due to persistent ischemia in the territory of the anterior cerebral artery (ACA). Several procedures targeting the ACA territory have been reported later. Thus, Kinugasa et al inserted the pedicle of the galea on both sides into the interhemispheric fissure in addition to EDAMS (ribbon EDAMS). Kawaguchi et al developed multiple burr hole surgery to induce neovascularization through indirect bypass, using one to four burr holes.[7] Yoshida et al inserted the dural pedicles into the epiarachnoid space to enlarge the revascularized area around craniotomy. For the same purpose, Kim et al also developed EDAS with bifrontal encephalogaleo(periosteal) synangiosis.[8] Subsequently, Kamiyama and colleagues developed STA–MCA/ACA anastomosis and pan-synangiosis, which consists of EDMAS and EGS for the MCA and ACA territories through two different craniotomies, respectively.[9] Kuroda et al further advanced indirect bypass procedure that can provide collateral blood flow to the whole territory of the internal carotid artery (ICA). For this purpose, a large frontal pericranial flap was employed to widely cover the frontal lobe through one craniotomy.[10,11]

Alternatively, the omentum has been employed as a donor tissue for indirect bypass and shown an aggressive neovascularization into the brain, but there are no reports on omental transplantation for these 20 years probably because of its invasiveness.[12–16]

## 3.3 Pathophysiology

As aforementioned, indirect bypass surgery induces spontaneous and aggressive neovascularization between the vascularized donor tissues and brain surface, which is almost specific for moyamoya disease. According to previous observations, the elevated levels of angiogenic factors in the cerebrospinal fluid (CSF) may play an important role in neovascularization between them. These angiogenic factors include basic fibroblast growth factor (bFGF) and hepatocyte growth factor (HGF). The concentrations of bFGF in the CSF significantly elevates in

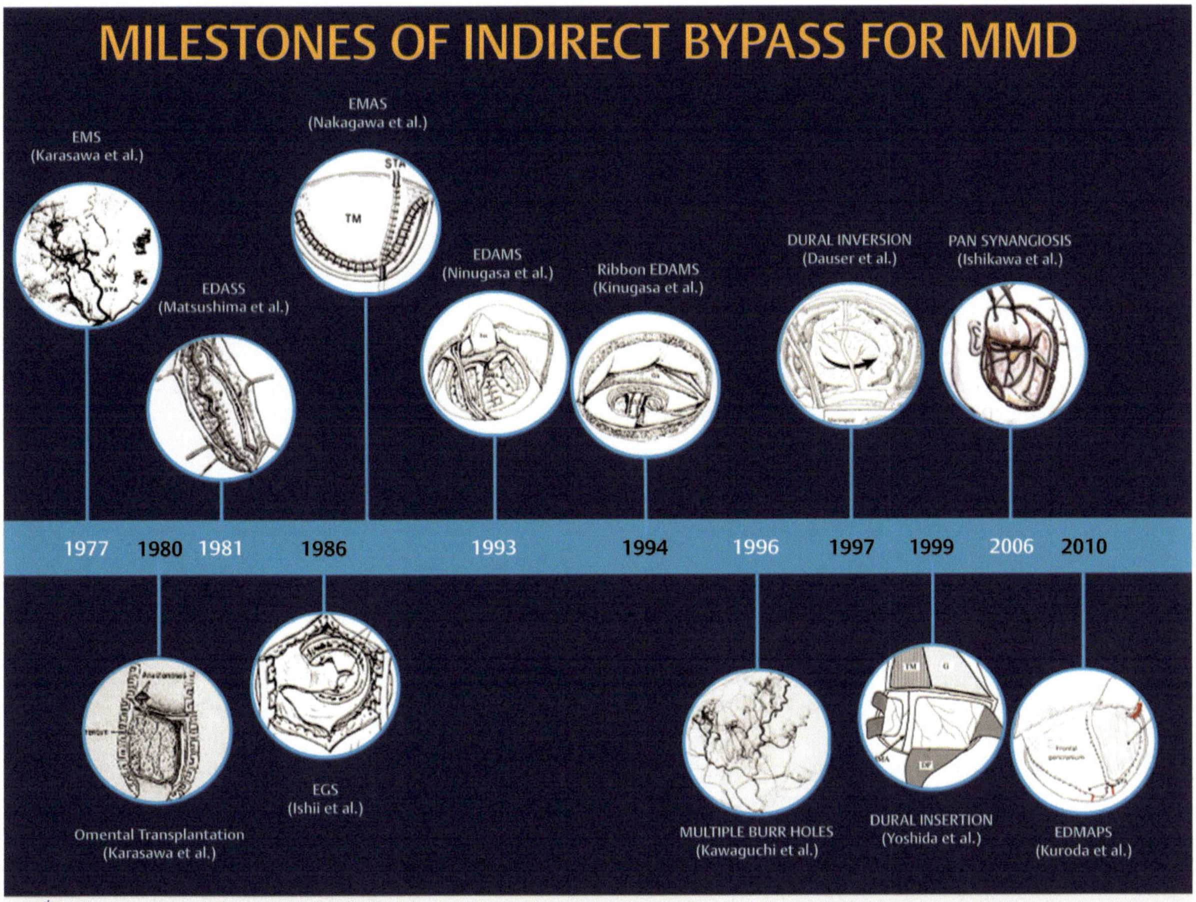


**Fig. 3.1** History of indirect bypass surgery.

the CSF of patients with moyamoya disease, when compared with the controls.[17] Interestingly, the concentration of bFGF is reported significantly higher in patients with good development of surgical collaterals via indirect bypass than in those without, strongly suggesting that bFGF are playing an important role in neovascularization after indirect bypass.[18,19] However, the concentration of bFGF does not correlate with patients' age, gender, and Suzuki's angiographical stage. The elevation of bFGF concentration in the CSF may not be specific for moyamoya disease because it is confirmed in patients with Chiari malformation, arteriovenous malformation (AVM), brain tumor, and hydrocephalus.[19] Pediatric patients with moyamoya syndrome also exhibit significantly elevated CSF levels of vascular cell adhesion molecule type 1 (VCAM-1), intercellular adhesion molecule type 1 (ICAM-1), E-selectin, and cellular retinoic acid-binding protein (CRABP)- I.[20,21] However, the biological roles of these soluble factors are not known precisely. On the other hands, the concentration of HGF significantly elevates up to twofold of the controls in patients with moyamoya disease. Interestingly, HGF and its receptor, c-Met are highly expressed in the media and thickened intima of the involved carotid fork.[22] Theses angiogenic factors may play a key role in not only disease onset but also the specific neovascularization after indirect bypass surgery.

## 3.4 Concept of Indirect Bypass Surgery

Previously reported donor tissues include the dura mater, temporal muscle, galea aponeurotica, and pericranium. These tissues can easily be used as the vascularized donors for indirect bypass, because they are surrounding the cranium. Surgical procedures are not difficult for the well-trained neurosurgeons. Alternatively, the omentum has also been reported to supply efficient blood flow to the ischemic brain as a surgically anastomosed flap or long vascularized flap.

However, the neurosurgeons should be aware of several important issues about indirect revascularization for moyamoya disease. First, indirect revascularization functions as effective collaterals in a majority of pediatric patients, but in only 50 to 70% of adult patients.[23,24] Therefore, direct revascularization such as STA–MCA

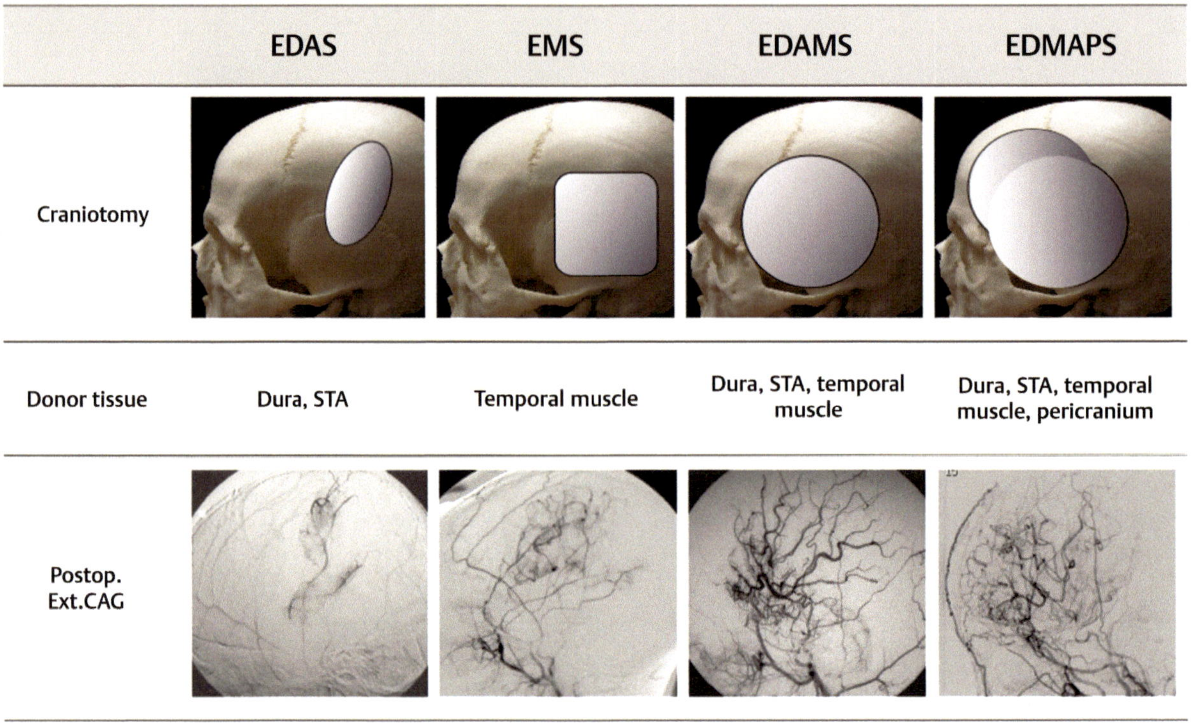


**Fig. 3.2** The extent of craniotomy and dural opening determines the extent of surgical collateral developments.

anastomosis should simultaneously be indicated especially in adult patients. Second, indirect revascularization requires 3 to 4 months to complete the development of effective collaterals, and thus carries the risk for ischemic stroke during and just after surgery, especially in patients with dense cerebral ischemia.[25] Therefore, proper anesthetic management is essential to prevent perioperative ischemic complications.[26–28] Third, the extent of craniotomy and dural opening largely determines the extent of surgical collaterals development, which means that surgical design should be determined according to the extent of cerebral ischemia in each patient (▶ Fig. 3.2).[29–32]

# References


[1] Matsushima Y, Fukai N, Tanaka K, et al. A new surgical treatment of moyamoya disease in children: a preliminary report. Surg Neurol. 1981; 15(4):313–320

[2] Karasawa J, Kikuchi H, Furuse S, Sakaki T, Yoshida Y. A surgical treatment of "moyamoya" disease "encephalo-myo synangiosis". Neurol Med Chir (Tokyo). 1977; 17(1 Pt 1):29–37

[3] Nakagawa Y, Sawamura Y, Abe H, Gotoh S, Shimoyama M. Revascularization surgery for 28 patients with moyamoya disease—operative methods, outcome and postoperative angiography. Hokkaido Igaku Zasshi. 1987; 62(1):133–144

[4] Kinugasa K, Mandai S, Kamata I, Sugiu K, Ohmoto T. Surgical treatment of moyamoya disease: operative technique for encephalo-duro-arterio-myo-synangiosis, its follow-up, clinical results, and angiograms. Neurosurgery. 1993; 32(4):527–531

[5] Ishii R. Surgical treatment of moyamoya disease. No Shinkei Geka. 1986; 14(9):1059–1068

[6] Dauser RC, Tuite GF, McCluggage CW. Dural inversion procedure for moyamoya disease. Technical note. J Neurosurg. 1997; 86(4):719–723

[7] Kawaguchi T, Fujita S, Hosoda K, et al. Multiple burr-hole operation for adult moyamoya disease. J Neurosurg. 1996; 84(3):468–476

[8] Kim SK, Wang KC, Kim IO, Lee DS, Cho BK. Combined encephaloduroarteriosynangiosis and bifrontal encephalogaleo(periosteal)synangiosis in pediatric moyamoya disease. Neurosurgery. 2002; 50(1):88–96

[9] Ishikawa T, Kamiyama H, Kuroda S, Yasuda H, Nakayama N, Takizawa K. Simultaneous superficial temporal artery to middle cerebral or anterior cerebral artery bypass with pan-synangiosis for moyamoya disease covering both anterior and middle cerebral artery territories. Neurol Med Chir (Tokyo). 2006; 46(9):462–468

[10] Kuroda S, Houkin K. Moyamoya disease: current concepts and future perspectives. Lancet Neurol. 2008; 7(11):1056–1066

[11] Kuroda S, Houkin K, Ishikawa T, Nakayama N, Iwasaki Y. Novel bypass surgery for moyamoya disease using pericranial flap: its impacts on cerebral hemodynamics and long-term outcome. Neurosurgery. 2010; 66(6):1093–1101, discussion 1101

[12] Goldsmith HS. Patients with moyamoya disease who had not fully benefited from encephaloduro-arterio-synangiosis (EDAS). Acta Neurochir (Wien). 1991; 111(1–2):68–69

[13] Karasawa J, Kikuchi H, Kawamura J, Sakai T. Intracranial transplantation of the omentum for cerebrovascular moyamoya disease: a two-year follow-up study. Surg Neurol. 1980; 14(6):444–449

[14] Karasawa J, Touho H, Ohnishi H, Miyamoto S, Kikuchi H. Cerebral revascularization using omental transplantation for childhood moyamoya disease. J Neurosurg. 1993; 79(2):192–196

[15] Ohtaki M, Uede T, Morimoto S, Nonaka T, Tanabe S, Hashi K. Intellectual functions and regional cerebral haemodynamics after extensive

omental transplantation spread over both frontal lobes in childhood moyamoya disease. Acta Neurochir (Wien). 1998; 140(10):1043–1053, discussion 1052–1053
[16] Touho H, Karasawa J, Tenjin H, Ueda S. Omental transplantation using a superficial temporal artery previously used for encephaloduroarteriosynangiosis. Surg Neurol. 1996; 45(6):550–558, discussion 558–559
[17] Takahashi A, Sawamura Y, Houkin K, Kamiyama H, Abe H. The cerebrospinal fluid in patients with moyamoya disease (spontaneous occlusion of the circle of Willis) contains high level of basic fibroblast growth factor. Neurosci Lett. 1993; 160(2):214–216
[18] Yoshimoto T, Houkin K, Takahashi A, Abe H. Angiogenic factors in moyamoya disease. Stroke. 1996; 27(12):2160–2165
[19] Malek AM, Connors S, Robertson RL, Folkman J, Scott RM. Elevation of cerebrospinal fluid levels of basic fibroblast growth factor in moyamoya and central nervous system disorders. Pediatr Neurosurg. 1997; 27(4):182–189
[20] Soriano SG, Cowan DB, Proctor MR, Scott RM. Levels of soluble adhesion molecules are elevated in the cerebrospinal fluid of children with moyamoya syndrome. Neurosurgery. 2002; 50(3):544–549
[21] Kim SK, Yoo JI, Cho BK, et al. Elevation of CRABP-I in the cerebrospinal fluid of patients with Moyamoya disease. Stroke. 2003; 34(12):2835–2841
[22] Nanba R, Kuroda S, Ishikawa T, Houkin K, Iwasaki Y. Increased expression of hepatocyte growth factor in cerebrospinal fluid and intracranial artery in moyamoya disease. Stroke. 2004; 35(12):2837–2842
[23] Mizoi K, Kayama T, Yoshimoto T, Nagamine Y. Indirect revascularization for moyamoya disease: is there a beneficial effect for adult patients? Surg Neurol. 1996; 45(6):541–548, discussion 548–549
[24] Uchino H, Kim JH, Fujima N, et al. Synergistic interactions between direct and indirect bypasses in combined procedures: the significance of indirect bypasses in moyamoya disease. Neurosurgery. 2017; 80(2):201–209
[25] Ishikawa T, Houkin K, Kamiyama H, Abe H. Effects of surgical revascularization on outcome of patients with pediatric moyamoya disease. Stroke. 1997; 28(6):1170–1173
[26] Iwama T, Hashimoto N, Tsukahara T, Murai B. Peri-operative complications in adult moyamoya disease. Acta Neurochir (Wien). 1995; 132(1–3):26–31
[27] Iwama T, Hashimoto N, Yonekawa Y. The relevance of hemodynamic factors to perioperative ischemic complications in childhood moyamoya disease. Neurosurgery. 1996; 38(6):1120–1125, discussion 1125–1126
[28] Kim SH, Choi JU, Yang KH, Kim TG, Kim DS. Risk factors for postoperative ischemic complications in patients with moyamoya disease. J Neurosurg. 2005; 103(5) Suppl:433–438
[29] Kuroda S, Houkin K, Ishikawa T, et al. Determinants of intellectual outcome after surgical revascularization in pediatric moyamoya disease: a multivariate analysis. Childs Nerv Syst. 2004; 20 (5):302–308
[30] Matsushima T, Inoue T, Katsuta T, et al. An indirect revascularization method in the surgical treatment of moyamoya disease—various kinds of indirect procedures and a multiple combined indirect procedure. Neurol Med Chir (Tokyo). 1998; 38 Suppl:297–302
[31] Matsushima T, Inoue T, Suzuki SO, Fujii K, Fukui M, Hasuo K. Surgical treatment of moyamoya disease in pediatric patients—comparison between the results of indirect and direct revascularization procedures. Neurosurgery. 1992; 31(3):401–405
[32] Takahashi A, Kamiyama H, Houkin K, Abe H. Surgical treatment of childhood moyamoya disease—comparison of reconstructive surgery centered on the frontal region and the parietal region. Neurol Med Chir (Tokyo). 1995; 35(4):231–237

# Part 2

## Indirect Revascularization



2

# 4 Multiple Burr Holes

*Thomas Blauwblomme, Philippe Meyer, and Christian Sainte-Rose*

**Abstract**
Thirty years after its princeps description, multiple burr hole surgery is yet not recognized as a first-line revascularization procedure in moyamoya angiopathy. Here, we describe the indications, technique, and pitfalls, emphasizing pediatrics patients. Complication rate of this indirect procedure is remarkably low, and efficacy to restore cerebral blood flow, as assessed by imaging and clinical outcome, is at least comparable to other indirect techniques in children.

*Keywords:* moyamoya angiopathy, multiple burr hole, indirect revascularization

## 4.1 History and Initial Description

Using cranial burr holes for cerebral revascularization is the consequence of serendipity more than a Cartesian, scientific approach. Spontaneous neovascularization through a burr hole in a child with moyamoya was first observed by Endo et al in 1984.[1] A 10-year-old boy with intraventricular hemorrhage was treated with two frontal external ventricular drains. Bilateral encephalo-myo-synangiosis (EMS) was performed 3 months later, and postoperative digital subtraction angiography (DSA) showed marked bilateral neovascularization through the burr holes. This single "burr-hole" technique was therefore performed in five other pediatric cases along with EMS, with excellent clinical and angiographic results.[1]

Seven years after this princeps publication, Kawaguchi et al published their experience with multiple burr holes, as the sole revascularization supply in a series of 10 adult patients with moyamoya.[2] One to four burr holes were drilled on each hemisphere, bilaterally in 8 out of 10 cases. Neovascularization was found in 41/43 burr holes on postoperative angiography performed 3 to 23 months after surgery, along with improvement in cerebral hemodynamics on SPECT studies, and cessation of transient ischemic attacks (TIAs) in 6/6 patients with preoperative ischemic attacks.

Eight years later, results of indirect cerebral revascularization with multiple burr holes were reported in a pediatric series of 14 children.[3] The authors increased the number of burr holes to cover the entire cranial vault, through 10 to 24 holes per case. Excellent clinical outcome was observed after surgery, as no child suffered from recurrent ischemic strokes. Postoperative angiography showed good neo vascularization, and the complication rate was low.

Since these pioneer studies, and despite good results, multiple burr holes were rarely reported in the literature,[4] and this procedure is more considered as a salvage procedure, or as an adjunct to other direct or indirect techniques.[5]

## 4.2 Indications

There is currently no class A-B evidence in the literature to demonstrate the superiority of direct revascularization on indirect revascularization in pediatric moyamoya. Among indirect revascularization procedures, outcome is comparable between EMS, encephalo-duro-arterio-synangiosis, and burr holes as more than 85% of children are stroke free after surgery.

In our pediatric neurosurgical department, Necker–Enfant Malades in Paris, multiple burr hole surgery is *the first-line surgical option for pediatric moyamoya angiopathy.* We choose this approach regardless of the underlying etiology, age of the patient, or modality of revelation of the disease.

## 4.3 Key Principles

Although no basic science research has demonstrated how pial anastomosis occur in multiple burr hole surgery, vasculogenesis and angiogenesis are believed to occur at each burr hole because of chronic brain ischemia and vascular growth factor secretion. The principle of the technique is to facilitate the communication between the external (donor) and internal carotid (recipient) arteries systems through bone and meningeal opening. Increasing the number of burr holes increases the surface of brain to be revascularized, in particular the junctional areas (PCA/MCA or ACA/MCA) in the frontal poles, near the midline and parietoccipital area.

## 4.4 SWOT Analysis

### 4.4.1 Strengths

This surgical technique is simple and safe. It does not require transient clipping of the arterial vessels, as needed in bypass surgery, and there is no cosmetic defect associated to temporalis muscle transposition, as with EMS or EDAMS. The complication rate is very low, as we report no permanent neurological deficit or death related to the procedure in our cohort of 64 operated children (transient subcutaneous effusion, $n = 5$; meningitis, $n = 1$; superficial skin infection, $n = 1$).

This approach allows extensive revascularization of the hemispheres. Indeed, burr holes can be placed all over the cranial vault, and revascularization of the frontal pole, occipital lobe, and junctional areas is therefore possible.

Bilateral revascularization is easy during the same procedure, through a unique cosmetic incision, without increasing the morbidity related to the surgery.

This technique does not preclude further revascularization in case of stroke relapse, as the superficial temporal artery (STA) is respected, and other indirect (burr holes, EMS, EDAMS, omentum transposition) and direct techniques (STA–MCA bypass) can be performed despite the initial procedure.

### 4.4.2 Weakness

Multiple burr hole surgery is an indirect technique and, as such, revascularization is efficient only a few weeks after the surgery. Therefore, patients with frequent TIAs may undergo ischemic events during the postoperative period. In our cohort of 64 patients, 4 patients had TIAs that resolved spontaneously after a mean delay of 79 days.

### 4.4.3 Opportunities

As imaging evolves, brain hemodynamics can be studied with magnetic resonance imaging (MRI) techniques. Cerebral blood flow (CBF) can be measured with arterial spin labeling (ASL) MRI,[6] along with cerebrovascular reserve with blood oxygen level-dependent (BOLD) MRI, and oxygen extraction fraction. Targeted cerebral reperfusion may therefore be possible, with neuronavigation, to increase CBF where it is needed.

### 4.4.4 Threats

Thickness of the cranial vault can make the surgery challenging in case of sickle cell disease, but is never a formal contraindication. Cerebral atrophy is a concern, as the distance between the brain and the dura makes it difficult for the angiogenesis to occur, and pericerebral fluid collection can be a complication in very atrophic patients.

## 4.5 Contraindications

There is no absolute contra indication to this technique in patients with moyamoya and cerebral hemodynamics impairment.

However, as in all indirect techniques, cortical atrophy is a bad prognosis factor for revascularization, and is associated with an increased risk of complications, like subdural effusion. In case of major atrophy, the balance between risk and benefit shall be carefully weighted.

## 4.6 Special Considerations

### 4.6.1 Imaging

In order to avoid perioperative complications, preoperative imaging shall be analyzed carefully. Spontaneous transosseous anastomosis need to be localized on the angiography. They must be respected during the subgaleal dissection, the drilling of the burr holes, and the meningeal opening, to avoid perioperative ischemic events.

Delineating areas with cortical atrophy is important, as the burr holes may not be targeted on these areas.

Identification of areas with hemodynamic impairment is crucial, as they are the target of the procedure.

### 4.6.2 Patient

Patients with sickle cell disease deserve special attention among other moyamoya patients. A systemic evaluation is mandatory, as these patients may suffer from cardiac failure, or complications from chronic blood exchanges. Preoperative blood exchange may be necessary, as preoperative hemoglobin levels need to be higher than 10 g/dl. Careful analysis of the blood group is required, as these patients may have alloimmunization that needs to be anticipated if perioperative transfusion is required. During surgery, cautious hemostasis of the burr hole is mandatory with bone wax, as the cranial vault may be particularly thick because of the hematopoiesis process.

Avoiding hypoxia and hypothermia is essential to avoid vaso-occlusive crisis.

## 4.7 Pitfalls, Risk Assessment, and Complications

In our cohort of 64 patients operated with the multiple burr holes techniques, neither mortality nor permanent neurological morbidity was noted.

Possible complications included: transient subdural effusion ($n = 5$), meningitis ($n = 1$), and superficial scar infection ($n = 1$).

Information to the patient must mention that indirect techniques are efficient only a few weeks after the procedure, and therefore ischemic events are possible after the surgery. In our cohort, with a mean follow-up of 270.6 patient years, 89.1% of the patients had no postoperative ischemic events, and a second surgery because of recurrent TIA was required in 3 out of 64 patients.

## 4.8 Special Instructions, Position, and Anesthesia

### 4.8.1 Anesthesia

During anesthesia and recovery, acute and revolving episodes of decreased cerebral perfusion pressure, exposing these patients to a major risk of silent ischemic events, should be strictly avoided. The first imperative is to maintain a stable arterial pressure with a mean arterial pressure level as close as possible from usual measurements in each patient. Continuous invasive arterial pressure monitoring should therefore be initiated during anesthesia and maintained in the immediate postoperative. Excessive vasoplegia with anesthetic drugs should be avoided, and blood losses strictly compensated.

The second imperative is to insure a stable normoventilation during anesthesia and recovery. Since hypocapnia could be a major source of harmfully decreased CBF in these patients, careful continuous monitoring of end tidal carbon dioxide ($ETCO_2$) is critical, and all episodes of hyperventilation should be avoided. A permissive moderate hypoventilation with an $ETCO_2$ in the range of 40 to 45 mm Hg could be a safe goal to attain during mechanical ventilation. In the postoperative period, painful stimulations could generate episodes of relative hyperventilation in children, resulting in decreased arterial $CO_2$, and decreased CBF. Careful staged analgesia should be therefore maintained during recovery, and in the immediate postoperative period.

### 4.8.2 Position

The patient is positioned supine in a horseshoe headrest, with the head flexed in a neutral position for bilateral approach, or with the head turned on the contralateral side for unilateral procedures.

## 4.9 Skin Incision and Key Surgical Steps

Subcutaneous infiltration with a saline solution can be used to facilitate the dissection, but is not mandatory.

A bitragial retrocoronal "zigzag" incision is performed for bilateral revascularization, allowing exposure of the entire vault (▶ Fig. 4.1), and a T-shaped incision is done for unilateral approaches (coronal incision and a posterior parietal incision). Section with the monopolar coagulation reduces the blood loss in the pediatric population, and careful hemostasis is required at each step of the procedure.

Subgaleal dissection is performed gently, with particular attention to preserving the subcutaneous vascularization, and notably the STA and its branches. The periosteum is not elevated to preserve the vessels.

The burr holes are made 3 cm apart from each other on the entire exposed vault. Three lines can be determined: 3 cm from the midline (to avoid any bleeding from the bridging veins during the dural opening), above the linea temporalis, and bellow the temporalis muscle.

For each burr hole, the procedure is the same. A 3 cm triangular periosteal flap is elevated, with the tip facing the midline. A burr hole is made with a 1 cm high speed drill. Under the operative microscope, the dura is widely opened in order to avoid cutting the meningeal arterial branches. The arachnoid layer is opened. Cautious hemostasis is obtained with cottonoid patties and gentle irrigation of saline. Cautery is avoided as much as possible to preserve the potential anastomotic vessels. The periosteal flap is then positioned over the brain in the subdural space.

Two-layer watertight closure of the skin and galea is then done with absorbable sutures, and a subcutaneous drainage is left. A compressive head draining is positioned for 5 days, in order to avoid subcutaneous effusion.

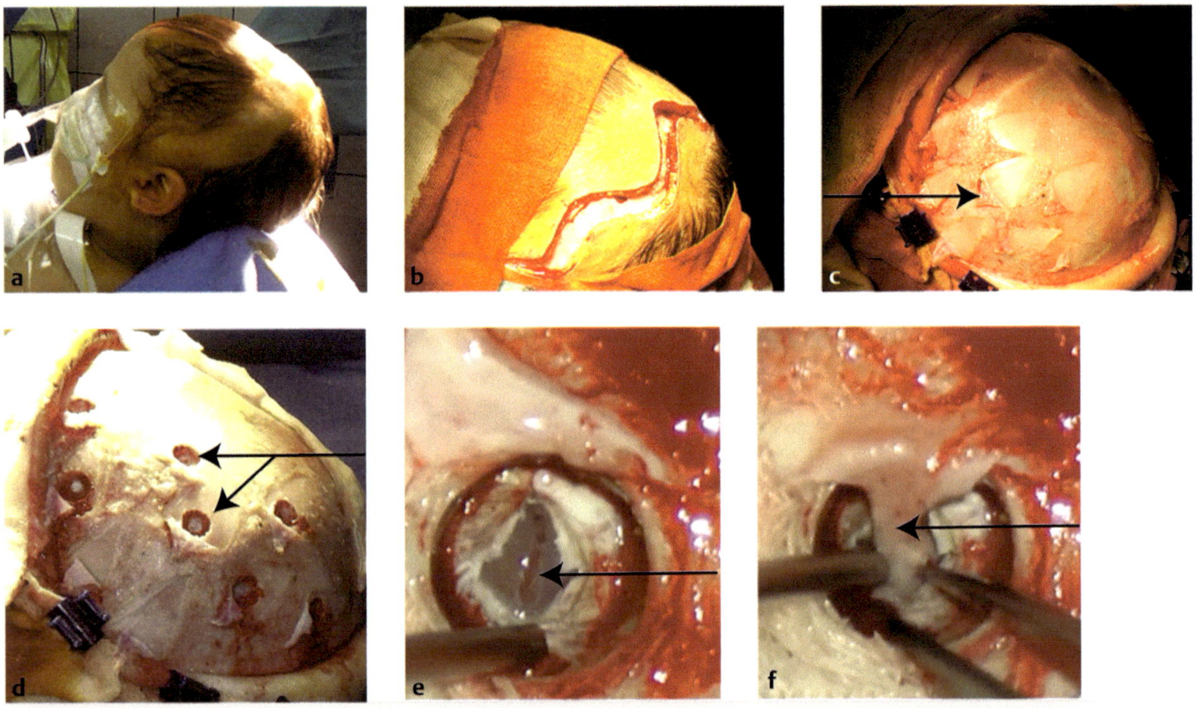


Fig. 4.1 (a) Patient postionning for a bilateral approach. (b) Bitragialretrocoronal skin incision, (c) subgaleal dissection, and periostel flaps elevated. (d) Burr holes. (e) Dural and arachnoidal layers are opened. (f) Periosteal flap is inserted in the subdural space.

## 4.10 Difficulties Encountered

No major difficulties may be encountered intraoperatively, as drilling a burr hole is a standard procedure in neurosurgery.

## 4.11 Bailout, Rescue, and Salvage Maneuvers

In case of failure of the revascularization procedure, when ischemic events are still reported by the patient more than 3 months after the surgery, further imaging studies are needed. MRI allows the visualization of the transosseous collateral with tetralogy of Fallot studies, and brain hemodynamics can be assessed with perfusion studies (ASL MRI) or BOLD studies. DSA is also necessary to observe if and where pial anastomosis have occurred, and if some burr holes failed to develop collaterals (▶ Fig. 4.2).

A second procedure is then possible, and needs to be targeted to the areas where no collateral developed. Multiple small linear skin incision permits to drill additional burr holes on the ischemic regions, and in our cohort succeeded in two out of two cases to resolve the clinical symptoms. It is important not to reopen the bitragial coronal incision, as it would disrupt some collateral circulation.

If no collateral circulation is noted in any of the burr holes, another revascularization procedure needs to be considered. This was necessary in 1 of the 64 cases in our cohort, and dissection of the STA is possible, and therefore direct (STA–MCA bypass) or indirect procedures are still possible (EDAMS).

## 4.12 Tips, Pearls, and Lessons Learned

The key issue in multiple burr hole surgery is the selection of the patient, as in all direct or indirect revascularization procedure. Careful morphological imaging and hemodynamic studies are necessary to identify the patients who will develop collateral circulations through the burr holes. Indeed, when surgery is offered too late, after ischemic stroke, at the stage of cortical atrophy, functional improvement is minor, and risk of failure and complications is significant. On the other hand, revascularization at a very early stage, without hemodynamic compromise may lead to the impossibility of the brain to develop collateral vessels through the burr holes.

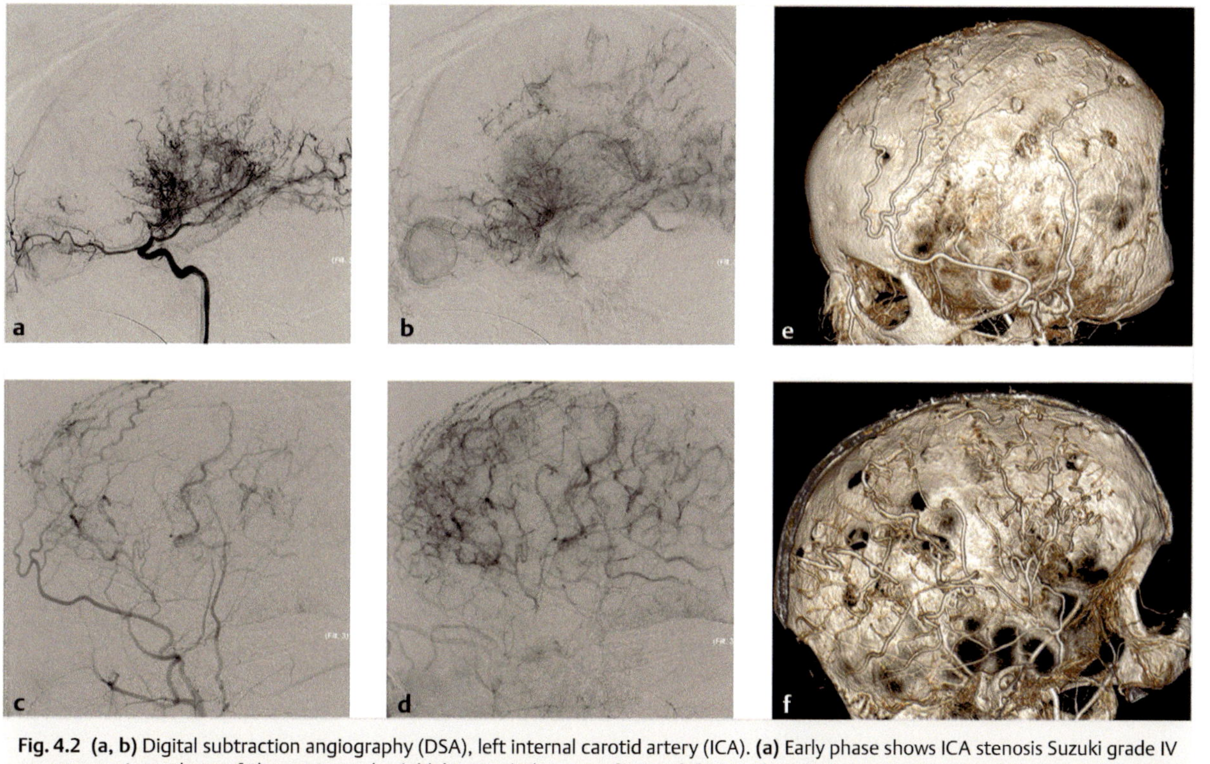


**Fig. 4.2 (a, b)** Digital subtraction angiography (DSA), left internal carotid artery (ICA). **(a)** Early phase shows ICA stenosis Suzuki grade IV moyamoya. Late phase of the angiography (phlebogram) shows perfusion defect in the whole hemisphere. **(c, d)** Postoperative DSA performed 1 year after revascularization. Selective left external carotid opacification shows collateral through the burr holes at the early stage of the angiography, and a good perfusion of the whole hemisphere on the phlebogram. **(e, f)** Three-dimensional angiography with selective injection of the external carotid artery (ECA) shows marked dilatation of the superficial temporal artery **(e)**, with collateral through the burr holes, and intracranial vessels opacification through the ECA–ICA anastomosis **(f)**.

Even if the surgical principle is simple, a meticulous technique is mandatory, and in particular, avoiding excessive coagulation on the dura/arachnoid layers is important.

# References

[1] Endo M, Kawano N, Miyasika Y, Yada K. Cranial burr hole for revascularization in moyamoya disease. J Neurosurg. 1989; 71(2):180–185

[2] Kawaguchi T, Fujita S, Hosoda K, et al. Multiple burr-hole operation for adult moyamoya disease. J Neurosurg. 1996; 84(3):468–476

[3] Sainte-Rose C, Oliveira R, Puget S, et al. Multiple bur hole surgery for the treatment of moyamoya disease in children. J Neurosurg. 2006; 105(6) Suppl:437–443

[4] Oliveira RS, Amato MCM, Simão GN, et al. Effect of multiple cranial burr hole surgery on prevention of recurrent ischemic attacks in children with moyamoya disease. Neuropediatrics. 2009; 40(6):260–264

[5] McLaughlin N, Martin NA. Effectiveness of burr holes for indirect revascularization in patients with moyamoya disease-a review of the literature. World Neurosurg. 2014; 81(1):91–98

[6] Blauwblomme T, Lemaitre H, Naggara O, et al. Cerebral blood flow improvement after indirect revascularization for pediatric moyamoya disease: a statistical analysis of arterial spin-labeling MRI. AJNR Am J Neuroradiol. 2016; 37(4):706–712

# 5 Encephalo-myo-synangiosis

*Nils Hecht and Peter Vajkoczy*

**Abstract**

An encephalo-myo-synangiosis (EMS) describes a form of indirect revascularization, where a vascularized pedicle graft of the temporalis muscle is placed directly onto the surface of the brain, which results in spontaneous sprouting of transpial extracranial–intracranial collaterals in patients suffering from moyamoya vasculopathy. Compared to a direct bypass, the advantages of an EMS are its technical simplicity and lower perioperative stroke risk. On the other hand, current research focuses on how to improve the hemodynamic efficacy and overall effectiveness of an EMS. Against this background, this chapter reviews and focuses on the indication and technical aspects of an EMS as well as its pearls, pitfalls, and limitations.

*Keywords:* cerebral revascularization, encephalo-myo-synangiosis, indirect revascularization, moyamoya vasculopathy

## 5.1 History and Initial Description

Surgical treatment of hemodynamic compromise typically uses the external carotid artery (ECA) as a source of new blood flow to the ischemic hemisphere. The two general methods of revascularization are as follows: (1) direct, where an extracranial to intracranial (EC–IC) bypass anastomosis between a donor vessel (typically the frontal or parietal branch of the superficial temporal artery [STA]) and a cortical recipient vessel (typically an M4-segment branch of the middle cerebral artery [MCA]) is grafted, or (2) indirect, where a vascularized, autologous graft supplied by the ECA is placed in direct contact with the surface of the brain, which results in spontaneous transpial vessel sprouting from the vascularized graft into the hypoperfused brain. The earliest attempt of indirect revascularization in humans was reported in 1942 by Kredel, who placed a vascularized pedicle graft of the temporalis muscle directly onto the surface of the brain after removal of the underlying bone and opening of the dura.[1] However, Kredel was discouraged by the high rate of perioperative seizures and abandoned the procedure until it was revived in 1977 by Karasawa, who termed the procedure encephalo-myo-synangiosis (EMS).[1] In 1981, Kobayashi used cerebral angiograms to confirm patent EC–IC collaterals at the muscle/brain interface of an EMS.[2] Later, Perren and colleagues nicely showed that a patent EMS not only results in transpial collateralization, but that these EC–IC collaterals also carry functional hemodynamic efficacy.[3] Meanwhile, several other procedures for indirect revascularization exist, such as encephalo-duro-arterio-synangiosis (EDAS), encephalo-myo-arterio-synangiosis (EMAS), pial synangiosis, dural inversion, and the drilling of burr holes without vessel synangiosis.[4–8] However, most experts agree that usage of the temporalis muscle as a vascularized graft probably provides the best prerequisite for successful indirect revascularization due to its rich blood supply and large surface area.

## 5.2 Indications

The key factor for compensation of hemodynamic compromise is endogenous flow augmentation through outgrowth of preexisting collaterals.[9] This requires an active proliferation of endothelial and perivascular cells, which is naturally limited. In cases of hemodynamic failure, surgical revascularization is a recognized treatment option. However, there remains considerable debate about the merits and shortcomings of direct versus indirect revascularization. In certain cases, however, the grafting of a direct bypass is technically more challenging and sometimes not feasible due to the small caliber and fragile cortical vasculature, such as in moyamoya vasculopathy, where vascular remodeling of the tunica muscularis renders the cortical vessels prone to rupture during suturing of the anastomosis. Also, there are situations where direct grafting of a standard STA–MCA bypass is not possible due to lack of a suitable STA donor vessel. In these cases, an EMS has the advantage of being less complex and safer than a direct bypass with proven benefit in pediatric patients with moyamoya vasculopathy.[10–13] Sometimes, even a combination of a bypass with an EMS may be indicated, for example, above the symptomatic hemisphere in pediatric patients with moyamoya vasculopathy. On the other hand, compared to a direct bypass, an EMS has the main disadvantages that (a) it offers no immediate ischemic protection and (b) that it is characterized by lower hemodynamic effectiveness and inconsistent revascularization results in adults and patients suffering from arteriosclerotic disease.[14] Therefore, we recommend that an EMS *alone* as the primary revascularization option should only be considered for treatment of the asymptomatic hemisphere in pediatric patients with moyamoya vasculopathy.

## 5.3 Key Principles

The general principle of an EMS is to transpose a vascularized pedicle graft of the temporalis muscle onto the surface of the underlying brain after performing a craniotomy and opening the dura. In all cases, the following key principles need to be considered in order to ensure successful indirect revascularization and limit the risk of complications:

1. The size of the craniotomy should match the size of the temporalis muscle to provide the largest possible contact surface between the muscle and the brain.
2. The sylvian fissure should be at the center of exposure so that the temporal and frontal regions of the brain are equally able to receive transpial collaterals.
3. Meticulous hemostasis of the dura border and at the surface of the muscle is imperative to minimize the risk of postoperative subdural hemorrhage.
4. Compression of the muscle with the bone flap at the base of the craniotomy should be avoided so that perfusion of the graft is not compromised.

# 5.4 SWOT Analysis

## 5.4.1 Strengths

Compared to direct revascularization, an EMS is a technically simple, safe and quick procedure, which provides a large surface for spontaneous transpial EC–IC collateralization.

## 5.4.2 Weaknesses

The muscle surface and border of the dura are potential sources of postoperative subdural hemorrhage. Also, hemodynamic effectiveness is inconsistent and does not occur immediately after surgery.

## 5.4.3 Opportunities

The current challenge in EMS surgery is to improve functional and morphological collateralization across all patient populations, for example, by local boosting of proangiogenic activity with continuous delivery of vascular growth factors at the muscle/brain interface.[15,16]

## 5.4.4 Threats

The indirect EC–IC collaterals of an EMS may be ineffective in restoring hemodynamic compromise in some cases. Further, certain steps of the surgical preparation, such as the craniotomy and durotomy may injure spontaneously formed middle meningeal artery (MMA) collaterals, which are termed "vault moyamoya vessels" and frequently encountered in patients with moyamoya vasculopathy.

# 5.5 Contraindications

Although an EMS offers a technically simple alternative to direct revascularization, the following contraindications need to be considered in order to ensure safety and effectiveness of the procedure. First, patients should not have a history of coagulopathy or platelet dysfunction because hemorrhage from the dissected surface of the temporalis muscle is one of the most feared postoperative complications. Prior to EMS surgery, we therefore recommend pausing anticoagulants or platelet inhibitors that may be required for treatment of the underlying vascular pathology. Second, EMS revascularization should not be performed in patients with brain atrophy because direct contact between the surface of the temporalis muscle and the brain is essential to ensure sprouting and ingrowth of transpial collaterals. Third, the angiograms of the patient should be studied for signs of preexisting EC–IC collaterals from the MMA because although EMS revascularization with sparing the MMA and its branches is technically feasible, this requires advance planning of the craniotomy and dural opening (i.e., with image guidance) in order to avoid perioperative ischemia due to iatrogenic transection of preexisting MMA collaterals.

# 5.6 Special Considerations

When planning for an EMS, specific details need to be considered. Despite the recent advances of 7 Tesla magnetic resonance imaging (MRI), digital subtraction angiography (DSA) remains the gold standard in the preoperative workup of moyamoya patients planned for cerebral revascularization.[17,18] Here, a DSA with an external carotid injection is required not just for identification of a suitable donor vessel in the case of a direct revascularization, but also to identify vault moyamoya vessels.[19] These preformed EC–IC collaterals at the surface of the brain typically feed off branches from the MMA, superficial temporal or occipital artery or from branches of tentorial arteries or the anterior falx and need to be preserved during dissection in order to avoid ischemic complications. Also, a recent MRI scan is needed to identify the extent of brain atrophy and exclude extensive preexisting postischemic tissue damage in the cortical region below the intended EMS. Further, patients scheduled for an EMS require an in-depth hemostasiological analysis to exclude coagulopathies and platelet dysfunction and any anticoagulant or antiplatelet therapy should be discontinued perioperatively. To further optimize the revascularization result, the EMS can be combined with additional inversion of a frontal dural pedicle graft (encephalo-duro-synangiosis).

# 5.7 Pitfalls, Risk Assessment, and Complications

At present, there are no reports regarding the risk of perioperative complications following an EMS. However, most experts agree that the main specific surgical risk of an EMS is subdural hemorrhage and/or hemorrhagic swelling of the temporalis muscle that requires revision in approximately 5% of all cases. Another typical complication in patients undergoing cerebral revascularization is ischemic stroke, which was shown to occur in up to 15% after direct bypass revascularization.[20] Even in highly specialized centers this perioperative stroke risk rarely drops below 5%,[10,21,22,23] against which the estimated perioperative stroke risk of 1 to 2% after an EMS alone compares favorably.

## 5.8 Special Instructions, Position, and Anesthesia

The key element of neuroanesthesia is to maximize brain relaxation ("slack brain") in order to avoid swelling and venous congestion of the cerebral veins at the border of the durotomy. For this purpose, anesthetic agents that lower the cerebral metabolic rate, neuronal activity, and cerebral blood volume, such as propofol and remifentanil are commonly used.[24,25] Barbiturates may be administered up to burst suppression on electroencephalography (EEG). Osmotic agents (i.e., mannitol) may gain additional brain relaxation. Hyperventilation should be avoided in order to prevent further reduction of the already compromised cerebral perfusion. Most importantly, blood pressure should be maintained at high normal level with a mean arterial pressure (MAP) targeted between 80 and 90 mm Hg at all times. Next to anesthesia, positioning of the patient is equally important to prevent jugular venous congestion and subsequent cerebral swelling, since there is usually no relevant amount of cerebrospinal fluid to be gained from the sulci and fissures of the juvenile brain with moyamoya vasculopathy. For an EMS, we generally recommend a horizontal surgical field orientation similar to a standard STA–MCA bypass, particularly in cases where a combined revascularization is planned and feasibility of a bypass cannot be anticipated.

## 5.9 Key Surgical Steps

### 5.9.1 Patient Position and Skin Incision

To avoid excessive head rotation, the ipsilateral shoulder should be supported with the patient secured to the operating table. Final 90-degree positioning is then accomplished by the following two measures:

- Head rotation of 50 to 60 degrees.
- Tilting of the operating table to 30 to 40 degrees.

▶ Fig. 5.1 describes patient positioning and head rotation.

### 5.9.2 Pterional Skin Incision

An extended pterional skin incision (▶ Fig. 5.2) is planned according to the required dimensions of the craniotomy along the insertion border of the temporalis muscle and to expose an equally large frontal–temporal surface area including the end of the sylvian fissure, which can be identified with the help of the target point described by Peña and colleagues.[26]

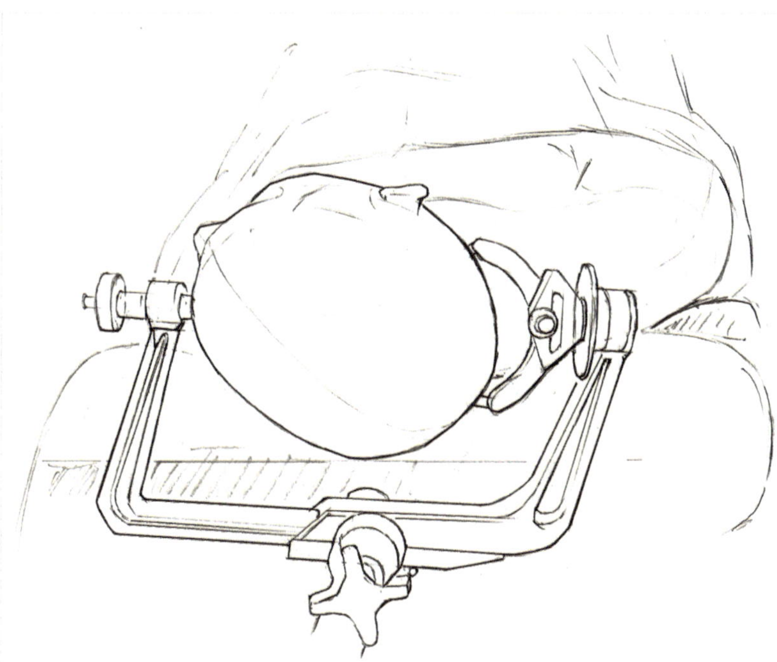

**Fig. 5.1** Patient positioning with 50- to 60-degree head rotation. Horizontal positioning of the surgical field is accomplished by 30 degrees tilting of the operating table.

## 5.9.3 Separate Skin and Muscle Flaps

To allow transposition of the temporalis muscle below the underlying bone, the skin is dissected from the outer fascia of the temporalis muscle to create separate skin and muscle flaps (▶ Fig. 5.3). The insertion of the temporalis muscle at the superior temporal line is cut with monopolar cautery. Importantly, monopolar cautery should only be used to cut the insertion line of the muscle and not to dissect the muscle from the bone (see Chapter 5.9.4).

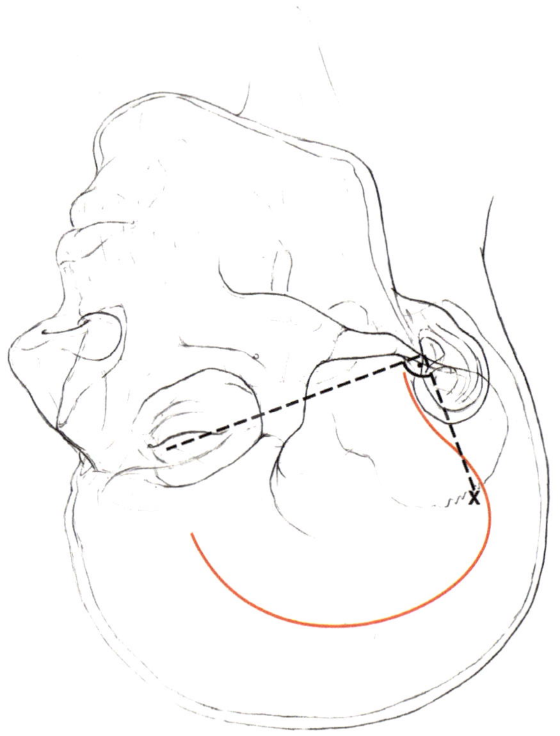


**Fig. 5.2** Extended pterional skin incision beyond the end of the sylvian fissure (*red line*).

## 5.9.4 Mobilization of the Temporalis Muscle

To spare the blood supplying vessel branches and limit dissection trauma to the muscle fibers, the temporalis muscle should be mobilized from proximal to distal along the course of the muscle fibers with the help of a curved raspatorium (▶ Fig. 5.4). Caution should be exercised to preserve the integrity of the inner muscle fascia.

## 5.9.5 Elevation of the Muscle Flap

After mobilization, the muscle flap is elevated and turned towards the base of the exposure (▶ Fig. 5.5). The muscle is then held back over the skin as a separate flap by gentle retraction.

## 5.9.6 Craniotomy and Drilling of the Sphenoid Wing

After retraction of the muscle pedicle graft, the lateral sphenoid wing should be spared when performing the craniotomy to preserve potential MMA collaterals. After removal of the bone flap, the lateral sphenoid wing is drilled down to spare potential MMA collaterals (see ▶ Fig. 5.6).

## 5.9.7 Opening of the Dura and Encephalo-duro-synangiosis

The dura is opened along the border of the MMA using a window technique to preserve potential vault moyamoya vessels beyond the area of exposure (▶ Fig. 5.7). The dural flaps are then inverted as an encephalo-duro-synangiosis to provide an additional surface for spontaneous EC–IC collateralization beyond the border of the craniotomy.

## 5.9.8 Suturing of the Muscle Fascia to the Edge of the Dural Opening

To complete the EMS, the muscle graft is placed onto the surface of the brain after final hemostasis and the muscle

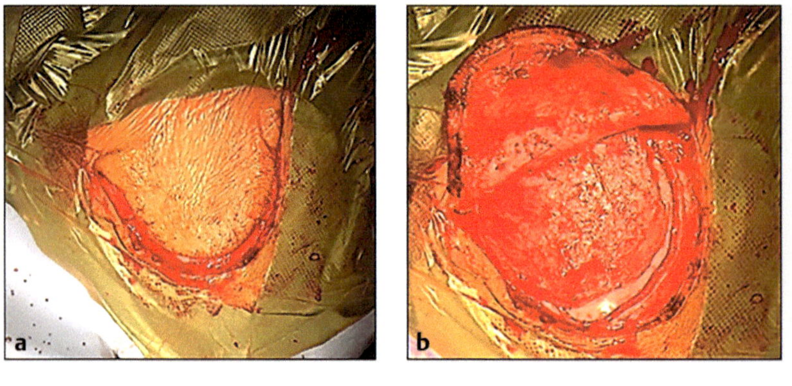


**Fig. 5.3 (a, b)** Following the skin incision, separate skin and muscle flaps are dissected before cutting the insertion of the temporalis muscle along the superior temporal line.

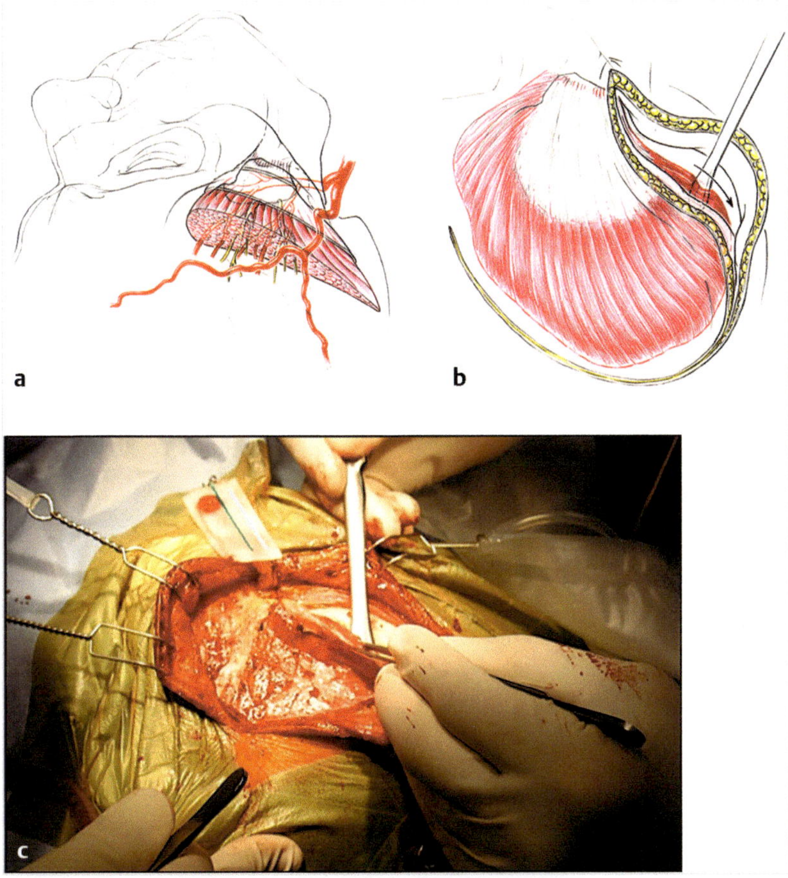

Fig. 5.4 (a–c) Anatomy of the vessel branches of the external carotid artery (ECA) supplying the temporalis muscle and illustration of graft mobilization.

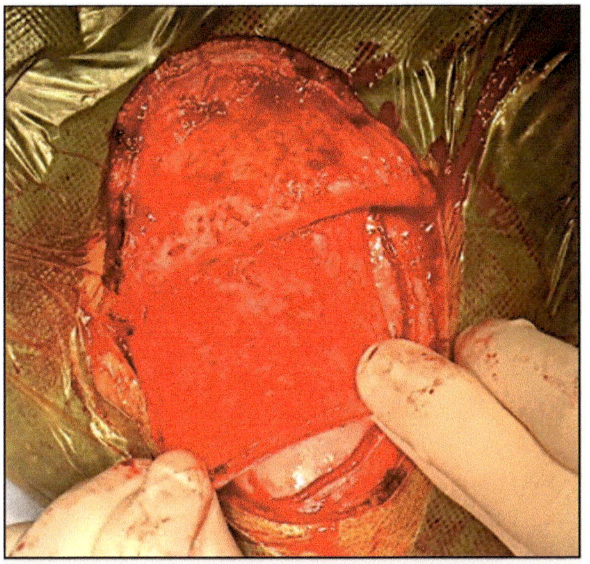

Fig. 5.5 Elevation of the muscle pedicle graft from the underlying bone.

fascia is sutured to the outer edge of the dural opening with a nonabsorbable 3–0 running suture (see ▶ Fig. 5.8).

### 5.9.9 Bone Flap Reimplantation

After completion of the EMS, the bone flap is reimplanted and secured with titanium pins. To avoid compression of the graft, it is important to leave sufficient space for the muscle to pass through at the base of the craniotomy by removal of excess bone (see ▶ Fig. 5.9).

## 5.10 Difficulties Encountered

Frequently, the MMA is very adhesive to the bone and/or has a prolonged course within the flap, which may result in unintentional injury to the MMA during turning of the flap. As outlined above, this can be avoided by drilling the lateral sphenoid wing with a diamond burr and careful elevation of the flap under visual inspection. In case intramuscular hemorrhage or swelling occurs prior to suturing the fascia to the dural edges, the bone flap should be left out to avoid compression of the brain. Further, compression of the muscle at the base of the craniotomy during flap reimplantation may result in venous stasis and additional swelling of the graft, which can be prevented by removing excess bone from base of

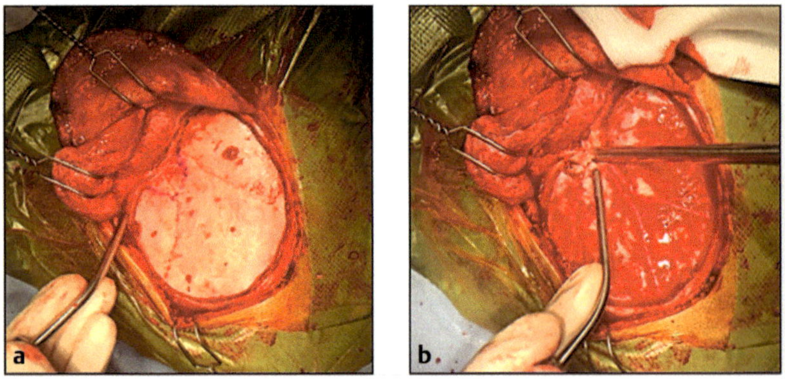


**Fig. 5.6 (a, b)** The lateral sphenoid wing is identified and spared from the craniotomy in order to preserve middle meningeal artery (MMA) collaterals. After turning of the bone flap, the sphenoid wing is drilled down and removed with the help of Kerrison punches.

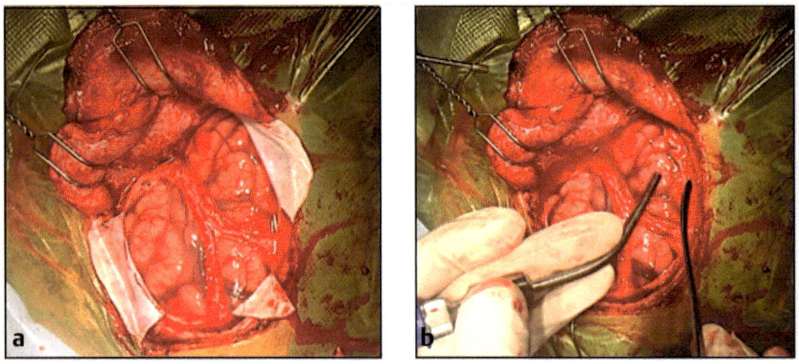


**Fig. 5.7 (a, b)** Opening of the dura with sparing of the middle meningeal artery (MMA) and dural inversion.

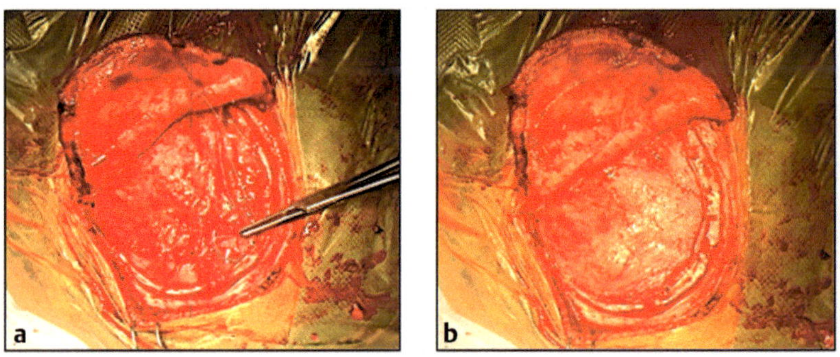


**Fig. 5.8 (a, b)** The fascia of the temporalis muscle is sutured to the outer edge of the dura.

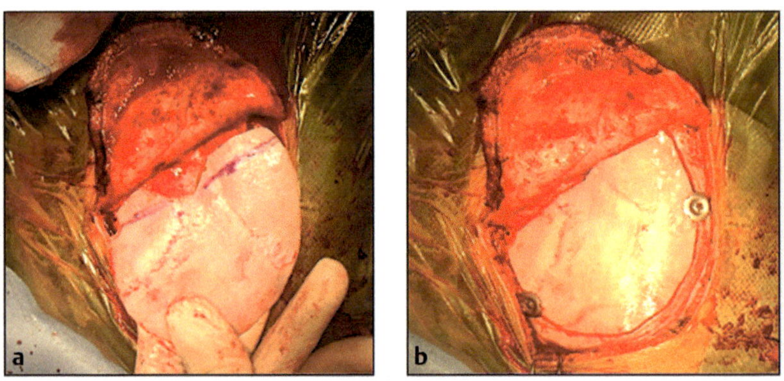


**Fig. 5.9 (a, b)** Excess bone is removed from the base of the bone flap before final reimplantation.

the craniotomy. If a subdural hematoma is noted on routine postoperative imaging, revision surgery may be required for hematoma evacuation. In addition, the surgeon should steer clear of the following typical pitfalls:

- Inadequate (too small) size of the craniotomy.
- Inadequate hemostasis.
- Antiplatelet therapy continued.
- Injury to vault moyamoya (MMA) collaterals.
- Injury to the cortical surface during suturing.

## 5.11 Bailout, Rescue, and Salvage Maneuvers

For utilization of the maximum surface area for endogenous EMS collateralization, the craniotomy should be enlarged if the sylvian fissure and both opercula are not well exposed. Coincidentally, patient safety is ensured by management of coagulation disorders or platelet dysfunction.

## 5.12 Tips, Pearls, and Lessons Learned

In conclusion, an EMS poses an effective alternative to a direct bypass procedure in juvenile patients with moyamoya vasculopathy. Most importantly, simplicity and safety of an EMS remain ensured if the following technical aspects are observed:

1. The craniotomy should be large enough to expose the whole sylvian fissure.
2. Temporal–basal muscle retraction should be gentile to avoid facial nerve palsy.
3. Avoid monopolar cautery to spare the muscle fascia and vasculature.
4. The temporalis muscle should be mobilized from proximal to distal.
5. The lateral sphenoid wing should be spared during the craniotomy.
6. Thorough hemostasis should be performed at the muscle surface.
7. The EMS should be combined with dural inversion (encephalo-duro-synangiosis).
8. The muscle fascia should be stitched to the dura using the operating microscope.
9. Sufficient bone should be removed at the base of the craniotomy.

After surgery, we recommend overnight postoperative intensive care unit monitoring for adults and 24-hour observation in a neurological/neurosurgical intensive care unit (NICU) for pediatric patients. On the day after surgery, a noncontrast computed tomography is performed to rule out procedure related hemorrhage or ischemia. At 12 months, morphological function of the graft in terms of transpial EC–IC collateralization is assessed by conventional DSA.

## References


[1] Karasawa J, Kikuchi H, Furuse S, Sakaki T, Yoshida Y. A surgical treatment of "moyamoya" disease "encephalo-myo synangiosis". Neurol Med Chir (Tokyo). 1977; 17(1 Pt 1):29–37

[2] Kobayashi K, Takeuchi S, Tsuchida T, Ito J. Encephalo-myo-synangiosis (EMS) in moyamoya disease -with special reference to postoperative angiography (author's transl). Neurol Med Chir (Tokyo). 1981; 21 (12):1229–1238

[3] Perren F, Meairs S, Schmiedek P, Hennerici M, Horn P. Power Doppler evaluation of revascularization in childhood moyamoya. J Neurol. 2005; 64(3):558–560

[4] Dauser RC, Tuite GF, McCluggage CW. Dural inversion procedure for moyamoya disease. Technical note. J Neurosurg. 1997; 86(4):719–723

[5] Sencer S, Poyanli A, Kiriş T, Sencer A, Minareci O. Recent experience with moyamoya disease in Turkey. Eur Radiol. 2000; 10(4):569–572

[6] Matsushima T, Inoue T, Katsuta T, et al. An indirect revascularization method in the surgical treatment of moyamoya disease—various kinds of indirect procedures and a multiple combined indirect procedure. Neurol Med Chir (Tokyo). 1998; 38 Suppl:297–302

[7] Scott RM, Smith JL, Robertson RL, Madsen JR, Soriano SG, Rockoff MA. Long-term outcome in children with moyamoya syndrome after cranial revascularization by pial synangiosis. J Neurosurg. 2004; 100 (2) Suppl Pediatrics:142–149

[8] Matsushima T, Fujiwara S, Nagata S, et al. Surgical treatment for paediatric patients with moyamoya disease by indirect revascularization procedures (EDAS, EMS, EMAS). Acta Neurochir (Wien). 1989; 98 (3–4):135–140

[9] Schaper W. Collateral circulation: past and present. Basic Res Cardiol. 2009; 104(1):5–21

[10] Guzman R, Lee M, Achrol A, et al. Clinical outcome after 450 revascularization procedures for moyamoya disease. Clinical article. J Neurosurg. 2009; 111(5):927–935

[11] Kim S-K, Cho B-K, Phi JH, et al. Pediatric moyamoya disease: an analysis of 410 consecutive cases. Ann Neurol. 2010; 68(1):92–101

[12] Fung L-WE, Thompson D, Ganesan V. Revascularisation surgery for paediatric moyamoya: a review of the literature. Childs Nerv Syst. 2005; 21(5):358–364

[13] Czabanka M, Peña-Tapia P, Scharf J, et al. Characterization of direct and indirect cerebral revascularization for the treatment of European patients with moyamoya disease. Cerebrovasc Dis. 2011; 32(4):361–369

[14] Komotar RJ, Starke RM, Otten ML, et al. The role of indirect extracranial-intracranial bypass in the treatment of symptomatic intracranial atheroocclusive disease. J Neurosurg. 2009; 110(5):896–904

[15] Hecht N, Marushima A, Nieminen M, et al. Myoblast-mediated gene therapy improves functional collateralization in chronic cerebral hypoperfusion. Stroke. 2015; 46(1):203–211

[16] Marushima A, Nieminen M, Kremenetskaia I, et al. Balanced single-vector co-delivery of VEGF/PDGF-BB improves functional collateralization in chronic cerebral ischemia. J Cereb Blood Flow Metab. 2019; 271678X18818298 [Epub ahead of print]

[17] Deng X, Zhang Z, Zhang Y, et al. Comparison of 7.0- and 3.0-T MRI and MRA in ischemic-type moyamoya disease: preliminary experience. J Neurosurg. 2016; 124(6):1716–1725

[18] Oh BH, Moon HC, Baek HM, et al. Comparison of 7 T and 3 T MRI in patients with moyamoya disease. Magn Reson Imaging. 2017; 37:134–138

[19] Kodama N, Fujiwara S, Horie Y, Kayama T, Suzuki J. Transdural anastomosis in moyamoya disease—vault moyamoy (author's translation). No Shinkei Geka. 1980; 8(8):729–737

[20] Powers WJ, Clarke WR, Grubb RL, Jr, Videen TO, Adams HP, Jr, Derdeyn CP, COSS Investigators. Extracranial-intracranial bypass surgery for stroke prevention in hemodynamic cerebral ischemia: the Carotid Occlusion Surgery Study randomized trial. JAMA. 2011; 306(18):1983–1992

[21] Yasargil MG, Yonekawa Y. Results of microsurgical extra-intracranial arterial bypass in the treatment of cerebral ischemia. J Neurosurg. 1977; 1(1):22–24

[22] Hecht N, Woitzik J, König S, Horn P, Vajkoczy P. Laser speckle imaging allows real-time intraoperative blood flow assessment during neurosurgical procedures. J Cereb Blood Flow Metab. 2013; 33(7):1000–1007

[23] Sandow N, von Weitzel-Mudersbach P, Rosenbaum S, et al. Extra-intracranial standard bypass in the elderly: perioperative risk, bypass patency and outcome. Cerebrovasc Dis. 2013; 36(3):228–235

[24] Cole CD, Gottfried ON, Gupta DK, Couldwell WT. Total intravenous anesthesia: advantages for intracranial surgery. J Neurosurg. 2007; 61 (5) Suppl 2:369–377, discussion 377–378

[25] Kaisti KK, Långsjö JW, Aalto S, et al. Effects of sevoflurane, propofol, and adjunct nitrous oxide on regional cerebral blood flow, oxygen consumption, and blood volume in humans. J Anesthesiol. 2003; 99(3):603–613

[26] Peña-Tapia PG, Kemmling A, Czabanka M, Vajkoczy P, Schmiedek P. Identification of the optimal cortical target point for extracranial-intracranial bypass surgery in patients with hemodynamic cerebrovascular insufficiency. J Neurosurg. 2008; 108(4):655–661

# 6 Encephalo-duro-arterio-synangiosis: Pediatric

*Edward Smith*

**Abstract**
Pediatric moyamoya is typically treated with surgical revascularization. In this chapter, we review variations of surgical treatments of this disease, with a specific focus on methods of encephalo-duro-arterio-synangiosis. This approach employs vascularized tissue supplied by the external carotid artery to serve as a graft to ischemic territories of the brain. Surgical indications, preoperative evaluation, perioperative management, and technical nuances—with relevant illustrations—will be discussed.

*Keywords:* encephalo-duro-arterio-synangiosis, pial synangiosis, moyamoya, indirect, pediatric, revascularization, stroke

## 6.1 History and Initial Description

Indirect procedures for moyamoya syndrome tend to be reserved for pediatric patients where there is more successful collateralization, when compared with direct revascularization and where direct procedures are difficult due to the small size of the arteries. Indirect procedures include encephalo-myo-synangiosis, encephalo-galeo-myo-synangiosis, encephalo-duro-arterio-synangiosis, pial synangiosis, omental transplant (encephalo-omental synangiosis), and multiple burr holes. All are based on the observation that vascularized tissue placed on the brain induces vascular collateralization from the graft to the brain. Encephalo-duro-arterio-synangiosis (EDAS) involves the use of the dura and a branch of the superficial temporal artery (STA) to revascularize the brain. Originally described by Matsushima, the technique uses a branch of the STA to revascularize the brain by suturing the vessel in between two leaves of dura. A variant of this procedure, pial synangiosis, was developed by R. Michael Scott and differs by (1) affixing the STA to the brain surface with pial sutures and (2) widely opening the arachnoid to facilitate ingrowth of new vessels in response to growth factors elaborated by the ischemic brain. Pial synangiosis has become widely used in the pediatric population in the United States.

## 6.2 Indications

With caveats, the analysis from American Heart Association (AHA) concluded that "the data from the medical literature suggest that surgical revascularization is a safe intervention for pediatric moyamoya syndrome and most treated patients derive some symptomatic benefit." The authors offer revascularization for patients with radiographic evidence of moyamoya, as defined by Suzuki grade II-VI on angiogram (or comparable findings on magnetic resonance angiogram/computed tomography angiogram [MRA/CTA] in the rare cases when catheter angiography is not possible), typically coupled with evidence of diminished or limited brain perfusion (most commonly the presence of "ivy sign"—hyperintense sulcal signal on axial fluid-attenuated inversion recovery (FLAIR) MRI, but also with evidence from other perfusion studies when necessary). This radiographic evidence is paramount, but clinical examination is important for decision making. Symptomatic patients are usually offered surgical treatment, but asymptomatic children are also operated if the imaging findings indicate severe perfusion deficits or progression of disease over time. In contrast, contraindications to surgery include evidence of preexisting neurologic devastation or very early disease (Suzuki I or II without perfusion problems) in an asymptomatic patient.

Surgical procedure selection is predicated on the symptom presentation, patient age, and anatomy. In most cases, there is a predilection to choose pial synangiosis over direct bypass, because of the data supporting the long-term durability of these grafts, and the ability to offer this operation to any age group. In patients without suitable vessels, myosyangiosis (using temporalis muscle) or pericranium with dura are suitable alternatives. Direct bypass is typically reserved for patients with vessels large enough for anastomosis (often teens or older), coupled with acute presentation of rapidly progressive strokes.

Regarding timing, the general principle of minimizing the time between diagnosis and revascularization is supported.

- Delays may be reasonable to schedule experienced anesthetic/intensive care unit (ICU).
- Medical contraindications may mandate delays (such as recent infarction, infection, or hemorrhage) (Class IIb C).

## 6.3 Key Principles

The surgical technique of EDAS is unique in the focus on creating a direct connection between the recipient brain and donor tissue. This principle is best exemplified by the most common subtype of EDAS used in the United States for children, pial synangiosis. In this procedure, an indirect anastomosis of the parietal branch of the superficial temporal artery is made to the cerebral cortex. Like other indirect operations, it also benefits from the recruitment of collateral vasculature from adjacent tissue, such as the dura and middle meningeal vessels. It differs from other EDAS procedures because pial sutures and the aggressive approach of a wide arachnoidal opening are used. The principle of the pial sutures rests on the concept that the normal pulsatile nature of the brain and donor vessel might inhibit growth of new vasculature, but suturing them together reduces relative motion and facilitates better growth.

The wide arachnoidal opening is perhaps the biologically most important aspect of the surgery, as recent data have revealed the significant role of angiogenic growth factors in the spinal fluid and embedded in the extracellular matrix of the pia as contributors to new vessel growth. Opening the arachnoid offers the double benefit of removing a mechanical barrier to ingrowth while also facilitating improved contact between nascent vasculature and growth factors.

# 6.4 SWOT Analysis

Assessment of EDAS using SWOT analysis is summarized below.

## 6.4.1 Strengths

- EDAS can be applied with any age group and any size artery.
- No concerns with proximal vessel stenoses that might limit retrograde filling with direct bypass.
- It is technically less challenging than a direct bypass, with no clamping time or potential ischemic period.
- It can be used in any vascular territory and can be expanded to cover as much cortex as wanted, with a broader area of revascularization.

## 6.4.2 Weaknesses

- It takes time for the donor vessels to grow in, thereby not providing immediate protection.
- Preexisting spontaneous transdural collaterals may limit surgical exposure.

## 6.4.3 Opportunities

- Indirect bypasses can sometimes be combined with direct procedures (although committing donor vessels to direct bypass necessarily limits distal revascularization).
- Laboratory data suggest that angiogenesis can be accelerated with biological agents, offering opportunities to enhance the speed and effectiveness of this approach in the future.

## 6.4.4 Threats

- Donor vessels may not grow if there is no underlying brain ischemia to drive angiogenesis.
- Patient selection needs to be tailored to surgical approach.

# 6.5 Contraindications

There are a number of contraindications to EDAS. These can be divided into general contraindications for revascularization surgery of any sort with moyamoya and specific contraindications to EDAS.

## 6.5.1 General Contraindications to Revascularization Surgery

- Unclear angiographic (or MRI) evidence of moyamoya.
- Medically unstable for operating room (OR).
- Recent stroke (may increase risk of general anesthesia and might consider 4–6 week delay).

## 6.5.2 Specific Contraindications to EDAS

- May not produce robust collateral growth if poor ischemic drive, so EDAS may not be suitable for early-stage, asymptomatic moyamoya (Suzuki I/II).
- Rapid, repeated strokes in a short period of time may suggest a role for direct bypass if a proper vessel and anatomy is favorable, given the delay inherent to EDAS revascularization.

# 6.6 Special Considerations

Several special considerations are worth reviewing while performing EDAS. Given the importance of underlying ischemia to drive surgical collateral vessel growth, the presence of radiographic evidence of ischemia (such as ivy sign on axial FLAIR imaging in MRI) is important. In some cases, arterial spin labeling (ASL) may be a useful adjunct to document ischemia if other studies, such as single-photon emission computed tomography (SPECT), are not available or practical in a pediatric population.

Aspirin is generally used in all cases, typically with doses adjusted for weight. For practical purposes, 41 mg/day is given to children 3 years of age and younger, 81 mg/day is given to all others (including adults), but some obese patients (100 kg or more in weight) or those with limited aspirin resistance may require higher doses (up to 325 mg twice a day). Some patients may exhibit varying degrees of innate aspirin resistance, in which case some institutions perform specific testing to assess the degree of impairment. In other cases, children may experience side effects from the aspirin, such as bruising or stomach upset. In these cases, adjusting the dose of aspirin often solves the problems, but alternatives exist in the use of low-molecular-weight heparin or other antiplatelet agents, if necessary. Consultation with hematology may be helpful in these circumstances.

Lastly, pediatric moyamoya has a high percentage of children who have arteriopathy in association with other systemic disorders (neurofibromatosis, sickle cell disease, Down's syndrome, etc.). In these complex medical cases, multidisciplinary consultation is often important to coordinate care and reduce risk of surgical intervention.

## 6.7 Pitfalls, Risk Assessment, and Complications

The overall perioperative stroke rate is reported at about 4.5% per hemisphere (during the operation and subsequent 30 days postoperatively). This rate varies in different populations, with higher risk associated with younger age (under 3 years of age), syndromic cases (Down's syndrome and sickle cell disease in particular), and history of recent stroke (within 1 month prior to surgery). Another known risk factor for perioperative stroke is the presence of transdural collateral vessels. It is particularly important to consider a full catheter angiogram (including the selective injection of the internal carotids, external carotids, and vertebrobasilar system) to fully detail the extracranial circulation. This allows identification of any preexisting, spontaneous transdural collateral vessels that may be supplying the cortex, thereby reducing the risk of inadvertently interrupting these vessels during surgery. This is particularly important in children who have already undergone any cranial operations (ventricular shunt, tumor, etc.).

## 6.8 Special Instructions, Position, and Anesthesia

The technical aspects of the surgery include several unique steps. Preoperatively, the patient is admitted the day before surgery for overnight intravenous hydration and aspirin therapy is continued right up to, and including, the day before surgery.

On the day of surgery, intraoperative electroencephalographic (EEG) monitoring may be used to help identify real-time changes in cerebral blood flow, as indicated by EEG slowing, allowing anesthesia to adjust blood pressure, carbon dioxide ($CO_2$) levels, and medications. Positioning is important, keeping the neck as neutral as possible with the use of a shoulder roll and bed turning, in order to prevent kinking of vessels in the neck and concomitant reductions in cerebral blood flow. Keeping the STA course flat relative to the floor and seating on opposite sides of the vessel with the microscope will aid an easy dissection for both the surgeon and assistant.

During the initial dissection of the STA, the risk of vessel injury can be minimized by exposing the vessel in small segments. Arachnoidal opening is critical and spending time to widely open as much area as possible is important. Use of an arachnoid knife, linear openings along cortical vessels, and sharp dissection with microscissors are helpful techniques. At closure, the risk of cerebrospinal fluid (CSF) leak can occur if there is inadequate galea closure. Careful inspection of the wound prior to skin suture placement can reveal areas that may need additional sutures.

Immediate postoperative care should be administered in the ICU, with the goals of avoiding hypotension and hypocarbia. Generally patients are extubated, awake and have an arterial line (for blood pressure management) and a bladder catheter (for monitoring volume status). Antibiotics are used for 24 hours. Aspirin is administered on postoperative day #1. Antiepileptics are not routinely prescribed. Intravenous fluids are run at 1 to 1.5 times maintenance and slowly decreased as the ability to take oral fluids recovers. Pain control is important and frequent neurological examinations are critical to detect any changes in examination. The patient is encouraged to ambulate as soon as possible and children are managed to minimize pain and anxiety (as crying can cause vasoconstriction and potentially increase the risk of stroke).

## 6.9 Patient Position with Skin Incision and Key Surgical Steps

- The patient is placed supine in the Mayfield head holder or on a headrest with a roll placed under the ipsilateral shoulder. The head is turned to the contralateral side (▶ Fig. 6.1).
- The STA is marked by Doppler ultrasonography, and a linear incision is made over it. The artery is skeletonized with perivascular tissue using the microscope (▶ Fig. 6.2).

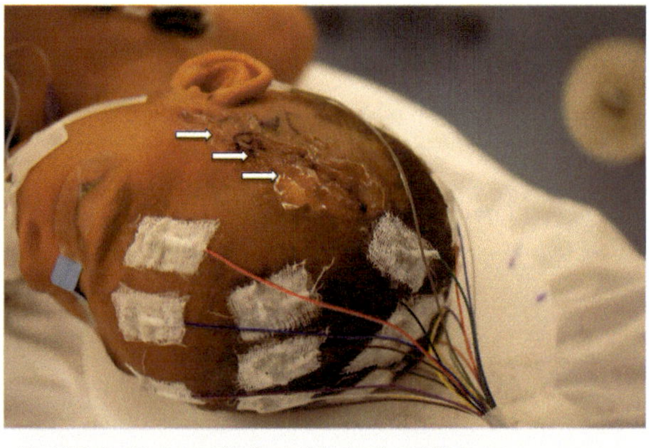

**Fig. 6.1** Patient positioning with the head flat, electroencephalographic (EEG) leads out of the way of the superficial temporal artery (STA) and the course of the STA marked out using ultrasound (*arrows*). The young age of this child led to the use of a headrest rather than pins.

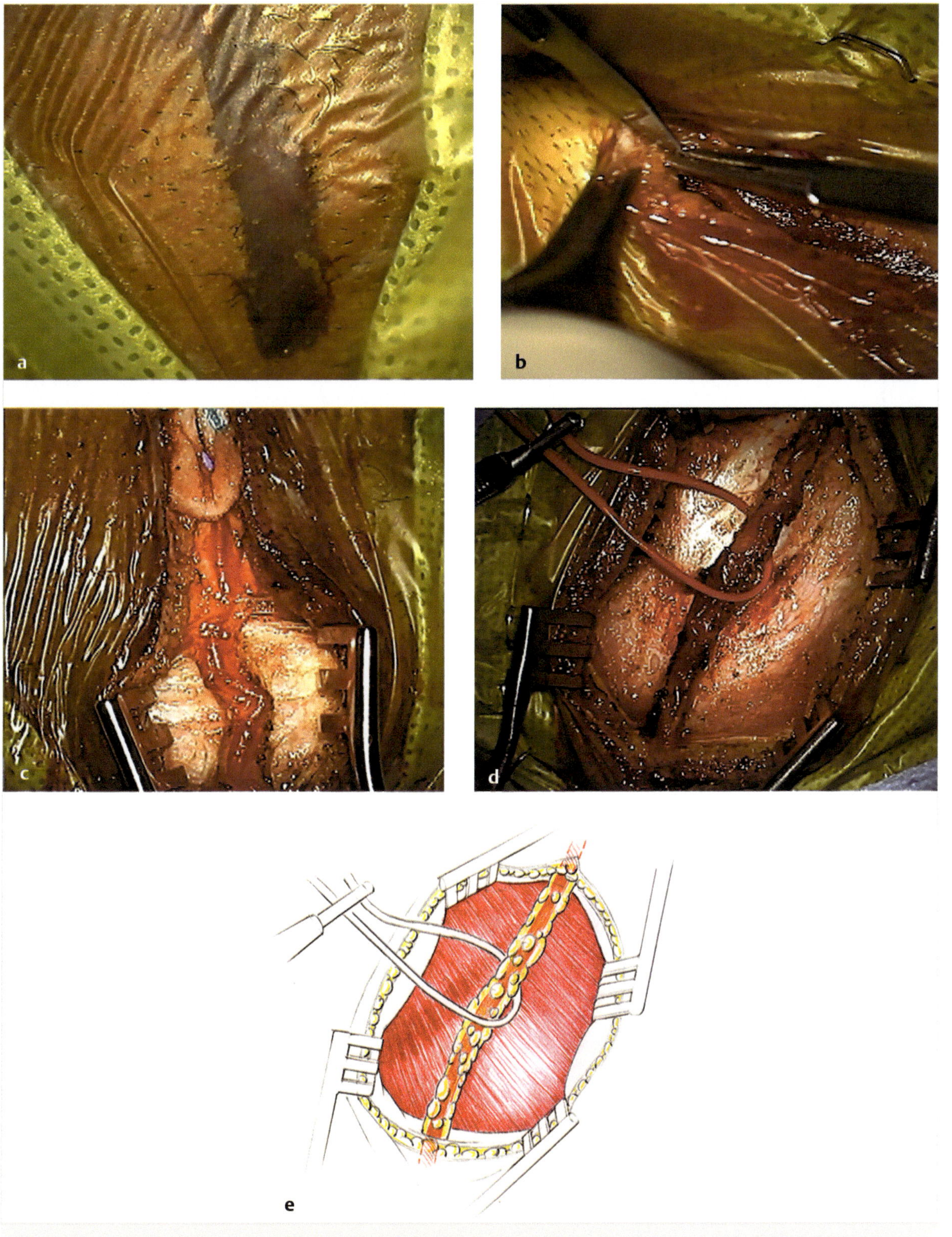


**Fig. 6.2** **(a)** Dissection of the superficial temporal artery (STA) takes place from the apex (near the top of the head) under the microscope. **(b)** The vessel is dissected free using fine curved snaps or forceps, with the assistant cutting on top of the closed tips. **(c)** A generous cuff of perivascular tissue is left along the sides of the vessel to encourage ingrowth. **(d, e)** At the conclusion of the vessel dissection, a loop is placed underneath the STA to facilitate mobilization during subsequent steps.

- The temporalis muscle is incised in a cruciate fashion and the craniotomy performed based on burr holes placed at either end of the arterial segment. The dura is incised along the artery and in flaps so as to allow retraction of the dura (▶ Fig. 6.3).
- The arachnoid is incised widely under the microscope. The superficial temporal artery is then placed on the pial surface and sutured to the pia using 10–0 monofilament sutures (▶ Fig. 6.4).

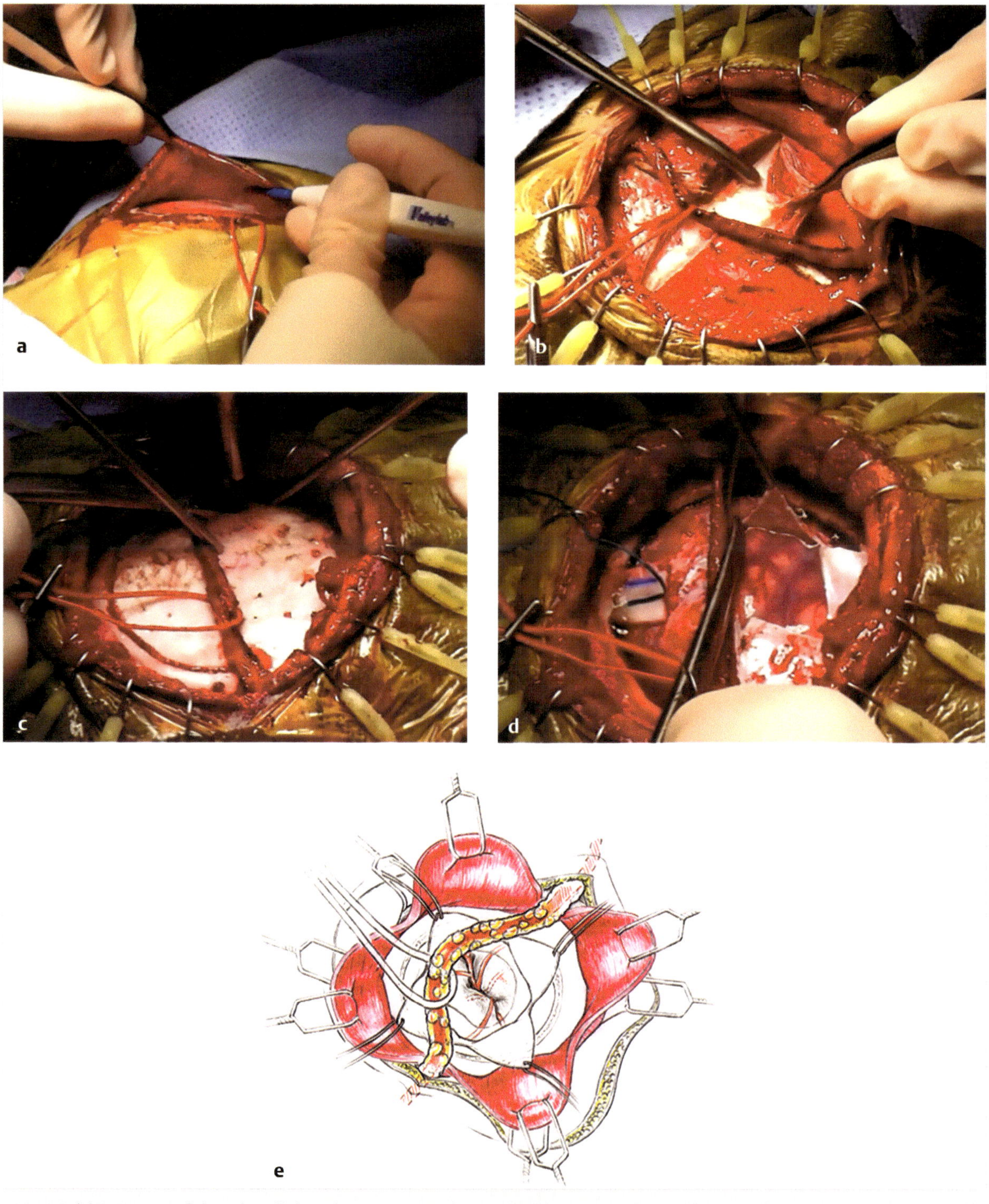

**Fig. 6.3 (a)** Dissection of the galea off the subjacent temporalis muscle. **(b)** Cruciate opening of temporalis muscle, with dissection off underlying bone. Note use of low profile retractors. **(c)** Craniotomy, with burr holes places at expected entry and exit of superficial temporal artery (STA). Care taken to drill away from the STA. **(d, e)** Stellate opening of dura to maximize exposure.

- Several sutures are placed to encourage tight approximation of the artery to the brain surface.
- When replacing the bone flap, care must be taken to prevent stretching the artery. The artery must enter and exit the burr holes in a gentle curve without tension (► Fig. 6.5).
- The temporalis muscle is loosely approximated so as not to kink or occlude the artery. The galea and skin are closed in the standard fashion, taking care not to injure the artery.

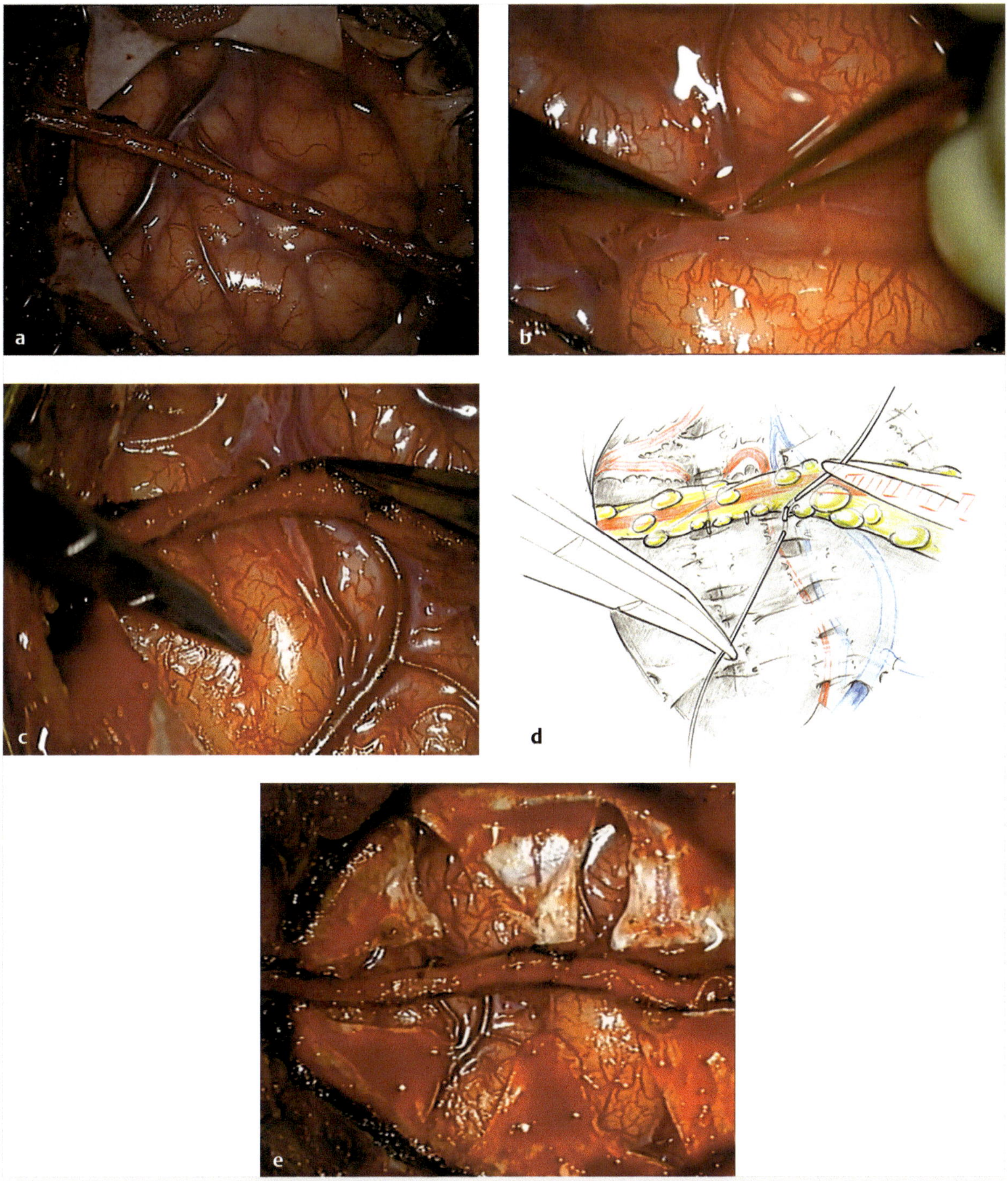

**Fig. 6.4 (a)** Exposure of cortex with maximal dural opening; dura tacked back with 4–0 sutures. **(b)** Careful opening of arachnoid, following along edges of vessels, then extending over cortical surface. Illustrated use of jeweler's forceps. **(c, d)** Initial 10–0 pial suture. **(e)** Conclusion of synangiosis with multiple sutures of superficial temporal artery (STA) to cortex. Note dural leaflets reflected back onto brain, but not closed in order to enable additional dural synangioses from dura.

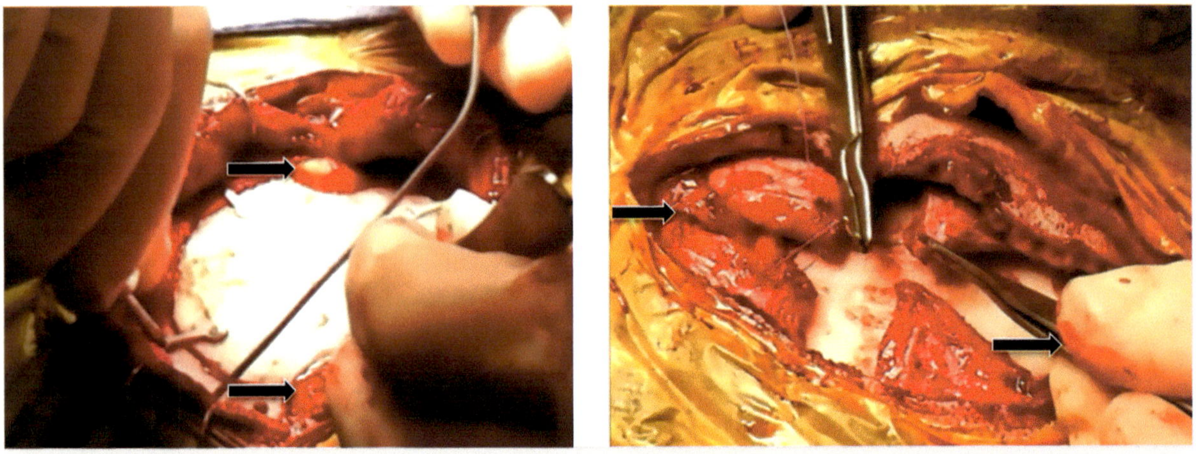

**Fig. 6.5** **(a)** Closure of craniotomy with entry and exit points of superficial temporal artery (STA) marked with arrows. **(b)** Temporalis closure in horizontal plane, avoiding closure along axis of artery in order to minimize compression of the donor vessel. Galea and skin are then closed after this layer, with resorbable sutures used on the skin layer.

## 6.10 Difficulties Encountered

There are general problems that can occur at any time during a moyamoya procedure.

- EEG slowing can herald reduced cerebral blood flow (possibly from spasm or blood pressure changes) and bolus administration of propofol may serve to reduce metabolic demand of the brain and thereby provide a neuroprotective effect.
- Bleeding is particularly troublesome and may be more pronounced if aspirin is used. Meticulous hemostasis is crucial, although "over-cautery" will only serve to deprive the brain from potential additional sources of blood supply.
- Brain swelling (unrelated to direct bypass) can create a cycle of reduced venous outflow—feeding more swelling. Elevation of the head of the bed, opening of arachnoid to drain CSF, and increased sedation are all tools to help. Hyperventilation and driving down $pCO_2$ should be avoided in moyamoya patients, as this may precipitate vasoconstriction and stroke in a brain with a tenuous blood supply.

The major risk of this surgery is perioperative stroke. Steps to mitigate this risk include:

- Preoperative hydration (admitting patients one day before surgery for intravenous fluids).
- Ongoing use of aspirin, including the day before and the day after surgery.
- Good pain control to minimize crying/hyperventilation (in order to avoid hypocarbic-related vasoconstriction).

Despite these measures (in addition to careful operative and anesthetic technique) a number of children will still experience strokes. Limitations of this technique include:

- Operator-independent capacity for stroke.
- Delayed ingrowth of collateral vessels, leaving a period of relative vulnerability to ischemia (for indirect procedures).

## 6.11 Bailout, Rescue, and Salvage Maneuvers

- Arterial injury: Can employ frontal branch, posterior auricular.
- No artery: Can use muscle, galea, dura as an alternative source of blood supply.
- EEG slowing/swelling: Anesthetic changes, including administration of propofol.

## 6.12 Tips, Pearls, and Lessons Learned

In bilateral cases, the dominant or most symptomatic side is generally done first, so that if there are intraoperative events that preclude continuing with the second side, the most important hemisphere has been treated. If the EEG and vital signs are stable, the patient is repositioned and the same operation is performed on the contralateral side in the same anesthesia.

- The most important aspects of this procedure may be nontechnical, including preoperative hydration and experienced anesthesia.
- Mapping as much STA as possible will increase potential collateral development.
- Wide opening of the arachnoid facilitates exposure of the donor vessel to growth factors present in the CSF, increasing the likelihood of better collateralization.
- Hemostasis at all stages of the operation is critical.

# Suggested Readings

Lin N, Baird L, Koss M, et al. Discovery of asymptomatic moyamoya arteriopathy in pediatric syndromic populations: radiographic and clinical progression. Neurosurg Focus. 2011; 31(6):E6

Scott RM, Smith JL, Robertson RL, Madsen JR, Soriano SG, Rockoff MA. Long-term outcome in children with moyamoya syndrome after cranial revascularization by pial synangiosis. J Neurosurg. 2004; 100(2) Suppl Pediatrics:142–149

Smith ER, Scott RM. Surgical management of moyamoya syndrome. Skull Base. 2005; 15(1):15–26

Smith ER, Scott RM. Spontaneous occlusion of the circle of Willis in children: pediatric moyamoya summary with proposed evidence-based practice guidelines. A review. J Neurosurg Pediatr. 2012; 9(4):353–360

# 7 Encephalo-duro-arterio-synangiosis: In Adults

*Hao Jiang, Michael Schiraldi, and Nestor R. Gonzalez*

**Abstract**

Encephalo-duro-arterio-synangiosis (EDAS) is a form of indirect bypass revascularization that was initially developed for the treatment of pediatric patients with moyamoya disease, but its application has now extended to adults. Although selection bias and lack of equipoise limit side-to-side comparisons with direct bypass, several clinical studies have shown that EDAS is a durable procedure, with excellent outcomes and low complication rates in adults with moyamoya disease. Scrupulous surgical technique is a key contributor for successful EDAS. In addition, judicious perioperative care is also crucial to prevent perioperative ischemia. Here, we systemically describe the EDAS technique, including its indications, surgical steps, operative challenges, surgical pearls of management, complications, and salvage maneuvers. Additionally, we present detailed EDAS-specific anesthesia and postoperative management protocols important in guaranteeing the success of the procedure.

*Keywords:* encephalo-duro-arterio-synangiosis (EDAS), adults, intracranial arterial steno-occlusive disorders, perioperative management and postoperative care, antiplatelets

## 7.1 History and Initial Description

Surgical approaches with direct external carotid to internal carotid bypass operations to treat moyamoya patients were introduced in the early 1970s by Kikuchi and Karasawa[1] in Japan and Krayenbühl[2] in Europe with the intention of providing additional blood supply to hypoperfused vascular territories. Despite initial successes with this technique, a direct bypass depends on patency and suitability of both donor and recipient vessels. In moyamoya patients, often the recipient or donor arteries are either small or fragile and pose significant challenges for direct vascular anastomosis; this is true in pediatric as well as adult patients. In 1964, Tsubokawa et al, reported successful cerebral revascularization in a 6-year-old female patient with use of a dural autograft containing the middle meningeal artery (MMA). Almost a decade later, Ausman et al reported the development of spontaneous anastomotic connections between the scalp and the cortical surface following direct superficial temporal artery (STA) to middle cerebral artery (MCA) bypass. Subsequent attempts at revascularization without a direct anastomosis led to the development of the encephalo-duro-arterio-synangiosis (EDAS) technique for the treatment of pediatric patients with moyamoya disease published by Matsushima et al in 1979. In 1980, Spetzler et al[3] were the first to report an "alternative method" for revascularization of the MCA, in which the STA was sutured to the cortical arachnoid in adults "in whom no adequate cortical recipient could be found." Subsequent angiography demonstrated neovascularization and the patient remained neurologically intact postoperatively. Since then, numerous authors[4–8] have reported good clinical results with the use of EDAS in adults with moyamoya.

### 7.1.1 Literature Support for the Use of EDAS in Adults

Although a paucity of literature comparing EDAS with direct bypass surgery exists, this technique has frequently been employed when the conditions do not permit a direct arterial anastomosis.[7,9] Thus, selection bias and lack of equipoise remain hurdles when comparing EDAS with direct bypass. Nevertheless, a literature search using the query "moyamoya disease AND surgery AND adult" yielded 646 references published between November 1971 and February 2015. Twenty-two of these references were clinical trials, of which 20 provided clinical outcome information; none were randomized.[9–25] A total of 1,862 patients were included in these 20 studies. Of all patients, 603 (32.4%) had a direct bypass, 814 (43.7%) had indirect revascularization, and 445 (23.9%) patients underwent combined procedures. An overview of these 20 studies appears in ▶ Table 7.1. Overall, the clinical outcomes indicate that both forms of surgical revascularization produce durable good outcomes, at least when performed in experienced centers. Interestingly, 4 of the 20 studies were performed with the intention of comparing direct bypass with indirect revascularization, but none showed statistically significant differences. The value of other studies is limited by utilization of perfusion imaging as an outcome measure, a diagnostic modality which lacks consistent correlation with clinical results. Until better surrogate markers are found, lack of postoperative ischemic stroke is the most adequate outcome to evaluate.

## 7.2 Indications

EDAS surgery is indicated for the management of all adult patients with intracranial arterial steno-occlusive disorders who present with symptoms of transient ischemic attack (TIA) or stroke in the territory of the affected vessel despite optimal medical management with antiplatelet agents. In our institution, and in a large number of

**Table 7.1** Studies on the use of EDAS in adults

| Author(s) | *n* | Surgery | Prospective | Independent outcome assessment | Term of follow-up (months) | Endpoint(s) | Result(s) |
|---|---|---|---|---|---|---|---|
| Baek et al[12] | 12 | Bypass | Yes | No | 3 | SNSB | NSD |
| Agarwalla et al[10] | 37 | Indirect | No | No | 6 | mRS | Improved $p = 0.002$<br>6% neurological deficit<br>2% hemorrhage |
| Cho et al[14] | 60 | Combined | No | No | 70 | mRS<br>Karnofsky | mRS: 0.4; SD: 0.7<br>Karnofsky: 96.2; SD 8.4<br>Stroke: 13%<br>4% permanent deficit<br>Seizures: 2.6%<br>Wound infection 1.3% |
| Jiang et al[18] | 113 | Combined | Yes | Yes | 30 | Stroke<br>Death<br>Hemorrhage | Stroke at 2y:1.9% Annual re-bleeding = 1.87% |
| Miyamoto et al[23] | 80 | Bypass | Yes | Yes | 52 | Composite: rebleeding or stroke | Rehemorrhage:<br>Surgical: 14.3%<br>Medical: 34.2%<br>Stroke:<br>HR 0.39 (95% CI 0.15–1.03) |
| Lin et al[26] | 36 | Indirect | No | No | 70 | Stroke<br>TIA<br>Death<br>Seizure<br>mRS | Stroke: 8.3%<br>TIA: 14%<br>Seizures: 5.5%<br>Death: 0<br>mRS 0–2: 90.6% |
| Sundaram et al[27] | 36/15 | Bypass or indirect vs. medical | No | No | 28 | mRS 0–2 | mRS 0–2:<br>Surgery: 75%<br>Medical: 94% |
| Mallory et al[22] | 75/7/60 | Bypass, indirect, and combined | No | No | 120 | Composite: stroke or death or hemorrhage | Event free survival (all techniques) at 5 years: 95%; at 10 years: 90% |
| Amin-Hanjani et al[11] | 13 | Combined | No | No | 18.6 | Stroke, seizure, NOVA flow | Stroke: 7.7%<br>Seizures: 15.4%<br>NOVA bypass flow decline: 68.8% |
| Abla et al[9] | 68/39 | Bypass vs. indirect | No | No | 25–36 | mRS | NSD<br>Bypass mRS improved: 0.39 (SD: 1.23)<br>Indirect mRS declined: 0.14 (SD: 1.86) |
| Liu et al[21] | 97/4/10 | Bypass vs. indirect vs. burr hole vs. | No | No | 85.2 | Rebleeding<br>Death | NSD |

**Table 7.1** (*Continued*) Studies on the use of EDAS in adults

| Author(s) | *n* | Surgery | Prospective | Independent outcome assessment | Term of follow-up (months) | Endpoint(s) | Result(s) |
|---|---|---|---|---|---|---|---|
| | | medical | | | | | |
| Bao et al[13] | 470 | Indirect | No | No | 26.5 | Stroke<br>mRS | Stroke rate at 2 years 10%<br>Stroke rate at 5 years 13%<br>mRS 0–1: 74.4%<br>mRS 0–3: 95% |
| Kim et al[19] | 96/62 | Indirect vs. combined | No | No | 38 | mRS | NSD |
| Fujimura and Tominaga[16] | 106 | Combined | Yes | No | 58.4 | Stroke<br>Hemorrhage<br>Hyperperfusion | Stroke: 1%<br>Hemorrhage: 1.8%<br>Hyperperfusion 25.5% (no permanent deficit) |
| Lee et al[20] | 169/67/29/18 | Bypass vs. indirect vs. combined vs. medical | No | No | 55 | Stroke | NSD |
| Czabanka et al[15] | 30 | Combined vs. indirect | Yes | No | 12 | Stroke | Combined: stroke: 10%; no significance was evaluated |
| Guzman et al[17] | 233 | Bypass (95.1% of cases) | No | No | 59 | mRS<br>Stroke<br>Hemorrhage<br>Death | Mean MRS: Preop = 1.62, postop=0.83 ($p$ < 0.0001)<br>Stroke rate: 3.8%<br>Hemorrhage rate: 3.4%<br>Death: 2.3% |
| Starke et al[25] | 43 | Indirect | No | Yes | 41 | mRS<br>Stroke | mRS deterioration 9%<br>5-year stroke free survival: 94% (95% CI 0.84–0.98) |
| Narisawa et al[24] | 49 | Bypass | No | No | NA | Stroke | No strokes |
| Mesiwala et al[28] | 39/4 | Bypass vs. indirect | No | No | 43 | Death | Bypass: 3<br>EDAS: 0 |

Abbreviations: CI, confidence interval; EDAS, encephalo-duro-arterio-synangiosis; HR, hazard ratio; mRS, modified ranking scale; NSD, no significant difference; SD, standard deviation; SNSB, Seoul Neuropsychological Screening Battery; TIA, transient ischemic attack.

centers in the United States, EDAS is the first choice of revascularization for any patient with intracranial arterial steno-occlusive disorders. For patients who have suffered stroke to be eligible for surgery, they need to have either functional independence (modified ranking scale < 3) or perfusion studies demonstrating tissue at risk for further ischemic damage in the territory of the stenoses. The diagnoses of the steno-occlusive disorder for which EDAS is indicated include:

- Moyamoya disease defined as bilateral stenoses of the terminal internal carotid artery and proximal anterior cerebral artery (ACA) or MCA, with different degrees of angiographically evident lenticulostriate, leptomeningeal, or dural collaterals, in patients without risk factors for intracranial atherosclerosis, vascular dissection, or vasculitis.
- Probable moyamoya disease defined as unilateral findings suggestive of moyamoya—as described above—in patients without risk factors for intracranial atherosclerosis, vascular dissection, or vasculitis.
- Intracranial atherosclerosis defined as intracranial arterial disease with evidence of vessel wall calcification plus atherosclerotic risk factors, including history of hypertension, dyslipidemia, diabetes mellitus, smoking, and/or coronary or peripheral vascular atherosclerotic disease, failing intensive medical management with antiplatelets, statins, and risk factor reduction may benefit also from indirect EDAS revascularization.[5]

## 7.3 Key Principles for the EDAS Surgery in Adults

Candidate patients for EDAS surgery are at risk for stoke during the perioperative period, both in the vascular territory to be treated and the contralateral hemisphere, if there is bilateral involvement. To reduce the risk of ischemic events associated with artery-to-artery embolisms, we recommend performing the operation under continuous antiplatelet therapy with aspirin. To reduce the risk of ischemia due to hypoperfusion, strict management of the patient's blood pressure and fluid balance status must be maintained.

A successful EDAS is most dependent on scrupulous surgical technique. As the patients continue antiplatelet therapy throughout the procedure, meticulous hemostasis needs to be achieved while balancing avoidance of excessive cauterization of the arterial cuff, dura mater, or any other tissue that is used as a donor angiogenesis. Fastidious surgical technique can further minimize vasospasm and tissue injury, thus preventing intra- and postoperative complications. Finally, to facilitate the desired intracranial angiogenesis, donor arteries are positioned and fixed in close proximity to the pial surface while avoiding excessive arterial cuffs, tissue injuries, or bleeding.

As patients remain at risk for untoward events during and after surgery, the intraoperative anesthesia and postoperative critical care management are crucial to prevent stroke in adults undergoing EDAS. A detailed description of the anesthesia management is provided elsewhere.[29] In brief, the goals of management include strict control of: (1) blood pressure, (2) fluid balance, (3) cerebral vascular reactivity, (4) platelet aggregation, (5) hematocrit, and (6) oxygenation. Some aspects of this management can seem unusual for a standard neurosurgical case; particularly the need to maintain a sufficiently high blood pressure at all times to avoid cerebral hypoperfusion in the territory of the stenosis may be overlooked with devastating consequences. Close coordination between the anesthesiologist and surgeon is therefore indispensable.

It is important to keep in mind that the surgery itself merely provides the starting point for revascularization, which may take several weeks to occur. Consequently, the perioperative care requires as much diligence as the surgical procedure. This includes continued adherence to anesthesia management goals in the immediate postoperative period until a stable and sufficient systolic blood pressure is reached. Thereafter, continued adherence to strict medical management is the key to obtain good clinical outcomes in adult patients undergoing EDAS.

## 7.4 SWOT Analysis

### 7.4.1 Strengths

- No ischemia time to perform anastomosis.
- Avoids manipulation of diseased arterial walls.
- Does not induce sudden hyperemia (reducing hemorrhage risk).
- Shorter surgical time than bypass.
- Revascularization occurs where needed.
- Prevents competing flow with stenotic segment (reducing proximal thrombosis).

### 7.4.2 Weaknesses

- There is no immediate improvement in cerebral perfusion.
- The process of neovascularization depends on individual ability to generate new vessels.
- Mainly produces neovascularization in the MCA but not ACA territory.
- Clinical outcomes do not correlate with surrogate current imaging markers.

### 7.4.3 Opportunities

- Manipulation of the individual angiogenic response may reduce the time necessary for neovascularization.
- The magnitude of neovascularization could also be regulated.

- Similar procedures with equivalent donors could be developed for ACA territory.
- Improvement of imaging tests may be more accurate to define physiologic impact.

### 7.4.4 Threats

- Surgeons may feel that a scrupulous surgical approach is not necessary if they view EDAS as technically simpler than direct bypass.
- EDAS requirements contradict instinctive operative management by most anesthesiologists.
- The success of the technique goes beyond surgeon control into anesthesiology, critical care, nursing, and support staff involvement.

## 7.5 Specific Adult EDAS Contraindications

### 7.5.1 Absolute

EDAS surgery is contraindicated for patients with completed strokes of the vascular territory of the involved artery, as in those patients no brain tissue can be salvaged or protected, and no expected benefits justify the risk of surgery. The same is true for patients with disabling strokes who do not have tissue at risk for further ischemic damage in the territory of the vascular stenosis. Furthermore, continued intensive medical management including antiplatelet therapy is necessary to prevent strokes due to the delayed revascularization following surgery. A foreseeable discontinuation of such medical management during and/or after surgery should therefore be considered a contraindication, as it acutely increases the risk of stroke and outweighs the potential benefits of the procedure.

### 7.5.2 Relative

In patients that are nonresponders to antiplatelet therapy with acetylsalicylic acid (ASA) and thus require Plavix or other agents, hemostasis is more difficult and the risk to benefit ratio must be considered carefully. A similar increased risk to benefit ratio is true in patients with innate presence of dural or STA collaterals that may be disturbed with the operation. Disruption of those collaterals may not in every case result in hypoperfusion and stroke, but leaves the patient at increased risk for these events before new vessels are formed. As EDAS results in the forming of new vessels with a consequent delay of increased perfusion, a complete occlusion or a lack of forward flow from collaterals into the distal vascular territory may not benefit in time from this procedure. In those cases, a direct bypass should be considered. The role of EDAS for hemorrhagic moyamoya is unknown, but one could argue that while preventing hyperemia which a bypass induces, the need for increased flow through the native collaterals will decrease as well, theoretically reducing the shear stress on those vessels and risk of rupture.[18]

### 7.5.3 Not Contraindications

Within sensible limits, advanced age is not a contraindication to EDAS surgery. Compared to direct bypass techniques, EDAS may reduce surgical risk in elderly and sick patients. However, the need for continuous intensive medical therapy, the consistent use of pressures during the operative and postoperative period with associated cardiac demand, the stress of the surgery itself, and the potentially delayed wound healing in the scalp due to the reduced blood supply should be considered when evaluating patients for EDAS.

While EDAS classically includes the intracranial rerouting of the STA, an absence or suboptimal appearance of this vessel on angiography is not a contraindication. That is, the STA might not be visible during angiography due to vasoconstriction but still suitable for EDAS, or the MMA might be used instead.[14,18]

## 7.6 Special Considerations

### 7.6.1 Care Beyond the Surgical Field

As indicated above, scrupulous intra- and postoperative management are the key to ensure successful outcomes. Such management should adhere to the following 11 *specific intra- and postoperative management rules:*

1. **ASA always:** aspirin, 81 to 325 mg the date of the surgery and for at least 3 days before the procedure.
2. **Strict blood pressure (BP) goal:** established in the clinic prior to surgery and defined as the average of three systolic blood pressure (SBP) measures at which the patient does not have symptoms. BP is managed with *intravenous continuous infusions* for rapid correction. *Avoid pro re nata (prn) orders.*
   - Minimum operative SBP = baseline (asymptomatic) SBP.
   - Maximum SBP goal is set at 200 mm Hg.
3. **Strict $CO_2$ goal:** avoid hyperventilation. End tidal $CO_2$ is kept between 35 and 45 mm Hg.
4. **Seizure prophylaxis:** administer 20 mg/kg phenytoin (slow infusion over 60 min).
5. **Mannitol should not be administered** before or during the procedure.
6. **Steroids are not necessary** during the procedure with the exception of a small dose of dexamethasone for nausea reduction. Their anti-inflammatory effects may hinder the process of angiogenesis required to form the new vessel connections to the intracranial circulation.
7. **Strict hematocrit goal:** greater than or equal to 30% and less than or equal to 50%.

8. **Strict intra- and immediate postoperative monitoring:** arterial catheter placed prior to induction of anesthesia and central venous catheter.
9. **Strict fluid management:** target euvolemia to 1.5 L hypervolemia. The patient should receive intravenous fluids to replace the calculated preoperative fluid balance deficit before the initiation of the surgery.
10. **Systemic hypothermia** and/or barbiturates are not routinely used.
11. **Target temperature** is normothermia.

# 7.7 Risk Assessment and Complications

EDAS surgery has low morbidity and mortality in adults. Based on our own published data, the risks and possible complications are[5]:

- Failure of the procedure to protect from stroke at 3 years (< 1%).
- Failure of the procedure to protect from persistent TIA at 3 years (< 2%).
- Seizures (3%).
- Wound dehiscence (3%).
- Mortality, intraoperative, or within 30 days from surgery. (We have not had operative deaths in more than 110 operations. In the consent, we include a statement for a general risk of death of less than 1%.)

# 7.8 Preoperative Workup

## 7.8.1 Specific Consideration with Anticoagulation

The patient is required to be on ASA (81–325 mg daily) as well as has to respond to ASA to be eligible for the treatment. If the patient is receiving other antiplatelet or anticoagulation agents, they are transitioned to ASA 7 to 10 days before the surgery. The EDAS surgery itself is performed while the patient receives full dose of ASA, which is to be continued postoperatively. If the patient cannot tolerate oral medications immediately after the surgery for more than 24 hours, ASA is administered rectally. Similarly, if a patient vomits within 1 hour of an ASA dose, rectal ASA is administered. In addition to ASA, patients receive standard deep venous thrombosis prophylaxis with subcutaneous heparin during and after surgery.

# 7.9 Patient Preparation

## 7.9.1 Patient Position with Skin Incision

- Patient is positioned with the operative side of the head up.
- Elevate the ipsilateral shoulder 45 degrees to avoid excessive head rotation.
- The hair on the side of the operation is clipped to allow for at least 2 cm of hair-free area around any surgical incision.
- No local anesthetic injections should be used as this introduces a potential source of damage to the STA.
- The skin of the scalp is cleaned with at least two scrubs of chlorhexidine or iodine before marking the incision. Do not use the brush part of the scrub sponges.
- Using the portable Doppler and a sterile-tip skin marking pen, the STA is marked in short intervals (▶ Fig. 7.1). The artery should be identified for a length of approximately 10 to 15 cm. In practice, several sterile-tip marking pens will be needed due to the required ultrasound gel. This step is the key for successful rapid dissection of the artery, and every effort is made to mark the artery with precision.
- The anesthesia provider will be notified prior to placement of the Mayfield head holder pins to allow for adjustments to anesthetic depth and/or administration of medications to optimize blood pressure. Evaluate the preoperative angiogram to identify potential spontaneous collaterals from the occipital arteries. If present, it is the key to avoid injuring the artery with the frame pins.
- The three-point Mayfield head holder is placed avoiding injury of the STA, the occipital after and avoiding interference with the operative field.
- The head is positioned above the level of the heart, maintaining the STA as parallel as possible to the floor while avoiding excessive head rotation.

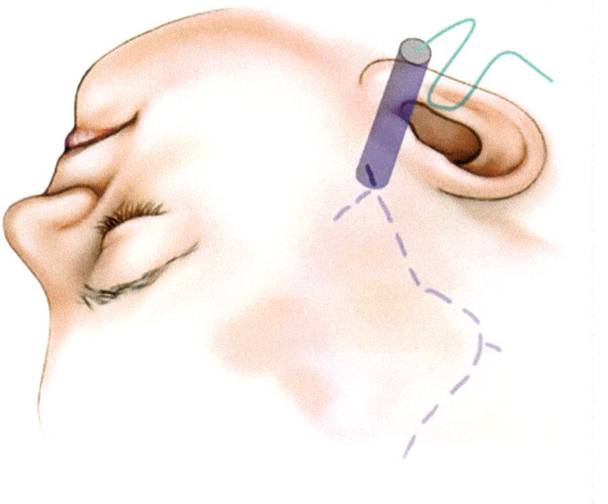

**Fig. 7.1** Using the portable Doppler and a sterile-tip skin marking pen, the superficial temporal artery (STA) is marked in short intervals. The artery should be identified for a length of approximately 10 to 15 cm. Every effort is made to mark the artery with precision.

- The skin is prepared with iodine using sterile technique.
- The surgical field is draped in sterile fashion. Do not use staples to secure any of the drapes (▶ Fig. 7.2).

# 7.10 Surgical Steps

## 7.10.1 STA Dissection

The STA is dissected using the operative microscope. The skin marking obtained during patient preparation indicates exactly the position of the artery, and the skin incision is performed along these markings using sharp dissection (▶ Fig. 7.3). Incision and artery isolation are performed stepwise from proximal to distal, elongating the epidermal cut once the vessel is dissected in the segment currently exposed (▶ Fig. 7.4). Note that from proximal to distal the artery is located increasingly superficial. Bleeding caused by the skin incision is controlled using a bipolar set at less than or equal to 20 W. Excessive cauterization of the skin edges or monopolar cauterization is avoided. After skin incision, the artery can be easily found with blunt dissection using sharp fine tip mosquitos.

During dissection of the STA, excessive coagulation of its branches is avoided and the anterior limb is preserved. Any necessary coagulation is limited to just the tip of the branches (facilitates sprouting). A small cuff of less than or equal to 2 mm is left on each side of the artery (▶ Fig. 7.5). This reduces the length of necessary new vessels, thus optimizing the gradient of pressure necessary for the maturation of the vessels (arteriogenesis) after the neoangiogenic connection with cerebral vessels is established. Once the artery is dissected within its cuff along the length of the planned incision, it can be separated from the galea, pericranium, and temporalis fascia with sharp or low power cautery (≤6 W) through the loose areolar connective tissue.

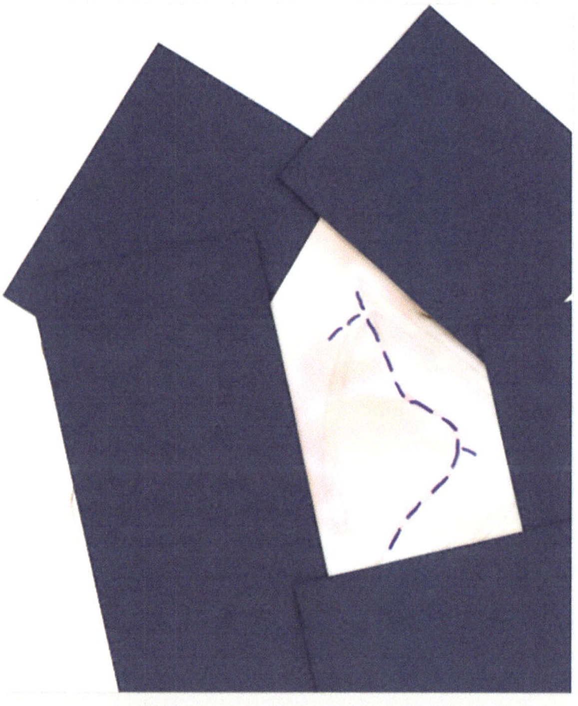

**Fig. 7.2** The surgical field is draped in sterile fashion. Do not use staples to secure any of the drapes.

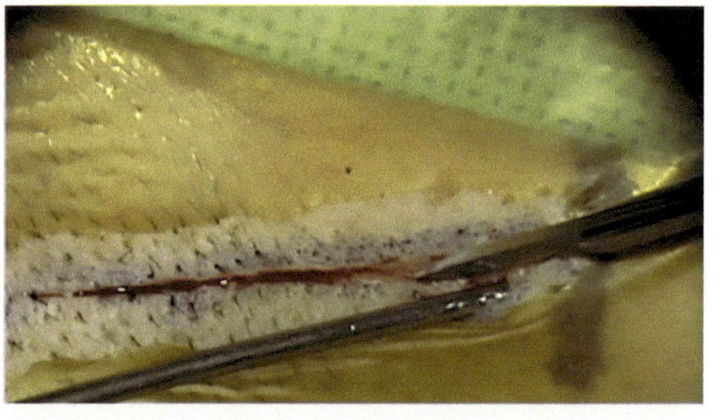

**Fig. 7.3** The operative microscope facilitates sharp dissection of the dermis.

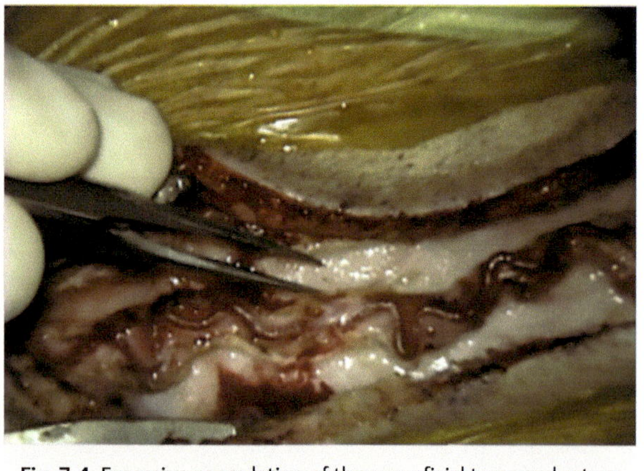

**Fig. 7.4** Excessive coagulation of the superficial temporal artery (STA) branches is also avoided and the anterior STA branch is preserved.

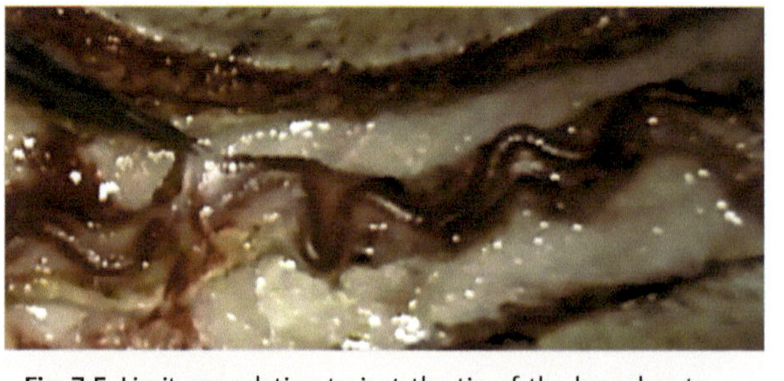

**Fig. 7.5** Limit coagulation to just the tip of the branches to facilitate sprouting and maintain a small perivascular cuff of approximately 2 mm.

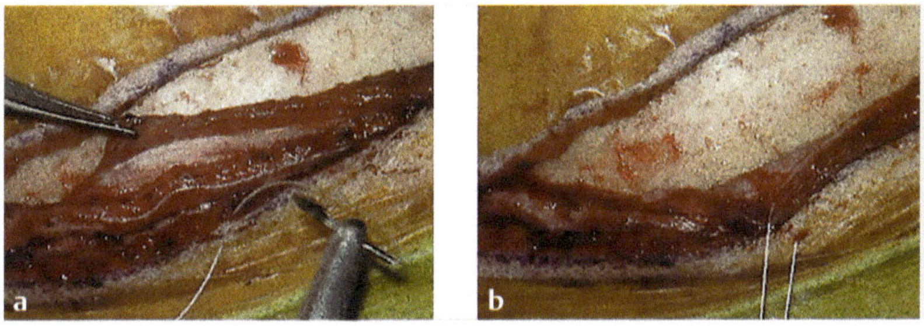


**Fig. 7.6 (a, b)** Protect the artery by wrapping it in a cuff of muscle and pericranium while periodically confirming vessel patency via Doppler.

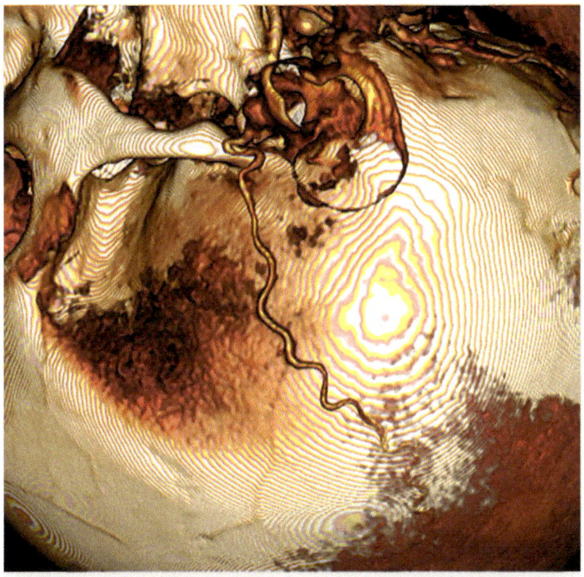

**Fig. 7.7** Perform an oval craniotomy with a longitudinal axis parallel to the exposed superficial temporal artery (STA) with care to protect the middle meningeal artery (MMA) during the process.

## 7.10.2 STA Care and Preservation

Once the artery is dissected and mobilized, it is particularly vulnerable. Protect the artery by wrapping it in a cuff of muscle and pericranium along one side of the incision (▶ Fig. 7.6). Do not use sharp fish-hooks on the side where the artery is located. It is highly recommended to check vessel patency with Doppler after every manipulation to immediately detect and correct arterial constriction.

## 7.10.3 Craniotomy

Once the STA is secured and the skull exposed, an oval craniotomy is performed (▶ Fig. 7.7). The longitudinal axis of the oval is determined by the length of exposed STA and marked by two burr holes. These two burr holes serve as the entry and exit points of the STA. During the craniotomy, protect the artery and its shielding cuff with vein retractors. Take care to protect the MMA during the elevation of the bone flap.

## 7.10.4 Middle Meningeal Artery Preservation

The dura is opened in a cruciate fashion with four resultant flaps. Approximately along the long axis of the craniotomy, these flaps provide space for the STA to be opposed to the brain. While opening the dura, take care to protect the MMA and its branches; avoid excessive coagulation of dural bleedings (▶ Fig. 7.8).

## 7.10.5 Cerebrospinal Fluid Release

After opening the dura and visualizing the arachnoid, opening of the arachnoid and gentle aspiration provides cerebrospinal fluid (CSF) release (▶ Fig. 7.9). This serves to reduce swelling as no mannitol is used during surgery. The use of mannitol may produce a reduction of the intravascular volume, which can affect the hypoperfused territories. The arachnoid opening is carefully extended to all exposed sulci. The goal is to minimize tissue and distance between STA/MMA branches and pial surface, as well as to remove the potential barrier that the arachnoid represents.

## 7.10.6 Dural Flaps Preparation and Superficial Temporal Artery Fixation

The inner layer of the dura is dissected and removed from each flap as it is fibrotic and prevents the spontaneous formation of connections between the meningeal arteries and pial intracranial vessels. Removing the inner layer of the dura increases the surface area for potential new vessels to form between the meningeal arteries and the cerebral vasculature (▶ Fig. 7.10). Thereafter, the STA cuff is attached to the arachnoid or dura with 8 or 9–0 sutures to minimize movement of the STA and dural flaps relative to the pial surface, thus facilitating the growth of new vessels (▶ Fig. 7.11).

## 7.10.7 Craniotomy Closure

It is recommended to check the blood flow within the STA regularly during the craniotomy and wound closures. Trim the burr hole openings and the inner table of the bone flap to avoid kinking and permit unrestricted

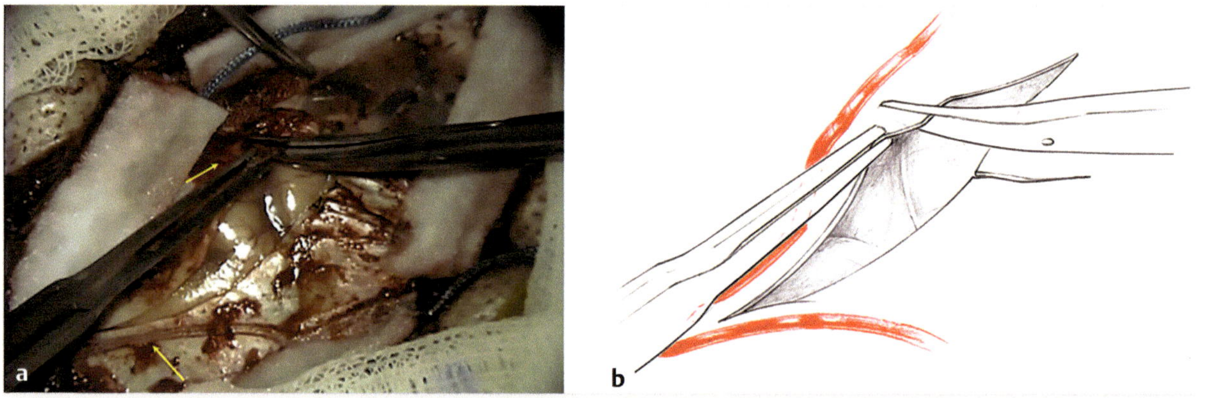


**Fig. 7.8 (a, b)** Protect the middle meningeal artery (MMA) branches while performing durotomy in close proximity to its branches.

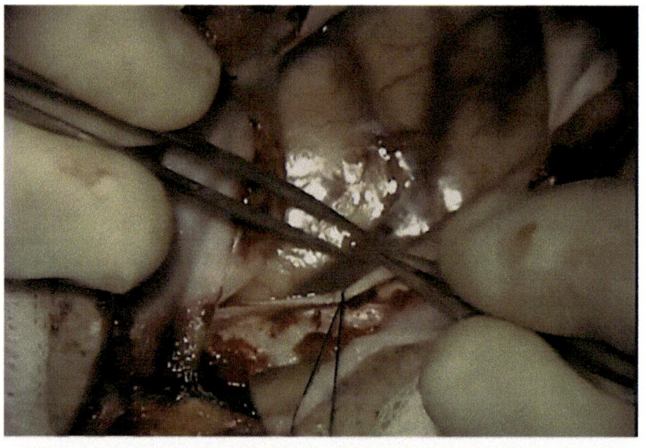

**Fig. 7.9** Opening of the arachnoid and gentle aspiration provides cerebrospinal fluid (CSF) release.

passage of the STA, and avoid excessively tight closure of muscle at the STA entry point. Keep all galeal sutures held with clamps before tying them to ensure visualization of proper purchase with every stitch. Once the muscle and galea are reconstructed and the patency of the STA confirmed using Doppler, the scalp is closed (▶ Fig. 7.12).

## 7.11 Difficulties Encountered and Pearls of Management

## 7.12 Pitfalls

The success of EDAS is directly dependent on the perioperative management and close communication between surgeon, anesthesia, postoperative care team, and operating room staff. It further requires careful planning and preparation of the procedure and perioperative care. Even in highly experienced and large neurosurgical centers, a lack of such communication and planning before and during each case can result in stroke and catastrophic outcome despite a "perfect" surgery. While EDAS is a relatively safe procedure, a series of misconceptions and pitfalls should be avoided:

- EDAS is not a direct bypass, however, that does not imply it requires less attention to detail.
- Never assume that the anesthesia team knows how to handle these cases. Time communicating with anesthesia is time well spent.
- A quick, not precise skin marking of the STA is not sufficient but can cause unnecessary problems and complications while finding and dissecting the artery in patients on ASA.
- Loupes are not as good as the microscope during the dissection of the STA. A perfectly dissected STA is one key to a successful outcome.
- Leaving a large cuff around the artery is safe and convenient for direct bypass, but not suitable for EDAS as it limits the formation of new functional collaterals.

| Difficulties (challenges) | Solution (tips of management) |
|---|---|
| Dissecting the artery on the left side for right handed surgeons | Position the patient always with the head toward the right of anesthesia. This allows for a dissection from proximal to distal for right handed surgeons. |
| Brain swelling after dura is open in absence of Mannitol | Do not hyperventilate the patient.<br>Perform the arachnoid dissection and aspirate CSF. |
| Compression of the STA at entry and exit points | Enlarge the burr holes in the bone flap. Do not use excessive amounts of collagen sponge. |
| Bowing of the STA after bone flap is placed | Trim the inner layer of thick bone flaps. Create a groove on the inner table of the bone flap in the anticipated location of the STA. |
| Galeal stitches | Pass each stitch in each side separately and use hemostats keeping them loosely ligated until all sutures are in place. |
| Wound healing problems | Keep sutures for 2 to 3 weeks. |

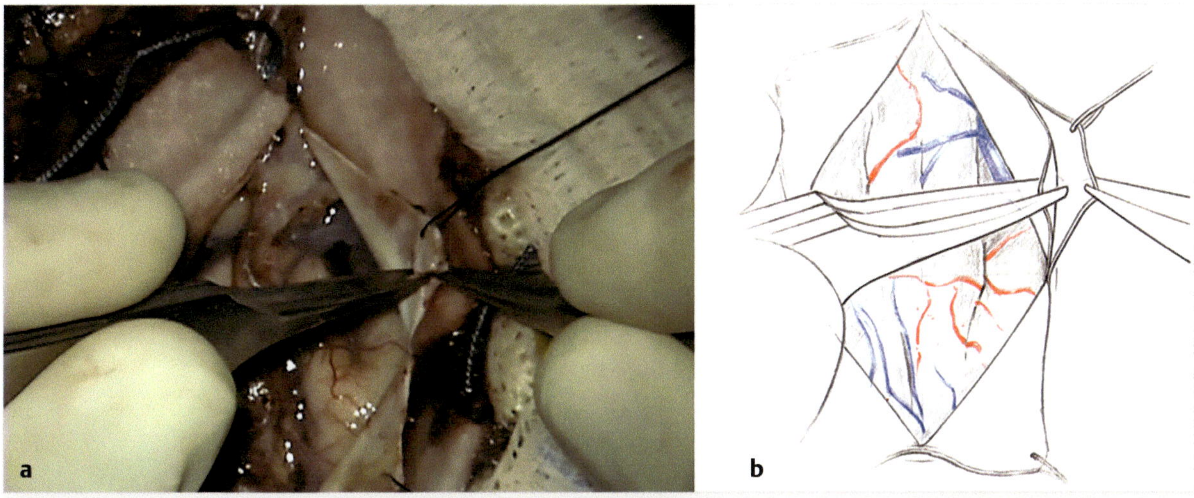


**Fig. 7.10 (a, b)** The inner layer of dura is dissected and removed from each flap.

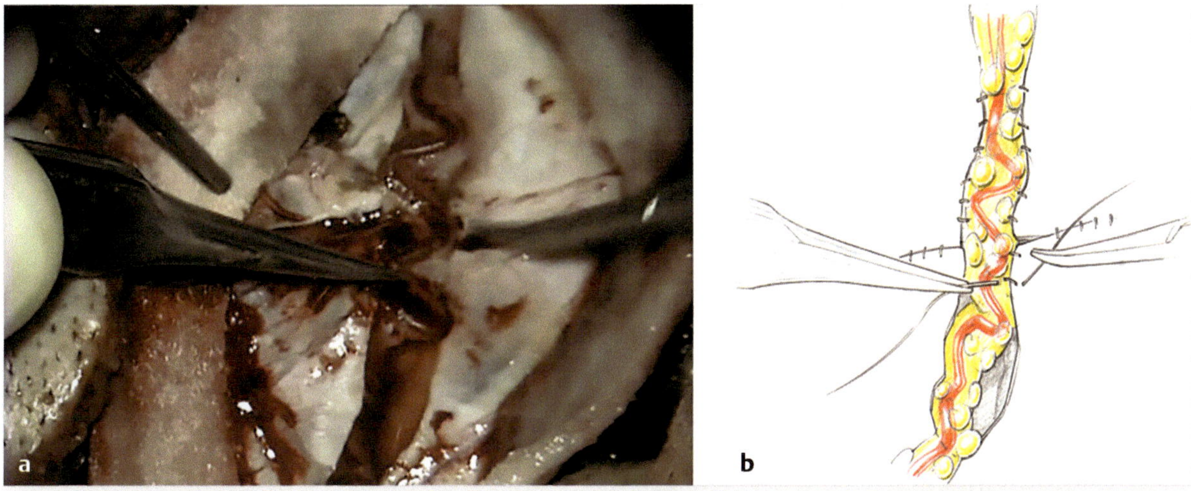


**Fig. 7.11 (a, b)** The perivascular cuff of the superficial temporal artery (STA) is attached to the arachnoid or dura with 8 or 9–0 sutures.

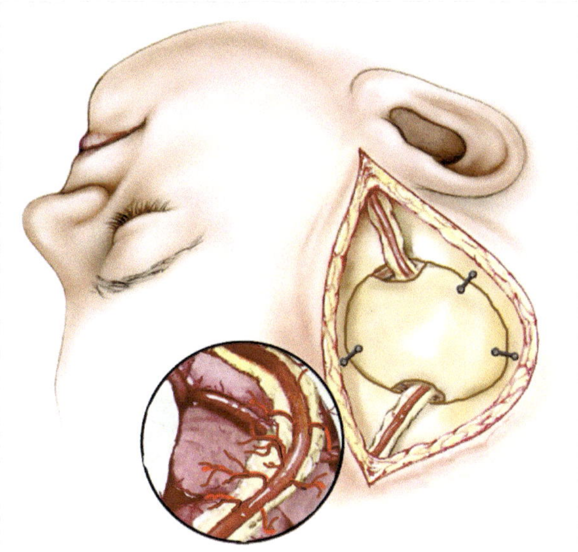

**Fig. 7.12** Trim the burr hole openings and the inner table of the bone flap to permit unrestricted passage of the superficial temporal artery (STA) while avoiding excessively tight closure of muscle at STA entry point. Keep all galeal stitches held with clamps before tying them to ensure the galea is taken on every stitch.

- Excessive cauterization of the arterial cuff or the dura matter may seem convenient for quick hemostasis but causes injury to the vascular stumps that yield new vessels.
- Skipping steps may save time during surgery, but results in complications or lack of success afterwards. This is particularly true for the meticulous STA dissection, the opening of the arachnoid for CSF release and exposure of the critical vessels, the dissection of the dural layers, or the suturing of the artery to the arachnoid or dura.
- Lack of attention to details during closure of galea and skin can easily result in wound dehiscence and/or compression of the STA with consequent loss of blood flow and a failed procedure.
- Use of PRNs for BP management. Delays in response to hypo- or hypertension increase the risk of bleeding or strokes in these patients.
- Failure to respond immediately to subtle postoperative neurological changes.

## 7.13 Bailout, Rescue, and Salvage Maneuvers

| Complications | Management |
|---|---|
| STA injury | Precise, short cauterization with very low power often is sufficient.<br>Use of topical papaverine.<br>Take advantage of collateral flow to the STA.<br>Reconstruct the artery (wall suture or primary reanastomose). |
| Pial injury during arachnoid dissection | Irrigate.<br>Mild pressure with a micro cottoned patty.<br>Do not coagulate. |
| Lack of Dopplerable pulse after closing | Confirm Doppler is functional.<br>Immediately reopen and correct cause.<br>It is better to Doppler few times after placing bone flap, closing muscle, and the skin. |
| Patient develops new symptoms after the surgery | Place head of the bed down, increase SBP lacing bone flap, closing mHct, check fluid balance. If no improvement after 30 minutes, activate "stroke" system. |
| Evidence of new stroke in imaging or no improvement of symptoms despite medical measures | Consider immediate endovascular interventions:<br>• Patients may develop vasospasm that responds to intra-arterial pharmacologic treatment.<br>• If a new occlusion of the previous stenotic vessels is seen, recombinant tissue plasminogen activator or mechanical retrieval is contraindicated after surgery. |

## 7.14 Postoperative Care

### 7.14.1 Patient Surveillance

As stated, the patient remains at risk for stroke postoperatively until sufficient new blood vessels have formed, and the principles of strict anesthesia management applied intraoperatively continue during the immediate postoperative period. Therefore, without exception, the patient is monitored in the neurocritical care unit after surgery. Due to the continued risk for cerebrovascular events and bleeding, nursing staff capable of identifying subtle neurological symptoms is required. All rules of preoperative management apply as explained before. Once the patient does not require support of BP for symptom control, s/he is ready to be transferred to the regular ward. No routine diagnostic images are performed in the immediate postoperative period.

### 7.14.2 EDAS Functional Assessment

The primary functional assessment of EDAS is the clinical examination. Often, perfusion studies fail to show resolution of asymmetric blood flow in asymptomatic patients even after years from the surgery. In addition, traditional perfusion measurement techniques using MRI and CT do not allow for actual comparison of cerebral blood flow over time. New techniques that are not dependent on relative measures, such as arterial spin labeling might be more useful, but may not detect local flow changes. Nevertheless, overall the goal of EDAS is to keep patient symptom free.

### 7.14.3 EDAS Angiographic Assessment

Angiographic assessment of neovascularization after EDAS is currently the gold standard to identify new collaterals. Early angiographic studies reveal Perren Grade 3 (Extensive neovascularization) in 80% of cases, and new vessels seen as early as 1.5 months after surgery. Although neovascularization is detectable early on, we initially follow-up in our practice with clinic visits and perform an angiographic study only at six months after surgery.[5]

### 7.14.4 Advanced Imaging

For research purposes, MRI dynamic susceptibility contrast data is optimized using the functional MRI of the brain (FMRIB) tool library, and a probabilistic independent component analysis is performed (multivariate exploratory linear optimized decomposition into independent components [MELODIC], FMRIB), modeling data into three components—categorized as arterial, venous, and capillary. In a first study this approach revealed functional results that matched the anatomy observed in the angiographic assessment after surgery.[30]

## References


[1] KJ K. STA-cortical MCA anastomosis for cerebrovascular occlusive disease. No Shinkei Geka. 1973; 1:5–15

[2] Krayenbühl HA. The moyamoya syndrome and the neurosurgeon. Surg Neurol. 1975; 4(4):353–360

[3] Spetzler RF, Roski RA, Kopaniky DR. Alternative superficial temporal artery to middle cerebral artery revascularization procedure. Neurosurgery. 1980; 7(5):484–487

[4] Dusick JR, Jr, Gonzalez NR, Martin NA. Clinical and angiographic outcomes from indirect revascularization surgery for Moyamoya disease in adults and children: a review of 63 procedures. Neurosurgery. 2011; 68(1):34–43, discussion 43

[5] Gonzalez NR, Dusick JR, Connolly M, et al. Encephaloduroarteriosynangiosis for adult intracranial arterial steno-occlusive disease: long-term single-center experience with 107 operations. J Neurosurg. 2015; 123(3):654–661

[6] Hänggi D, Mehrkens JH, Schmid-Elsaesser R, Steiger HJ. Results of direct and indirect revascularisation for adult European patients with moyamoya angiopathy. Acta Neurochir Suppl (Wien). 2008; 103: 119–122

[7] Isono M, Ishii K, Kobayashi H, Kaga A, Kamida T, Fujiki M. Effects of indirect bypass surgery for occlusive cerebrovascular diseases in adults. J Clin Neurosci. 2002; 9(6):644–647

[8] Sakamoto S, Ohba S, Shibukawa M, et al. Angiographic neovascularization after bypass surgery in moyamoya disease: our experience at Hiroshima University Hospital. Hiroshima J Med Sci. 2007; 56(3–4): 29–32

[9] Abla AA, Gandhoke G, Clark JC, et al. Surgical outcomes for moyamoya angiopathy at barrow neurological institute with comparison of adult indirect encephaloduroarteriosynangiosis bypass, adult direct superficial temporal artery-to-middle cerebral artery bypass, and pediatric bypass: 154 revascularization surgeries in 140 affected hemispheres. Neurosurgery. 2013; 73(3):430–439

[10] Agarwalla PK, Stapleton CJ, Phillips MT, Walcott BP, Venteicher AS, Ogilvy CS. Surgical outcomes following encephaloduroarteriosynangiosis in North American adults with moyamoya. J Neurosurg. 2014; 121(6):1394–1400

[11] Amin-Hanjani S, Singh A, Rifai H, et al. Combined direct and indirect bypass for moyamoya: quantitative assessment of direct bypass flow over time. Neurosurgery. 2013; 73(6):962–967, discussion 967–968

[12] Baek HJ, Chung SY, Park MS, Kim SM, Park KS, Son HU. Preliminary study of neurocognitive dysfunction in adult moyamoya disease and improvement after superficial temporal artery-middle cerebral artery bypass. J Korean Neurosurg Soc. 2014; 56(3):188–193

[13] Bao XY, Duan L, Li DS, et al. Clinical features, surgical treatment and long-term outcome in adult patients with Moyamoya disease in China. Cerebrovasc Dis. 2012; 34(4):305–313

[14] Cho WS, Kim JE, Kim CH, et al. Long-term outcomes after combined revascularization surgery in adult moyamoya disease. Stroke. 2014; 45(10):3025–3031

[15] Czabanka M, Peña-Tapia P, Scharf J, et al. Characterization of direct and indirect cerebral revascularization for the treatment of European patients with moyamoya disease. Cerebrovasc Dis. 2011; 32(4):361–369

[16] Fujimura M, Tominaga T. Lessons learned from moyamoya disease: outcome of direct/indirect revascularization surgery for 150 affected hemispheres. Neurol Med Chir (Tokyo). 2012; 52(5):327–332

[17] Guzman R, Lee M, Achrol A, et al. Clinical outcome after 450 revascularization procedures for moyamoya disease. Clinical article. J Neurosurg. 2009; 111(5):927–935

[18] Jiang H, Ni W, Xu B, et al. Outcome in adult patients with hemorrhagic moyamoya disease after combined extracranial-intracranial bypass. J Neurosurg. 2014; 121(5):1048–1055

[19] Kim DS, Huh PW, Kim HS, et al. Surgical treatment of moyamoya disease in adults: combined direct and indirect vs. indirect bypass surgery. Neurol Med Chir (Tokyo). 2012; 52(5):333–338

[20] Lee SB, Kim DS, Huh PW, Yoo DS, Lee TG, Cho KS. Long-term follow-up results in 142 adult patients with moyamoya disease according to management modality. Acta Neurochir (Wien). 2012; 154(7):1179–1187

[21] Liu X, Zhang D, Shuo W, Zhao Y, Wang R, Zhao J. Long term outcome after conservative and surgical treatment of haemorrhagic moyamoya disease. J Neurol Neurosurg Psychiatry. 2013; 84(3):258–265

[22] Mallory GW, Bower RS, Nwojo ME, et al. Surgical outcomes and predictors of stroke in a North American white and African American moyamoya population. Neurosurgery. 2013; 73(6):984–991, discussion 981–982

[23] Miyamoto S, Yoshimoto T, Hashimoto N, et al. JAM Trial Investigators. Effects of extracranial-intracranial bypass for patients with hemorrhagic moyamoya disease: results of the Japan Adult Moyamoya Trial. Stroke. 2014; 45(5):1415–1421

[24] Narisawa A, Fujimura M, Tominaga T. Efficacy of the revascularization surgery for adult-onset moyamoya disease with the progression of cerebrovascular lesions. Clin Neurol Neurosurg. 2009; 111(2):123–126

[25] Starke RM, Komotar RJ, Hickman ZL, et al. Clinical features, surgical treatment, and long-term outcome in adult patients with moyamoya disease. Clinical article. J Neurosurg. 2009; 111(5):936–942

[26] Laiwalla AN, Ooi YC, Van De Wiele B, et al. Rigorous anaesthesia management protocol for patients with intracranial arterial stenosis: a prospective controlled-cohort study. BMJ Open. 2016; 6(1):e009727

[27] Laiwalla AN, Kurth F, Leu K, et al. Evaluation of encephaloduroarteriosynangiosis efficacy using probabilistic independent component analysis applied to dynamic susceptibility contrast perfusion MRI. AJNR Am J Neuroradiol. 2017; 38(3):507–514

[28] Lin N, Aronson JP, Manjila S, Smith ER, Scott RM. Treatment of Moyamoya disease in the adult population with pial synangiosis. J Neurosurg. 2014; 120(3):612–617

[29] Sundaram S, Sylaja PN, Menon G, et al. Moyamoya disease: a comparison of long term outcome of conservative and surgical treatment in India. J Neurol Sci. 2014; 336(1–2):99–102

[30] Mesiwala AH, Sviri G, Fatemi N, Britz GW, Newell DW. Long-term outcome of superficial temporal artery-middle cerebral artery bypass for patients with moyamoya disease in the US. Neurosurg Focus. 2008; 24(2):E15

# 8 Bifrontal Encephalo-duro-periosteal-synangiosis Combined with STA–MCA Bypass

*Giuseppe Esposito, Annick Kronenburg, Jorn Fierstra, Kees P.J. Braun, Catharina J.M. Klijn, Albert van der Zwan, and Luca Regli*

**Abstract**
Augmentation of cerebral blood flow (CBF) of the frontal areas is of importance in symptomatic pediatric moyamoya population. Bifrontal hypoperfusion in fact plays a deleterious role in intellectual development and cognitive performance, and in lower extremity and sphincter function.

In this chapter, we describe a technique of combined flow-augmentation bypass for managing moyamoya in children. The particularity of this technique is the one-stage surgical approach, combining direct and indirect revascularization techniques in three different vascular regions: the middle cerebral artery (MCA) territory unilaterally and the frontal areas bilaterally.

The procedure consists of: (1) a direct superficial temporal artery-to-middle cerebral artery (STA–MCA) bypass with encephalo-duro-myo-synangiosis (EDMS) for unilateral MCA revascularization, and (2) a bifrontal encephalo-duro-periosteal-synangiosis (EDPS) for bifrontal revascularization.

Direct STA–MCA bypass increases flow immediately and EDMS promotes progressive neoangiogenesis over time in the MCA territory. Bifrontal EDPS aims at inducing progressive neoangiogenesis over the frontal lobes bilaterally.

The indication to perform the one-step combined revascularization procedure is in the presence of children with hemodynamic compromise (impaired CBF and/or cerebrovascular reserve [CVR]) and clinical symptoms involving concurrently both the MCA territory and the bifrontal areas.

Bifrontal EDPS by itself could also be used as a supplementary procedure in patients who already underwent previous revascularization procedures, in case of bifrontal hypoperfusion or progression of the moyamoya vasculopathy with symptoms referable to frontal lobe hypoperfusion.

*Keywords:* bypass, cerebral revascularization, children, frontal areas, moya, pediatric, periosteum, synangiosis

## 8.1 History and Initial Description

Although most flow-augmentation bypass techniques aim to revascularize the middle cerebral artery (MCA) territory, augmentation of cerebral blood flow (CBF) of the frontal areas is of importance, especially in the pediatric population affected by moyamoya vasculopathy (MMV). Bifrontal hypoperfusion plays a deleterious role in intellectual development and cognitive performance, and in lower extremity and sphincter function.[1,2]

In pediatric MMV, CBF in the bifrontal areas and in the anterior watershed territory as well as in the anterior MCA regions may continue to worsen despite good collateral formation or successful revascularization of the MCA territory. Therefore, it is important to consider timely revascularization of the frontal areas to prevent neurocognitive decline in pediatric patients.[2]

Besides the direct STA to anterior cerebral artery (STA–ACA) bypass,[3] indirect and combined bypass techniques have been proposed for bifrontal reinforcement of blood supply.[4]

We describe a technique of combined flow-augmentation bypass for managing MMV in children. This technique represents a modification of existing techniques[1,5].

In fact Kim et al reported in 2003 on unilateral encephalo-duro-arterio-synangiosis (EDAS) and bifrontal encephalo-galeo(periosteal)-synangiosis (EGPS) for treating pediatric moyamoya disease.[6] Two separate scalp incisions (one for EDAS and one for EGPS) and a bifrontal 4 × 8 cm craniotomy across the superior sagittal sinus were performed. The prepared galea was inserted deep in the interhemispheric fissure.

Park et al reported in 2007 on a modified EDAS with bifrontal EGPS.[1] The authors increased the area of synangiosis by the use of a dural flap (inserted in into each interhemispheric fissure) in addition to a galeoperiosteal flap (that was used to cover the paramedian anterior frontal lobe). Also in this case, two scalp incisions were performed.

The particularity of our technique is the one-stage surgical approach, combining direct and indirect revascularization techniques in three different vascular regions: the MCA territory unilaterally and the frontal areas bilaterally.

The procedure consists of: (1) a direct superficial temporal artery-to-middle cerebral artery (STA–MCA) bypass with encephalo-duro-myo-synangiosis (EDMS) for unilateral MCA revascularization, and (2) a bifrontal encephalo-duro-periosteal-synangiosis (EDPS) for bifrontal revascularization.[4,7]

Direct STA–MCA bypass increases flow immediately and EDMS promotes progressive neoangiogenesis over time in the MCA territory. Bifrontal EDPS aims at inducing progressive neoangiogenesis over the frontal lobes bilaterally.

We first described this technique in 2014.[7] In 2015 we reported on the early postoperative and short-term (within 30 days) results of eight consecutive children treated with this technique.[4] The results showed that the technique is feasible and safe for treating children with moyamoya. Data on long-term clinical, neuropsychological, radiological, and hemodynamic follow-up of the whole case series are currently being collected.[4]

## 8.2 Indications

We perform this one-step revascularization procedure in children with hemodynamic compromise (impaired CBF and/or cerebrovascular reserve [CVR]) and clinical symptoms involving concurrently both the MCA territory and the bifrontal areas.[4]

In addition to symptoms that can be ascribed to the MCA territory, children may present with lower extremity motor weakness and neuropsychological dysfunctions probably due to involvement of the frontal lobes.[1,2,8–10] In pediatric MMV, the CBF in the bifrontal areas as well as in the anterior watershed territory may continue to worsen despite good collateral formation or successful revascularization of the MCA territory.[1,2,9,10] Therefore, it is important to consider timely revascularization of the frontal areas to prevent neurocognitive decline in pediatric patients.[1,2,8–10]

Direct revascularization by STA–ACA anastomosis in children can be technically challenging due to a small caliber of the cortical recipient of the ACA and very distal preparation of the frontal branch of the STA.[4]

Preoperative workup includes magnetic resonance imaging (MRI), six-vessel digital subtraction angiography (DSA), $H_2O$-positron emission tomography (PET) with and without acetazolamide challenge to study CBF and CVR and neuropsychological evaluation.

## 8.3 Key Principles

Adequate CBF supply in the bifrontal areas is of importance, especially in pediatric moyamoya patients.[1,7] Cerebral ischemia in this region can in fact lead to lower extremity motor weakness and to intellectual and neuropsychological dysfunction.[1] Stepwise decline of neurocognitive performance has been described in 44% of the pediatric population.[11] There is also growing evidence that decreased CBF, especially in the frontal lobes, is correlated with diminished neurocognitive development.[12]

In theory, by surgically restoring blood flow in the bifrontal areas, one expects a beneficial effect on neurocognitive performance.[2] An analysis of neurocognitive profiles pre- and postoperatively on 65 pediatric patients with MMV operated by means of a combination of indirect bypass procedures was recently presented. Unilateral EDAS was performed in 12 patients, bilateral EDAS in 11 patients, and bilateral EDAS and bifrontal EGPS in 42 patients. This study showed a retained intelligence quotient (IQ) and a significant improvement in performance IQ after surgery.[11] The benefits of bifrontal revascularization on long-term cognitive outcome in children with MMV, however, remain to be established in larger clinical series.[4]

The use of frontal pericranial flaps to induce neoangiogenesis in patients with MMV has shown to be effective.[1,5] The use of periosteum (frontal pericranium) for bifrontal revascularization relies on the abundant blood supply.[1] The frontal pericranium receives from the supraorbital and supratrochlear arteries (as well as from frontal branches of the STA).[13]

## 8.4 SWOT Analysis

The strengths of this technique are as follows:

- Revascularization of both frontal areas with reduced risk of injuries to the superior sagittal sinus (SSS) and the parasagittal veins. This is obtained by the use of two separate parasagittal frontal craniotomies, located 2 cm away from the midline and the SSS. Similarly, this technique avoids exposure and opening of the interhemispheric fissure.[4,7]
- Expanding the area of synangiosis by inverting and reflecting dural flaps under the craniotomy edges. This expands thereby the cortical coverage area for neoangiogenesis.
- Good cosmetic results: the scalp is not incised separately for this combined procedure. The skin incision is located behind the hairline and requires no shaving. The use of a single skin incision (either curvilinear or in a zig-zag fashion) and three craniotomies gives excellent cosmetic results.
- No compromise of other revascularization strategies: the technique does not compromise eventual future contralateral MCA territory revascularization, as well as revascularization procedures in the posterior circulation territory.[4]
- Easy procedure: the EDPS is technically easy to perform. EDPS represents therefor a very useful alternative to the existing indirect procedures for frontal lobe revascularization or to direct STA–ACA bypass for revascularization of frontal areas.[1] STA–ACA bypass is known to be technically challenging, especially in pediatric patients. In fact the site of microanastomosis into the ACA territory needs a very distal preparation of the STA frontal branch and the cortical recipient of the ACA is generally also very small and often located in a sulcus. Furthermore, performing a direct STA–ACA bypass may be difficult in combination with a direct STA–MCA bypass.[4,7]

The opportunities offered by this technique are as follows:

- Revascularization in one session of three different vascular regions: the MCA territory unilaterally and the frontal areas bilaterally.

- Combination of direct and indirect revascularization procedures: direct STA–MCA bypass increases flow immediately and EDMS promotes progressive neoangiogenesis over time in the MCA territory. Bifrontal EDPS aims at inducing progressive neoangiogenesis over the frontal areas bilaterally.[4,7]

The main weaknesses and threats of this technique are as follows:

- Long duration of surgery: in 8 cases the mean duration of the procedure (from incision to closure of the skin) was 6 hours and 54 minutes (range, 5:10–9:35).
- Possibility of considerable blood loss (with three craniotomies) in children. However, the immediate postoperative and short-term (within 30 days) follow-up confirms the feasibility and safety of this technique.[4]

## 8.5 Contraindications

No contraindications for indirect revascularization of bifrontal areas via EDPS and of MCA territory via EDMS are reported. Direct revascularization via STA–MCA bypass may not be feasible if a suitable donor vessel (STA) is absent.

## 8.6 Special Considerations

Patients undergo surgery under aspirin. Intraoperatively, no heparin is used.

## 8.7 Complications

Besides all the classical risks of every neurosurgical procedures via craniotomy, the parents should be informed that, despite the above reported advantages, the procedure represents a long surgery, mostly for young children. Eventual necessity of blood transfusion must be mentioned. Classical risks connected with every direct revascularization procedure via bypass need also to be elucidated: bypass malfunction and eventual reoperation for bypass revision, hyperperfusion syndrome (epilepsy, etc.), postoperative hemorrhage and infarcts.

## 8.8 Special Instructions and Anesthesia

Children are encouraged to have a higher than normal fluid intake (according to their weight) overnight, until 1.5 hours before anesthesia. The environment is adapted to avoid preoperative stress and hyperventilation. Lines and routine laboratory examinations are performed after the child is anesthetized. Peri- and postoperatively we aim at normotension, normovolemia, normoventilation and normothermia.

After the operation, children are observed in an intensive care unit for the first night, before they move to the medium care unit and thereafter to the ward.

MRI–MRA of the child is performed postoperatively prior to discharge.[4]

MMV is a progressive disease; therefore, at 1-year follow-up, we perform the same workup as done preoperatively (described earlier in Chapter 8.2).

## 8.9 Patient Position with Skin Incision and Key Surgical Steps

The patient is placed supine, the head mildly extended and 30-degree rotated to the opposite side. In case of the use of any frame, take notion of the risk of damaging the STA on the other side as this would compromise future STA–MCA bypass on the opposite side. We do not shave the hair.[4]

### 8.9.1 Direct (STA–MCA) and Indirect (EDMS) Bypass for Unilateral MCA Territory Revascularization

The incision starts over the parietal branch of the STA. The STA–MCA bypass is performed according to the classic technique described elsewhere.[14] Shortly, the parietal branch of the STA branch is dissected and prepared with the microscope: the STA is kept intact up to the anastomotic procedure (▶ Fig. 8.1**a**). The temporal muscle is cut along the skin incision, and a craniotomy performed on the sylvian point. The dura mater is opened in a star shaped fashion: care has to be paid to preserve the main branches of the middle meningeal artery (▶ Fig. 8.1**b**). After meticulous hemostasis, the dural flaps are reflected subdurally under the bone window to obtain encephalo-duro-synangiosis (EDS). The largest cortical M4 recipient artery is selected as recipient artery. A segment with no or only few cortical side branches is chosen (one to two tiny side branches may need to be interrupted) (▶ Fig. 8.1**c**). A temporary nontraumatic microvascular clip is placed on the exposed STA proximally. The distal STA is cut in a fish mouth to increase the opening diameter of the donor vessel and prepared for the microanastomosis. A blue dye is applied onto the donor and recipient vessels to improve visualization during the anastomotic procedure (▶ Fig. 8.1**d**). A linear arteriotomy on the cortical recipient is performed so that the microanastomosis is at least 2.5 times the size of the diameter of the recipient vessel. Two 10–0 monofilament sutures are applied at the toe and the heel of the anastomotic site to anchor the donor and recipient vessel. The microanastomosis is performed with interrupted 10–0 monofilament sutures to allow anastomosis growth with time. Before knotting the last suture, the anastomosis is flushed to clear air. Flow is

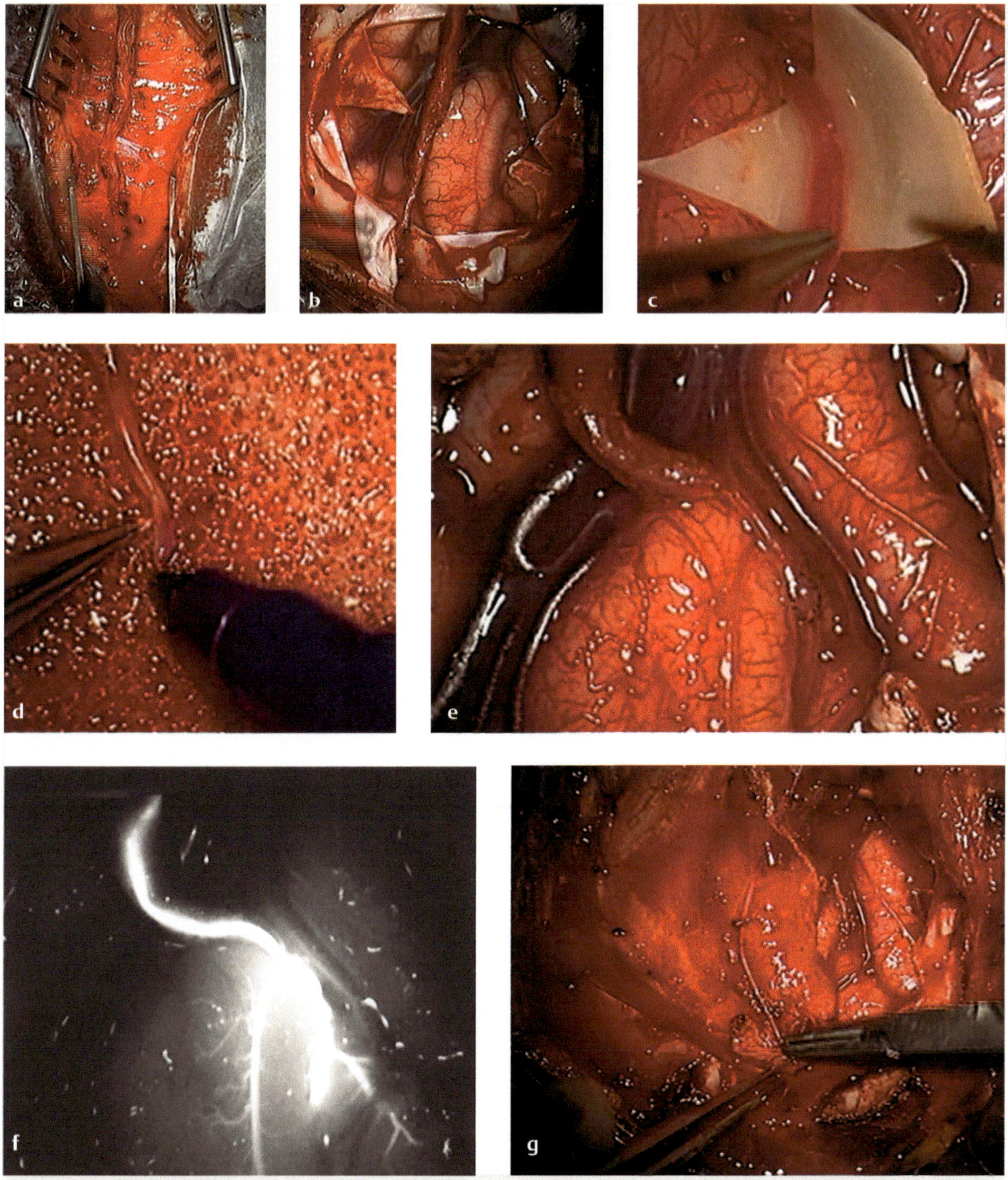


**Fig. 8.1** **(a)** The parietal branch of the superficial temporal artery (STA) branch is dissected. **(b)** After splitting the temporal muscle and performing a craniotomy over the sylvian point, the dura is opened in a star-fashion way. Thereafter the dural flaps are inverted on the cortex around the bone window (see *dotted lines*) in order to obtain encephalo-duro-synangiosis (EDS). **(c)** The cortex is inspected for the largest cortical M4 recipient artery, which is dissected by means of arachnoid opening. A segment with no or only few cortical side branches is chosen. A silicon triangle-shaped background sheets are inserted beneath the recipient artery. **(d)** A temporary nontraumatic microvascular clip is placed across the exposed STA proximally. The distal STA is cut in a fish mouth to increase the opening diameter of the donor vessel and prepared for the microanastomosis. A blue dye is applied onto the donor and recipient vessels to improve visualization during the anastomotic procedure. **(e)** Nontraumatic temporary microvascular clips are applied on the recipient vessel. A linear arteriotomy on the cortical recipient is performed so that the microanastomosis is at least 2.5 times the size of the diameter of the recipient vessel. Two 10–0 monofilament sutures are applied at the toe and the heel of the anastomotic site to anchor the donor and recipient vessel. The microanastomosis is performed with interrupted 10–0 monofilament sutures to allow anastomosis growth with time. Before knotting the last suture, the anastomosis is flushed to clear air. Flow is reestablished by removing first the distal and then the proximal temporary clips on the cortical middle cerebral artery (MCA) recipient artery, and finally the clip on the proximal STA. **(f)** Bypass patency is assessed with indocyanine green videoangiography. **(g)** Closure is performed by covering the exposed cortex with the temporal muscle and by suturing the muscle to the dural edges (to obtain encephalo-myo-synangiosis [EMS]). The bone flap is thereafter secured into place above the muscle. Attention is paid to avoid any compression of the bypass.

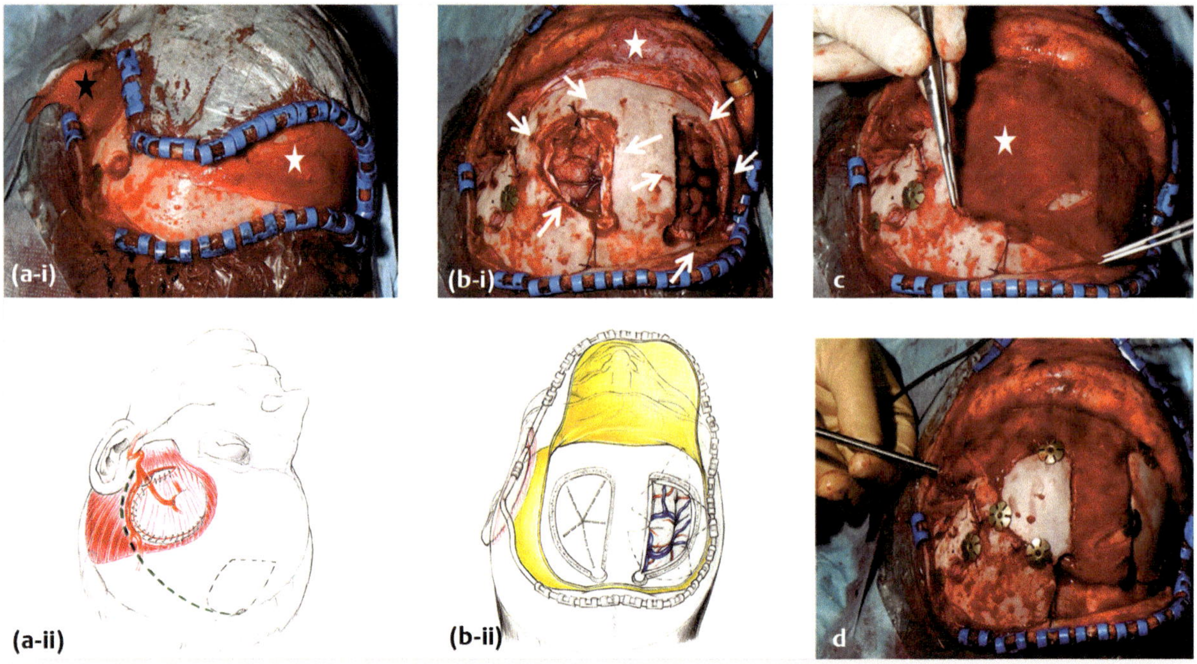


**Fig. 8.2** Intraoperative pictures. **(a-i, a-ii)** After having performed a left superficial temporal artery and middle cerebral artery (STA–MCA) bypass and encephalo-duro-myo-synangiosis (EDMS) (the *black asterisk* a cottonoid covering the bypass), the skin incision is extended 4-cm over the midline behind the hairline. All the skin incisions are performed behind the hairline. The *white asterisk* indicates the dissected frontal pericranial flap (*no-shaving technique*). **(b-i, b-ii)** The scalp flap is reflected anteriorly; the vascularized frontal pericranial tissue is further dissected and reflected on the scalp flap (see *white asterisk*); two symmetric bilateral frontal parasagittal craniotomies are performed; the underlying frontal dura is then opened in a star-fashion and the dural flaps are inverted onto the cortex around each frontal bone window, to obtain encephalo-duro-synangiosis (EDS) (see *multiple white arrows*). **(c)** The pericranial flap (*white asterisk*) is placed over the cortex surface and is sutured to dural edges to obtain encephalo-periosteal-synangiosis (EPS). **(d)** The bone flaps are repositioned. At the end of the procedure STA–MCA bypass plus EDMS has been performed unilateral for revascularization of a MCA territory, and bifrontal encephalo-duro-periosteal-synangiosis (EDPS) has been performed to revascularize the frontal areas bilaterally. (Reproduced with permission from Esposito G, Kronenburg A, Fierstra J, et al. STA-MCA bypass with encephalo-duro-myo-synangiosis combined with bifrontal encephalo-duro-periosteal-synangiosis as a one-staged revascularization strategy for pediatric moyamoya vasculopathy. Childs Nerv Syst 2015;31:765–772. Copyright © 2015, Springer-Verlag Berlin Heidelberg. Panels **(a-ii)** and **(b-ii)** are modified after Mr. Peter Roth; Department of Neurosurgery; University Hospital Zurich; Zurich, Switzerland.)

reestablished by removing first the distal and then the proximal temporary clips on the cortical MCA recipient artery, and finally the clip on the proximal STA (▶ Fig. 8.1**e**). Bypass patency is assessed with indocyanine green videoangiography (performed by the use of a commercially available microscope, OPMI Pentero, Carl Zeiss Co., Oberkochen, Germany) (▶ Fig. 8.1**f**). The flow in the bypass is quantitatively assessed using an intra-operative flow probe (Transonic Systems Inc., Ithaca, NY). In pediatric moyamoya patients, flow values are expected to be between 15 and 50 mL per minute, depending on patients' age, donor and recipient characteristics, and hemodynamic conditions. The microanastomosis is observed for 20 minutes to exclude decrease in flow.[4] Closure is performed by covering the exposed cortex with the temporal muscle and by suturing the muscle to the dural edges (to obtain encephalo-myo-synangiosis [EMS]) (▶ Fig. 8.1**g**). The bone flap is then secured into place above the muscle. Attention is paid to avoid any compression of the bypass.[4,7]

## 8.9.2 Bifrontal EDPS

After completing the direct (STA–MCA) and indirect (EDMS) revascularization for the MCA territory, the skin incision is extended frontally 4 cm over the midline, staying behind the hairline (▶ Fig. 8.2**a**). The scalp flap is reflected anteriorly and a vascularized bifrontal pericranial flap, consisting of the periosteum and the overlying loose areolar layer, is prepared (▶ Fig. 8.2**a, b**). This pericranial flap is kept pediculated toward the bitemporal and biorbital regions to maximize vascular supply. This pediculated pericranial flap will serve to perform the bifrontal encephalo-periosteal-synangiosis (EPS). Two separate frontal parasagittal craniotomies (4 × 5 cm) are performed, one on the left and one the right side. The craniotomies extend up to 2 cm away from the midline to avoid injuring the SSS and the parasagittal veins. The dura is then opened in a star-shaped fashion and, after meticulous hemostasis, the dural flaps are inverted and reflected under the edges of each frontal bone window to obtain EDS (▶ Fig. 8.2**b**). Small cortical arachnoidal openings are made. The periosteal flap is then positioned over the cortical convexity and sutured laterally to the dura (to obtain EPS) (▶ Fig. 8.2**c**). Both frontal bone flaps are repositioned and fixed (▶ Fig. 8.2**d**). The scalp flap is reapproximated and the skin incision closed in two layers taking care not to compromise the STA–MCA bypass.[4,7]

## 8.10 Difficulties Encountered

If the STA is not suitable for a direct bypass, another donor artery might be considered (posterior auricular artery), or the MCA territory has to be revascularized using an indirect technique only. We did not encounter technical difficulties for the bifrontal EDPS in our series.

## 8.11 Bailout, Rescue, and Salvage Manoeuvres

Intraoperatively, bypass occlusion/malfunction may need bypass reexploration, brain swelling may occur, and anemia may necessitate transfusion.

## 8.12 Tips, Pearls, and Lessons Learned

Bifrontal EDPS by itself could also be used as a supplementary procedure in patients who already underwent previous revascularization procedures, in case of bifrontal hypoperfusion or progression of the MMV with symptoms referable to frontal lobe hypoperfusion. Bifrontal EDPS itself is doable by means of a short bifrontal incision, from one superior temporal line to the contralateral one.

## References


[1] Park JH, Yang SY, Chung YN, et al. Modified encephaloduroarteriosynangiosis with bifrontal encephalogaleoperiosteal synangiosis for the treatment of pediatric moyamoya disease. Technical note. J Neurosurg. 2007; 106(3) Suppl:237–242

[2] Weinberg DG, Rahme RJ, Aoun SG, Batjer HH, Bendok BR. Moyamoya disease: functional and neurocognitive outcomes in the pediatric and adult populations. Neurosurg Focus. 2011; 30(6):E21

[3] Khan N, Schuknecht B, Boltshauser E, et al. Moyamoya disease and moyamoya syndrome: experience in Europe; choice of revascularisation procedures. Acta Neurochir (Wien). 2003; 145(12):1061–1071, discussion 1071

[4] Esposito G, Kronenburg A, Fierstra J, et al. "STA-MCA bypass with encephalo-duro-myo-synangiosis combined with bifrontal encephalo-duro-periosteal-synangiosis" as a one-staged revascularization strategy for pediatric moyamoya vasculopathy. Childs Nerv Syst. 2015; 31(5):765–772

[5] Kim CY, Wang KC, Kim SK, Chung YN, Kim HS, Cho BK. Encephaloduroarteriosynangiosis with bifrontal encephalogaleo(periosteal)synangiosis in the pediatric moyamoya disease: the surgical technique and its outcomes. Childs Nerv Syst. 2003; 19(5–6):316–324

[6] Kim SK, Wang KC, Kim IO, Lee DS, Cho BK. Combined encephaloduroarteriosynangiosis and bifrontal encephalogaleo(periosteal)synangiosis in pediatric moyamoya disease. Neurosurgery. 2002; 50(1):88–96

[7] Kronenburg A, Esposito G, Fierstra J, Braun KP, Regli L. Combined bypass technique for contemporary revascularization of unilateral MCA and bilateral frontal territories in moyamoya vasculopathy. Acta Neurochir Suppl (Wien). 2014; 119:65–70

[8] Festa JR, Schwarz LR, Pliskin N, et al. Neurocognitive dysfunction in adult moyamoya disease. J Neurol. 2010; 257(5):806–815

[9] Ibrahimi DM, Tamargo RJ, Ahn ES. Moyamoya disease in children. Childs Nerv Syst. 2010; 26(10):1297–1308

[10] Kim SK, Cho BK, Phi JH, et al. Pediatric moyamoya disease: an analysis of 410 consecutive cases. Ann Neurol. 2010; 68(1):92–101

[11] Lee JY, Phi JH, Wang KC, Cho BK, Shin MS, Kim SK. Neurocognitive profiles of children with moyamoya disease before and after surgical intervention. Cerebrovasc Dis. 2011; 31(3):230–237

[12] Kuroda S, Houkin K, Ishikawa T, et al. Determinants of intellectual outcome after surgical revascularization in pediatric moyamoya disease: a multivariate analysis. Childs Nerv Syst. 2004; 20(5):302–308

[13] Kuroda S, Houkin K, Ishikawa T, Nakayama N, Iwasaki Y. Novel bypass surgery for moyamoya disease using pericranial flap: its impacts on cerebral hemodynamics and long-term outcome. Neurosurgery. 2010; 66(6):1093–1101, discussion 1101

[14] Khan N, Luca R. STA-MCA microanastomosis: surgical technique. In: Abdulrauf S, ed. Cerebral Revascularization: Techniques in Extracranial-to-Intracranial Bypass Surgery. Philadelphia, PA: Elsevier; 2011:93–7

# Part 3

## Direct Revascularization

# 9 STA–MCA Bypass for Direct Revascularization in Moyamoya Disease

*Alessandro Narducci and Peter Vajkoczy*

**Abstract**

Superficial temporal artery (STA) to middle cerebral artery (MCA) bypass is one of the most widespread techniques to provide blood supply from external carotid to intracranial circulation. The procedure contemplates the microsurgical dissection of an STA branch in the scalp (donor vessel) and of a cortical MCA branch (recipient vessel) near to the end of Sylvian fissure, and their subsequent anastomosis. It represents a universal indication for moyamoya disease, since it lowers the risk of ischemic and hemorrhagic strokes, due to the immediate revascularization provided. For technical feasibility, the size of vessels to anastomose should not be inferior to 1 mm; thus, in pediatric patients, the procedure can be sometimes difficult or impossible.

The performance of this bypass requires specialized training and experience with the use of microvascular techniques. It is mandatory for a careful preoperative assessment (i.e., digital subtraction angiography, coagulation, and platelet function tests), as well as meticulous intraoperative attention to technical details because the risk of postoperative neurological deficits, hemorrhages, and ischemic stroke is non-negligible.

The major contraindication to STA–MCA bypass is represented by the presence of acute stroke; in such case it is recommended to postpone the procedure for a few weeks.

In this chapter we provide a detailed description of the surgical technique and patient care, basing on evidence and high-volume experience.

*Keywords:* moyamoya disease, bypass, superficial temporal artery, middle cerebral artery, direct revascularization, microvascular anastomosis

## 9.1 History and Initial Description

Superficial temporal artery (STA) to middle cerebral artery (MCA) nowadays represents an established technique for flow augmentation in chronic cerebral ischemic diseases. Yasargil was the first who described this procedure after technical development of microvascular anastomosis in dogs. He performed the first STA–MCA bypass in a human in 1967 to treat a patient with complete MCA occlusion,[1] carrying out an end-to-side anastomosis between a distal branch of STA and a cortical branch of MCA near the sylvian fissure. Variations of this procedure have been described, such as end-to-end anastomosis and double-limb STA–MCA grafts, but the original technique is still the most widespread.

One of the first applications in moyamoya disease was reported in 1980, by Holbach and coworkers, on a 41-year-old Libyan woman.[2] The authors evaluated the usefulness of direct revascularization through postoperative EEG (electroencephalography), which showed an "increase in the electrical brain activity."[2] The effectiveness of this procedure has been afterward evaluated through flow measurement tools[3] and imaging, such as magnetic resonance (MR) angiography,[4] even if angiography provided the clearest evidence in terms of improvement of intracranial circulation following bypass.

The value of STA–MCA bypass in moyamoya disease has been unclear for a long time, due to the scarcity of large series with long-term follow-up and the presence of patients largely treated with indirect revascularization techniques. In 2009, Steinberg and coworkers[5] reported a large cohort of patients with moyamoya treated at Stanford University, describing the benefit of direct bypass in terms of prevention of ischemic events and improvement of life quality.

Several studies have subsequently confirmed these findings and at present, STA–MCA bypass is well recognized as a useful treatment approach for moyamoya patients.

## 9.2 Indications

STA–MCA bypass, compared to indirect revascularization techniques, provides a great advantage of immediately increasing the blood flow in chronic hypoperfused brain. Its protective effect has been demonstrated both for ischemic and hemorrhagic moyamoya disease[6] because it implies a double result: improvement of cerebral perfusion and reduction of hemodynamic stress on collateral fragile moyamoya vessels, usually very prone to rupture. Medium term follow-up studies showed that the incidence of both ischemic and hemorrhagic strokes decreases, making STA–MCA bypass a universal indication for moyamoya disease, when technically feasible. The size of the vessels represents, in fact, the most important feature in decision making because a diameter of less than 1 mm makes the anastomosis technically difficult or even impossible. It is therefore deductible that in pediatric patients, indirect revascularization is sometimes the sole practicable surgical option.

Preoperative digital subtraction angiography (DSA) is the gold standard in assessing the caliber of STA;

nevertheless, the surgeon must keep in mind that, sometimes, the existent size of parietal and frontal branches observable during surgery is superior to the one expected according to imaging.

# 9.3 Key Principles

The classic and most widespread technique for STA–MCA bypass consists in performing a direct end-to-side anastomosis of one STA distal branch (parietal or frontal) with a cortical M3 branch, exposed through a small craniotomy ideally targeted on the distal portion of the sylvian fissure. The selection of the most prominent STA branch as well as an appropriate antiplatelet management are milestones for success.

# 9.4 SWOT Analysis

## 9.4.1 Strengths

- Immediate revascularization with subsequent immediate protection against stroke.
- Working horse of bypass surgery.
- Universally applicable.
- Proven efficacy against both ischemic and hemorrhagic strokes.

## 9.4.2 Weaknesses

- Technical complexity (good microsurgical skills required).
- Risk of intraoperative and postoperative graft occlusion.
- Risk of postoperative hyperperfision.

## 9.4.3 Opportunities

- Further reduction of invasiveness (navigation, augmented reality).

## 9.4.4 Threats

- Poor quality of vessels.
- Risk of hyperperfusion.
- Involvement of posterior cerebral artery in the disease.

# 9.5 Contraindications

Contraindications are few but significant. First, the presence of acute stroke with large restricted signal in diffusion weighted imaging represents a major contraindication; performing the procedure at least 6 weeks after the stroke can be considered safe. Second, it is possible that none of STA branches is suitable as a donor vessel or the artery is absent for different reasons (i.e., previous surgery); in this situation, alternative techniques must be considered. Lastly, the presence of substantial contribution to collateralization from STA needs to be evaluated in each patient prior surgery, weighting risks and benefits of the procedure.

# 9.6 Special Considerations

## 9.6.1 Preoperative Imaging

Preoperative imaging studies are fundamental for planning the correct strategy and include computed tomography (CT) scan, MR imaging, as well as six-vessel cerebral angiography. Lateral external carotid angiogram allows the evaluation of diameter, course, and tortuosity of STA, so that the prominent branch can be used as a donor vessel; it also provides information helpful in avoiding unexpected anatomical variations that can be encountered (i.e., atresia of parietal branch).

## 9.6.2 Anticoagulation

Optimal anticoagulation and antiplatelet therapy is still a matter of debate. Preoperative single dose of aspirin (100 mg) or clopidogrel (75 mg) or intraoperative administration of a bolus of aspirin seems to have no effect in increasing hemorrhagic risk; nevertheless, their efficacy in improving outcome is still unknown. Similar evidence regards administration of low molecular weight heparin. On the other hand, postoperative use of a single antiplatelet agent (aspirin 100 mg or clopidogrel 75 mg) is correlated with improved outcome, without increasing hemorrhagic risk. Double antiplatelet therapy does not offer additional benefits. Tests for platelet function and individual resistance to antiplatelet drugs can provide useful information for the best management.

## 9.6.3 Other Considerations

The concomitant exposure of both intracranial and extracranial vasculature gives the chance to perform further studies (i.e., evaluation of moyamoya-like change in external carotid circulation) by means of vessel biopsy (STA or MCA).

# 9.7 Pitfalls, Risk Assessment, and Complications

STA–MCA bypass carries non-negligible risk of complications. Steinberg and coworkers, in their large cohort, experienced postprocedural hemorrhagic strokes in 1.8% of treated patients, as well as 3.5% of neurological deficits. Schubert et al[7] reported an incidence of 8.5% of perioperative ischemic strokes, and a revision rate of 3.1%. General risks (i.e., infections, cerebrospinal fluid leak) are comparable to other neurosurgical procedures.

## 9.8 Special Instructions, Position, and Anesthesia

No special measures are required in terms of positioning and anesthesia, except for optimal intraoperative blood pressure management, since hypertension can be associated with decrease in bypass patency. Local anesthesia should be avoided, as it carries the risk of STA vasoconstriction or injuries.

## 9.9 Patient Position with Skin Incision and Key Surgical Steps

### 9.9.1 Preparation

The patient is placed in supine position with the ipsilateral shoulder elevated. The head, fixed by a Mayfield head holder, is rotated with almost 90 degrees to the opposite side, in such a way as to have the surgical field parallel to the floor. The donor vessel can be identified by palpation or with the aid of Doppler ultrasound, if needed. According with the STA branch chosen, the skin is marked directly along the course of the vessel (▶ Fig. 9.1). The craniotomy should be centered over the distal portion of the sylvian fissure. This relatively confined area, where several MCA branches emerge (▶ Fig. 9.2), is located approximately 6 cm above the external auditory canal. In our institution, for optimal location of craniotomy, we use a special designed template[8] (▶ Fig. 9.3), which allows the identification of the end of sylvian fissure with high accuracy. In our experience, a 3 cm craniotomy around the target point is sufficient to expose at least one suitable recipient MCA branch.

### 9.9.2 Surgical Technique

#### Donor Vessel Isolation

All surgical steps described are performed under microscope magnification. Isolation of donor vessel starts with incision through the skin and dermal fat. The initial steps carry the highest risk of STA injury; for this reason, it is advisable to begin the dissection distally, since if injury occurs, a substantial portion of vessel is still intact. Once STA is identified, a careful dissection is performed, cauterizing the side branches and releasing the artery from the surrounding tissue (▶ Fig. 9.4). Mechanical vasospasm is avoided by leaving a connective tissue cuff around the artery, which protects it from excessive manipulation and damage (▶ Fig. 9.5).

In cases in which parietal branch is used as a donor vessel, only 1 linear skin incision is needed, as it usually runs slightly in front of the target point for craniotomy,

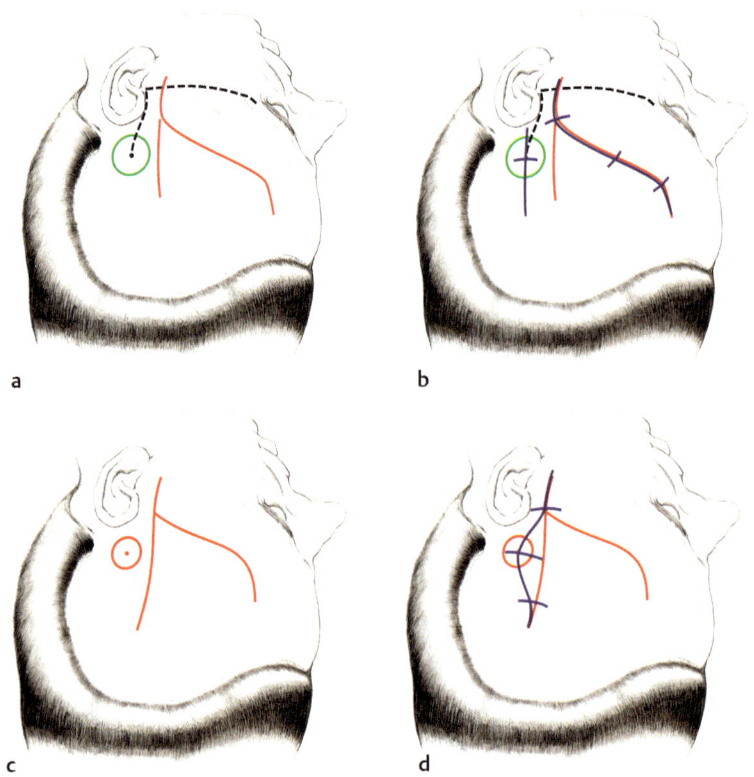

a b c d

**Fig. 9.1** Patient position and skin incision for left STA–MCA bypass. Localization of STA branches (*red mark*); targeted craniotomy (*green circle*); skin incisions (*blue marks*). **(a, b)** Double-skin incision in case of frontal branch used as a donor vessel. **(c, d)** Single-skin incision in case of use of parietal branch.

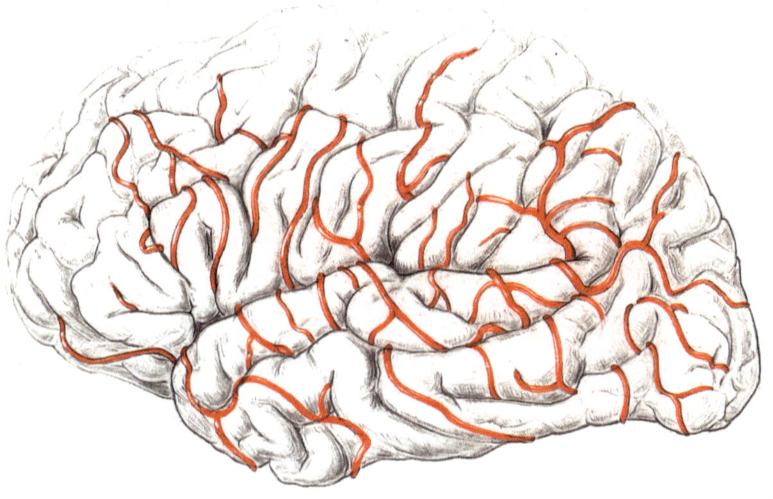

**Fig. 9.2** Left cerebral cortex in a cadaver specimen. Note the high number of M3 branches emerging from the end of sylvian fissure.

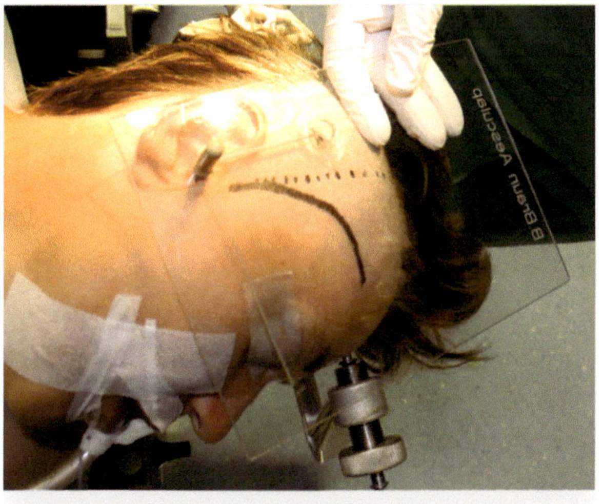

**Fig. 9.3** Rectangular shaped template for targeted craniotomy. The small handle that extends for 2 cm on both sides is placed in the outer external auditory canal. Two orthogonal lines intersect the handle. The horizontal one is used as reference, through alignment with the lateral canthus of the eye, while the 6-cm vertical one (with a small perforation at its end) allows to mark the targetpoint on the skin. The template can be used on both sides.

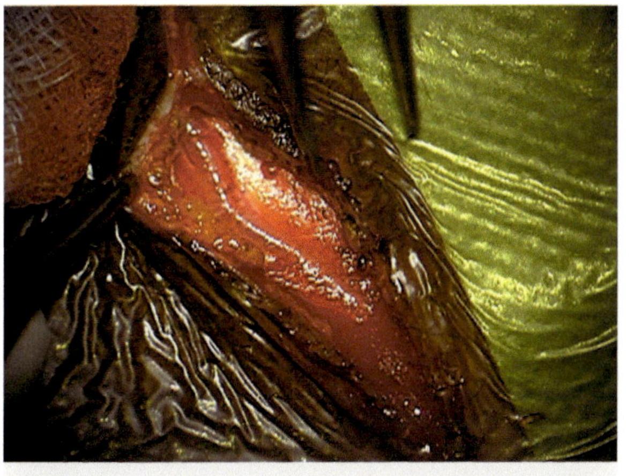

**Fig. 9.4** Skin incision along STA donor vessel and initial steps of dissection.

into the parietal scalp region (▶ Fig. 9.1**c, d**). On the other hand, when frontal branch is prominent and more suitable as a donor vessel, we use a double-skin incision technique (▶ Fig. 9.1**a, b**). A first linear cut is performed, starting in front of the ear and extending along the course of the artery into the lateral forehead. Next, a separate second 5 cm skin incision is made over the target point of craniotomy (▶ Fig. 9.6). After a sufficient length of artery is isolated, it is divided, distally clamped with a temporary clip, and subsequently tunneled under the skin which separates the two incisions, in order to reach the operative field. The donor vessel is then placed between cottonoids wet with papaverine.

## Craniotomy and Recipient Vessel Preparation

A 3 cm craniotomy is performed after division and lateral retraction of the temporalis muscle. It is advisable to place the burr hole caudally, in order to allow the passage of STA after bone flap replacement (▶ Fig. 9.7). The dura is opened in a U-shaped fashion, and turned cranially (▶ Fig. 9.8).

The cortical surface is inspected to identify the most suitable recipient vessel. It is important to select the most prominent one, evaluating also the absence of major side branches. After opening the arachnoid, minor collaterals

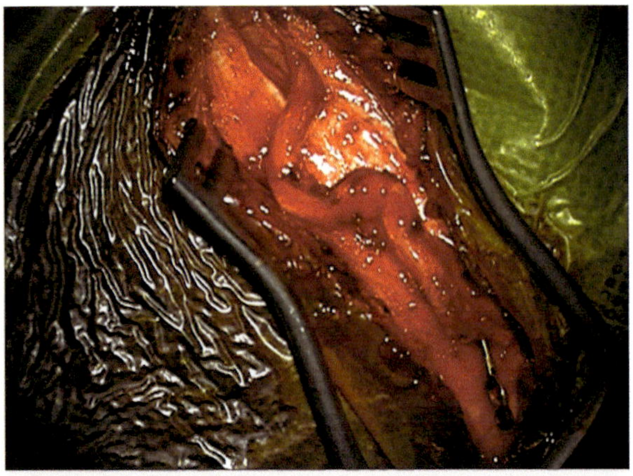

**Fig. 9.5** Mobilization of donor vessel. Note the connective tissue cuff left around it.

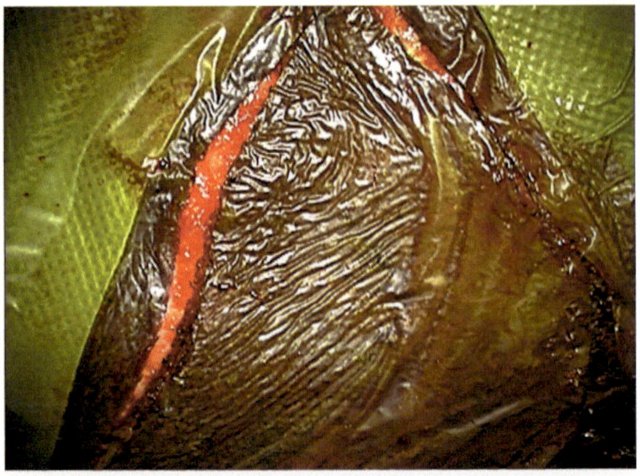

**Fig. 9.6** Second skin incision over targeted end of sylvian fissure.

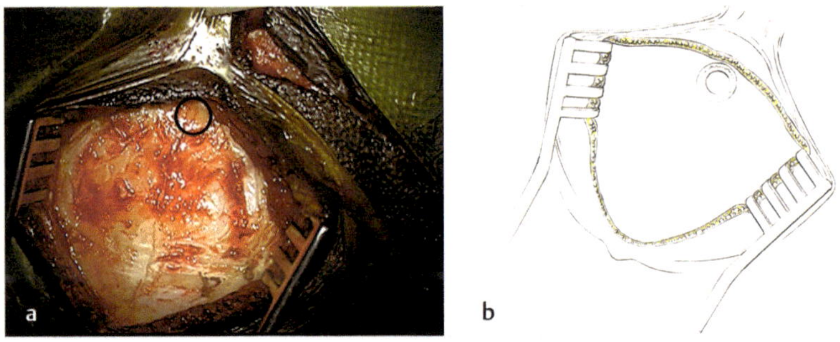

**Fig. 9.7 (a, b)** Exposure of bone. Ideal location of the burr hole (*black circle*).

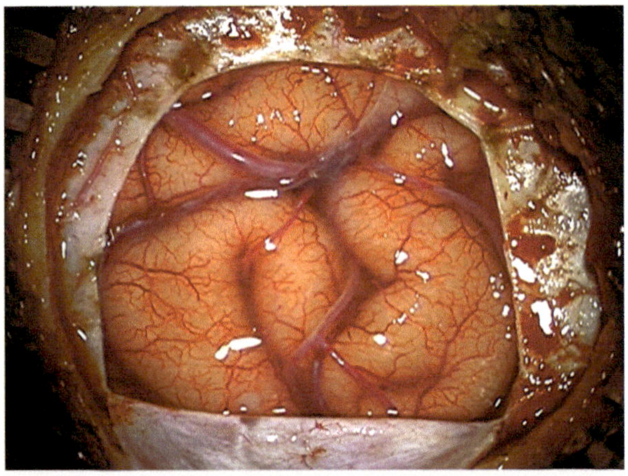

**Fig. 9.8** Craniotomy (3 cm) and dural opening. Note the dural flap turned cranially.

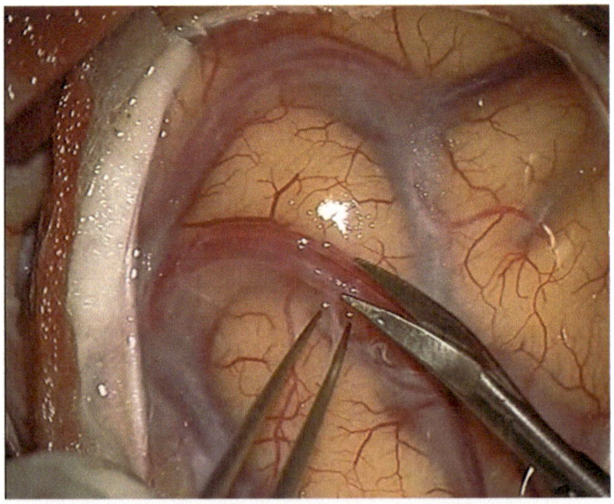

**Fig. 9.9** Mobilization of recipient vessel. Sacrifice of small perforators is sometimes required.

can be sacrificed without sequelae, in order to release tethering of M3 branch to cerebral cortex (▶ Fig. 9.9). After preparation of the recipient vessel, the cuff of connective tissue surrounding the distal end of STA is meticulously removed, and the vessel is irrigated with heparinized saline to prevent clot formation. The distal end is cut in oblique form and fish mouthed; this is fundamental because it allows obtaining a 4-times increase of cross-sectional area, so that the blood flow is ensured even if the anastomosis will provoke some degree of

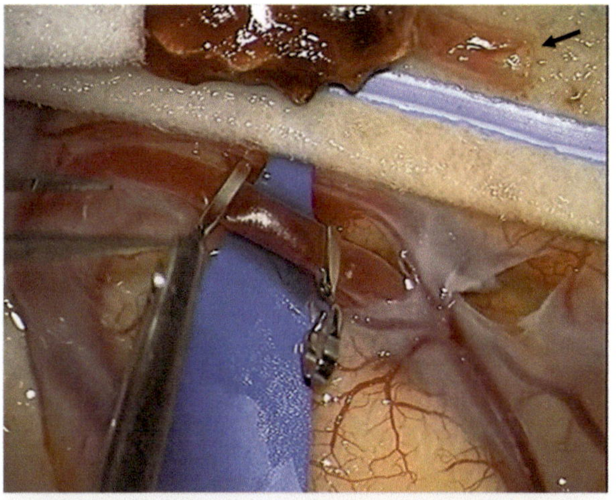

**Fig. 9.10** After fish-mouthing the end of STA branch (*arrow*), the recipient vessel is temporary occluded with small arteriovenous malformation clips (approximate distance: 5 mm).

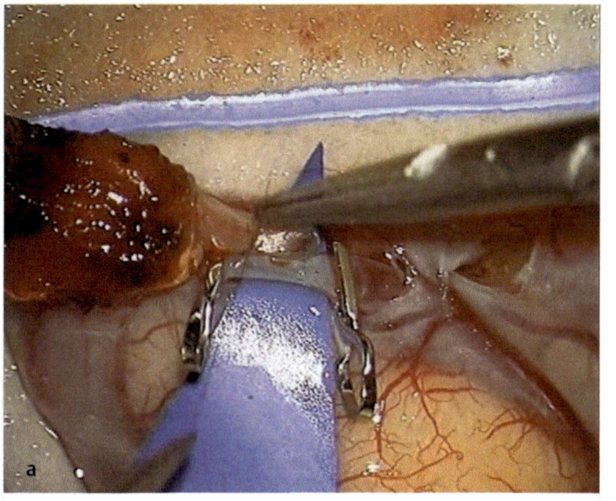

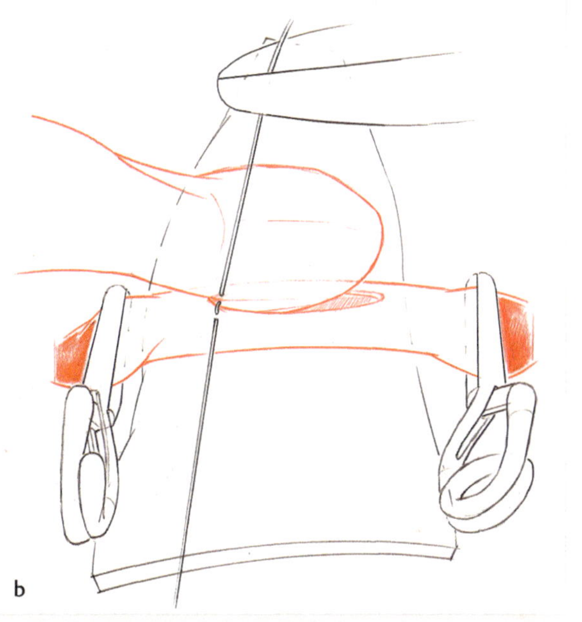

**Fig. 9.11 (a, b)** Beginning of anastomosis, suturing the heel of fish-mouth with one of the end of arteriotomy.

stenosis. The donor vessel should be adapted to the appropriate length in order to minimize intravascular resistance but at the same time ensure enough redundancy without tension.

A triangular-shaped plastic pad is placed under the recipient vessel and small arteriovenous malformation (AVM) clips are applied at a distance of about 5 mm to interrupt the blood flow within the recipient artery (▶ Fig. 9.10).

Arteriotomy can be performed in different ways. We place a 10–0 nylon stitch on the arterial wall parallel to the vessel course—this allows exerting a moderate traction in order to perform an easier arteriotomy using microscissors. The length of arteriotomy should ideally be twice the diameter of the recipient vessel, and match with the fish-mouthed donor vessel.

## Anastomosis

A 10–0 nylon microsuture is used to perform the anastomosis. The heel of the fish mouth is sawn to one of the two ends of the recipient artery, considering the flow direction (▶ Fig. 9.11). The toe of the donor vessel is then sutured to the second end of arteriotomy. Next, it is possible to start suturing the two walls, using interrupted or running technique. Suturing the back wall is more difficult, so it is advisable to perform it first (▶ Fig. 9.12); moreover, this strategy makes it possible to double-check the correct placement of sutures from the open front wall.

## Final Steps

After completion of the anastomosis, the clips are removed from recipient and donor vessels; during this step, some bleeding is commonly observable and somehow auspicable, witnessing the presence of blood flow. Small amount of bleeding is easily controlled applying cottonoids on the anastomosis with gentle pressure, and with the apposition of Surgicel or Gelfoam. Significant leaks can be closed with additional sutures. Direct revascularization can be supplemented with encephalo-duro-synangiosis, underturning the dural flap over the cortical surface; the remaining gap can be filled with a layer of Gelfoam (▶ Fig. 9.13).

Patency of the graft is intraoperatively assessed using different tools, such as indocyanine green videoangiography, micro Doppler probes, and DSA.

During closure, it is fundamental to allow graft to pass safely through the burr hole (▶ Fig. 9.14), and avoid too

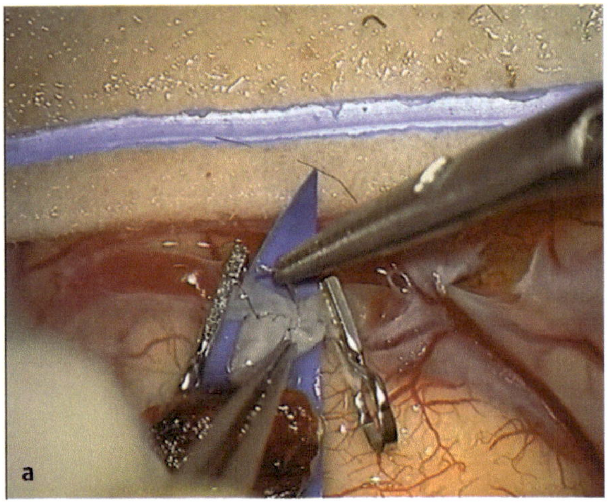


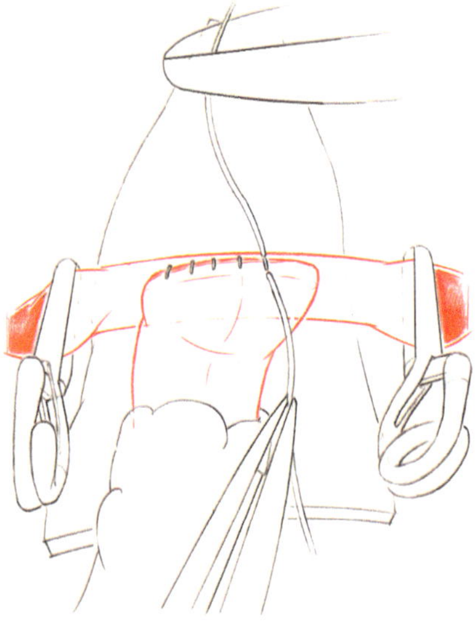

Fig. 9.12 (a, b) Suturing of the posterior wall.

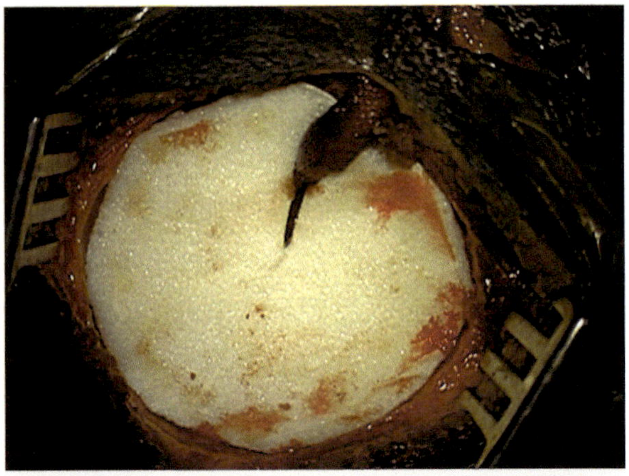

Fig. 9.13 Layer of gelfoam used to fill the dural gap left after encephalo-duro-synangiosis.

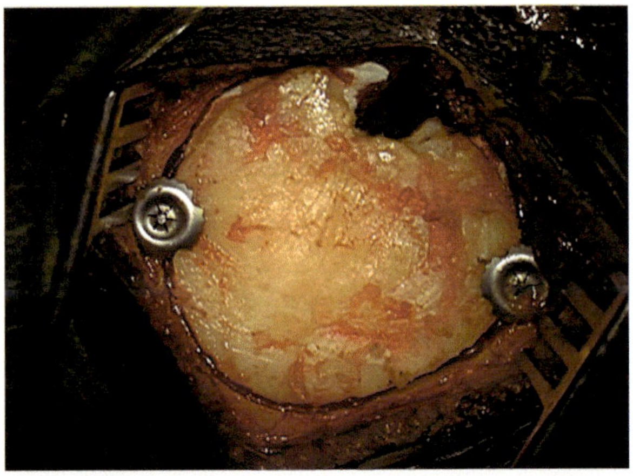

Fig. 9.14 Closure with bon flap allowing graft to pass safely through the burr hole.

tight closure of muscle, potentially leading to compressive effects and stenosis of STA. The graft is inspected for kinking or compression during all phases of the closure.

## 9.10 Difficulties Encountered

| Surgical step | Difficulty |
|---|---|
| Preparation of donor vessel | 1. Injury of STA branch<br>2. Low cut-flow in the STA/intraoperative STA occlusion |
| Craniotomy | 1. Absence of adequate recipient vessel in the exposed field |
| Anastomosis | 1. Short STA branch<br>2. Intraoperative detection of nonfunctioning bypass |

## 9.11 Bailout, Rescue, and Salvage Maneuvers

If the STA injury is small and clearly identifiable, it can be sutured, even if the vessel is completely broken off, performing an end-to-end reconstruction; conversely, if the damage is not recoverable, the use of the other branch needs to be considered.

Irrigation with heparinized saline can prevent or resolve clot formation, while the use of papaverine and hydrostatic dilation through saline flushing can decrease vasospasm.

Craniotomy must be enlarged in cases in which no adequate recipient vessels are detected in the surgical field. In case of short STA, it is possible to remedy, identifying a more proximal recipient vessel, splitting the sylvian fissure and using an infrasylvian recipient.

In cases of nonfunctioning bypass, it is mandatory a revision of anastomosis or, eventually, redo it choosing a different recipient vessel.

## 9.12 Tips, Pearls, and Lessons Learned

For a successful STA–MCA bypass, some precautions are of basic importance in preventing minimal and severe complications.

### 9.12.1 Preoperative Evaluations

Identification of hypercoagulable states, evaluation of coagulation parameters, as well as platelet function tests help to avoid thrombotic or hemorrhagic complications, which can badly affect the outcome.

Preoperative evaluation of STA course and detection of variation can alert the surgeon to a more mindful dissection, especially in case of tortuous artery, lowering the risk of injury.

### 9.12.2 Technical Tips

Minimizing skin incision decreases the incidence of wound-related problems, with a linear cut along the course of donor vessel. As mentioned earlier, it is safer to perform a distal to proximal dissection.

The distal portion of sylvian fissure (6 cm above the external auditory canal) represents an optimal location for craniotomy; adjunctive tools (i.e., navigation, augmented reality) could further increase the accuracy.

During anastomosis, it is fundamental to avoid excessive handling of arterial edges.

Marking the margins of donor and recipient arteries with ink, as well as keeping the surgical field dry and bloodless, improve visualization during suturing process. This is of particular importance in moyamoya disease, in which the thin wall of vessels may lead to collapse and difficult identification of arteriotomy edges.

Interrupted and running techniques for anastomosis provide the same level of efficacy, even if the latter is less time consuming. It is anyway advisable for beginners to start with interrupted technique because it allows fixing and redoing every single suture. Performing a running suture, in fact, requires a solid experience, since uncontrolled and unintentional movements may tear off the whole anastomosis.

Vasospasm is a common event during the procedure, particularly affecting recipient vessels: the frequent use of papaverine during all steps is helpful in tackling this issue.

Besides the strategies described in the previous paragraph to achieve a good final hemostasis at the suture line, a muscle patch could be helpful in the most troublesome cases. It is important to keep in mind that attempts in coagulation can lead to definitive opening.

In case of intraoperative detection of bypass failure, redo the anastomosis is safer than revising it, as revision carries higher risk of long-term occlusion.

### 9.12.3 Postoperative Care

STA–MCA bypass needs postoperative low intensity monitoring. One night in the intensive care is sufficient for adult patients, 48 hours for pediatric patients. The most important parameter to monitor is blood pressure, in order to avoid early graft failure (hypotension) or leakage from anastomosis leading to subdural hematoma (hypertension). Lowering the blood pressure is also important in management of postoperative hyperperfusion.

Postoperative radiological assessment contemplates CT scan to evaluate the presence of hemorrhagic complications, and DSA to assess bypass function.

## References


[1] Yaşargil MG. A legacy of microneurosurgery: memoirs, lessons, and axioms. Neurosurgery. 1999; 45(5):1025–1092

[2] Holbach KH, Wassmann H, Wappenschmidt J. Superficial temporal-middle cerebral artery anastomosis in moyamoya disease. Acta Neurochir (Wien). 1980; 52(1–2):27–34

[3] Moritake K, Handa H, Yonekawa Y, Nagata I. Ultrasonic Doppler assessment of hemodynamics in superficial temporal artery—middle cerebral artery anastomosis. Surg Neurol. 1980; 13(4): 249–257

[4] Horn P, Vajkoczy P, Schmiedek P, Neff W. Evaluation of extracranial-intracranial arterial bypass function with magnetic resonance angiography. Neuroradiology. 2004; 46(9):723–729

[5] Guzman R, Lee M, Achrol A, et al. Clinical outcome after 450 revascularization procedures for moyamoya disease. Clinical article. J Neurosurg. 2009; 111(5):927–935

[6] Miyamoto S, Yoshimoto T, Hashimoto N, et al. JAM Trial Investigators. Effects of extracranial-intracranial bypass for patients with hemorrhagic moyamoya disease: results of the Japan Adult Moyamoya Trial. Stroke. 2014; 45(5):1415–1421

[7] Schubert GA, Biermann P, Weiss C, et al. Risk profile in extracranial/intracranial bypass surgery—the role of antiplatelet agents, disease pathology, and surgical technique in 168 direct revascularization procedures. World Neurosurg. 2014; 82(5):672–677

[8] Peña-Tapia PG, Kemmling A, Czabanka M, Vajkoczy P, Schmiedek P. Identification of the optimal cortical target point for extracranial-intracranial bypass surgery in patients with hemodynamic cerebrovascular insufficiency. J Neurosurg. 2008; 108(4):655–661

# 10 Double-Barrel Bypass in Moyamoya Disease

*John E. Wanebo and Robert F. Spetzler*

**Abstract**

This chapter describes the use of two branches of the superficial temporal artery for direct anastomotic bypass in patients with moyamoya disease. Although some surgeons routinely perform a double-barrel bypass, it is typically used when significant superficial temporal artery ischemia is found in addition to middle cerebral artery ischemia. The technical features of the procedure are explained, including the ideal manner of harvesting both superficial temporal artery branches while minimizing wound issues. How to identify the best recipient middle cerebral artery branches for anastomoses is also discussed. Finally, specific perioperative management protocols and complication avoidance as well as management are reviewed.

*Keywords:* Anastomoses, middle cerebral artery, moyamoya disease, superficial temporal artery

## 10.1 History and Initial Description

Since the first superficial temporal artery (STA) to middle cerebral artery (MCA) bypass pioneered by Donaghy and Yaşargil et al in 1967, neurosurgeons have utilized multiple adaptations to augment cerebral blood flow.[1,2] Reichman was the first to use both STA branches in a bypass for ischemia in 1975. Sakamoto et al[3] applied the technique of using two STA branches for the treatment of pediatric moyamoya disease in 1997. Ishikawa et al[4] reported using one STA branch to revascularize the anterior cerebral artery (ACA) and the other for the MCA in 2005. Several reports from Hokkaido, Japan, describe large series of patients with moyamoya disease who routinely underwent a double-barrel bypass to the MCA cortical branches as part of a larger, combined, indirect revascularization procedure.[5,6] At Barrow Neurological Institute, like other centers, we use a double-barrel bypass in select patients, including those with moyamoya disease, intracranial occlusive cerebrovascular disease, and complex aneurysms.[7,8]

## 10.2 Indications

The basic indication for a double-barrel bypass in the setting of moyamoya disease is severe hemispheric hypoperfusion. This circumstance is usually the case when both the MCA and the ACA are involved and frequently when patients have severe bilateral disease. Rapid progression of the clinical course of the patient also lends support to performing a double-barrel bypass because these patients have not had time to develop sufficient collateral vascularization on their own. Since such patients have inadequate cerebral blood flow and rapid disease progression, they need STA branches and recipient cortical MCA arteries of sufficient quality to allow for a double-limbed bypass.

At Barrow Neurological Institute, we evaluate the cerebral blood flow in moyamoya patients using computed tomography (CT) perfusion imaging before and after a 1-g acetazolamide vasodilatory challenge. Patients with symptomatic moyamoya disease who have impaired cerebrovascular reserve on a CT perfusion study upon vasodilatory challenge are candidates for revascularization. In most cases, a six-vessel cerebral angiogram is performed to document the stage of moyamoya disease and to demonstrate donor suitability of the STAs. Patients with severe hemispheric hypoperfusion, usually including both STA and ACA territories, are those typically chosen for two direct anastomoses (▶ Fig. 10.1). The decision to

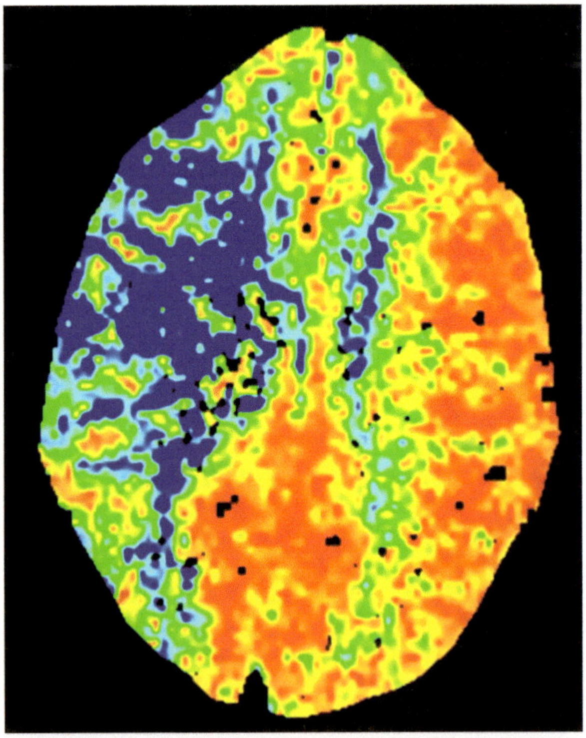

Fig. 10.1 Computed tomography perfusion image demonstrating severe reduction in cerebral blood flow and mean transit time in the anterior cerebral artery (ACA) and middle cerebral artery distributions on the right and in the ACA distribution on the left. (Used with permission from Barrow Neurological Institute, Phoenix, AZ.)

construct a double-barrel bypass depends, in part, on the philosophy of the surgeon managing the case. Some surgeons would argue for using one STA branch for an indirect onlay instead of using both for direct anastomoses. Others contend that a single direct bypass is sufficient to revascularize a patient. No single best method has been proven. As with moyamoya treatment in most centers, the specific treatment, such as a double-barrel bypass, is chosen for a particular patient on the basis of the clinical condition and specific cerebral blood flow deficits of that patient.

# 10.3 Key Principles of the Double-Barrel Bypass

The pattern of blood flow deficits on the CT perfusion scan and cerebral angiogram should guide the choice of the type of bypass. For a patient with broad hemispheric hypoperfusion, a double-limbed direct bypass with a frontal branch is used for the lower division of the MCA; above the sylvian fissure, the parietal STA branch is used for the upper MCA division. Since the posterior cerebral artery supply to the temporal lobe frequently augments the lower division MCA flow, it is common for the primary perfusion deficit to involve the upper MCA division; in such cases, both STA branches can be anastomosed to the cortical branches above the sylvian fissure. Although not used at our center, STA bypasses to both the MCA and ACA cortical branches remain options.[4] In addition to the appropriate targeting of the recipient artery, careful preparation of the STA grafts is crucial.

# 10.4 SWOT Analysis

## 10.4.1 Strength

- The double-barrel STA–MCA bypass provides immediate and robust cerebral blood flow to the ischemic hemisphere.

## 10.4.2 Weaknesses

- The procedure is more complex and requires more operating time than single-vessel bypass.
- Theoretical disadvantage is loss of use of one STA branch for an indirect encephalo-duro-arterio-synangiosis (EDAS) bypass, potentially reducing longer-term revascularization.

## 10.4.3 Opportunity

- A potential improvement in the execution of a double-barrel bypass would be the use of the cut flow index to assess the need for two grafts.[9]

## 10.4.4 Threats

- Use of two grafts might be more likely to cause hyperperfusion syndrome (not reported as a significant problem in one large series).[6]
- Two separate grafts might compete for blood flow, which could limit the benefit of a second graft or lead to an occlusion.

# 10.5 Contraindications

Moyamoya patients who have exceptionally small and fragile cortical MCA branches should not, and likely technically could not, undergo direct STA–MCA bypass. In clinical practice, this group represents about 10% of moyamoya patients who present for revascularization.

# 10.6 Special Considerations

A careful review of any preoperative CT angiography (CTA) and digital subtraction angiography images is required to ensure that both the frontal and the parietal STA branches are of sufficient size and quality for bypass use. Potential recipient MCA branches should also be assessed.

# 10.7 Risk Assessment and Complications

The perioperative risk of stroke is 3 to 5% in most large series. Rates of significant hemorrhage are greater than 1%, but they do occur, given the use of antiplatelet treatment and the potential for hyperperfusion. Infection and wound healing complications are less than 1%. Headaches and cosmetic issues such as temporalis wasting remain a possibility.

# 10.8 Special Instructions, Position, and Anesthesia

## 10.8.1 Preoperative Workup

A cerebral blood flow study and a catheter cerebral angiogram or a CTA must be evaluated preoperatively. Since patients with moyamoya angiopathy can have associated blood dyscrasias, it is important to verify each patient's response to antiplatelet therapy. We test patients to determine whether they are responsive to aspirin therapy (325 mg daily), which is our preferred antiplatelet agent before surgery and then for life. We avoid clopidogrel as an antiplatelet medication because of intraoperative bleeding issues. However, we did have a patient who did not respond to aspirin and who had a small stroke on discontinuation of clopidogrel. As a compromise, clopidogrel was withheld for 3 days prior to surgery, and the case proceeded without complication.

### 10.8.2 Patient Position

The patient is positioned supine with the head parallel to the floor and raised slightly above the heart. The courses of both the frontal and the parietal STA branches are insonated with Doppler ultrasonography and marked on the skin. The frontal STA is followed for at least 7 cm from its origin while the parietal branch is marked clear to the superior temporal line. The surgeon makes an incision along the parietal branch alone and shaves a 1-cm strip of hair along its path. An alternative incision is shaped like a hockey stick, with the parietal branch as the posterior limb and the second limb extending forward along the superior temporal line to the hairline. In addition to appropriate patient positioning, the proper instruments are critical to ensuring optimal technical results (▶ Table 10.1, ▶ Fig. 10.2).

### 10.8.3 Anesthesia

The anesthesiologist should have intravenous vasopressors and antihypertensives prepared for use before induction of anesthesia. Perhaps the single most important technique of surgery in these fragile patients is the maintenance of normal blood pressure, particularly during anesthesia induction. During temporary MCA occlusion, we routinely boost blood pressure to 10 mm Hg above baseline.

## 10.9 Skin Incision and Key Surgical Steps

### 10.9.1 Skin Incision and Dissection of STA

The STA resides in the deep dermal layer, and we follow the course of the parietal branch of the STA for the skin incision. The microscope is used from the outset, and we start at the junction of the superior temporal line over the parietal STA branch, making a 2-cm-long incision in the epidermis down to the fat with a number 15 blade. The STA is found just deep to the dermal fat between the superficial temporal fascia and the galea (▶ Fig. 10.3). The STA is dissected down to the zygoma, leaving a cuff of galeal tissue 5 mm on each side of the vessel. Small branches of the STA are cauterized 1 to 2 mm lateral to the main vessel with bipolar forceps set at 25 Malis units. This power level avoids injury to the STA.

The origin of the frontal branch of the STA, which is found 2 to 4 cm above the zygoma, is carefully preserved (▶ Fig. 10.4). An assistant then elevates the anterior edge of the scalp flap with a handheld retractor, and the frontal STA branch is dissected for 5 to 7 cm (▶ Fig. 10.5). Visualization of the frontal STA under the scalp is not difficult with angling of the microscope and, after temporary placement of a clip, it is divided obliquely at 5 to 7 cm. The STA is flushed with pure heparin, protected with a moist cotton sponge, and carefully retracted along with

**Table 10.1** Instruments and supplies for STA–MCA bypass

| Item |
|---|
| Small grasshopper retractors for STA dissection |
| Short nonstick bipolar with 0.5-mm tips |
| Short curved tenotomy scissors |
| Short curved iris scissors |
| Temporary microaneurysm clips (curved 5 mm) |
| Temporary microaneurysm clips (straight 5 mm) |
| Aneurysm clip applier |
| Straight tying forceps with platform tips, short |
| Curved microneedle holder, short |
| Straight microneedle holder, short |
| 10–0 monofilament nylon suture with BV-75–3 needle |
| 1-mL syringe with luer-lock connection |
| Blunt-tipped 25-gauge ophthalmic needle, angled 30 degrees |
| 3-F microvacuum suction catheter |

Abbreviations: STA–MCA, superficial temporal artery-to-middle cerebral artery.

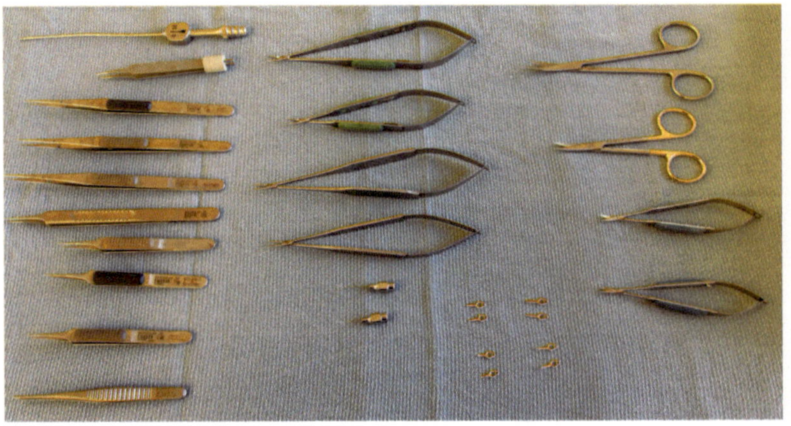

**Fig. 10.2** Photograph of key surgical instruments. (Used with permission from Barrow Neurological Institute, Phoenix, AZ.)

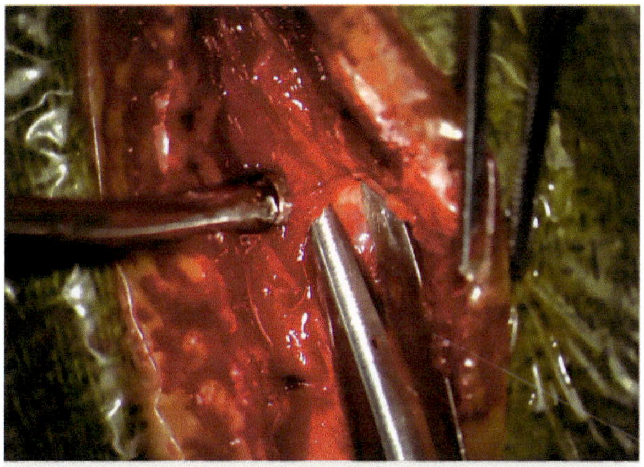

**Fig. 10.3** Close-up view of tenotomy microscissors spreading the epidermis off the subcutaneous fat, with visualization of the superficial temporal fascia encasing the superficial temporal artery in the layer below the subcutaneous fat. (Used with permission from Barrow Neurological Institute, Phoenix, AZ.)

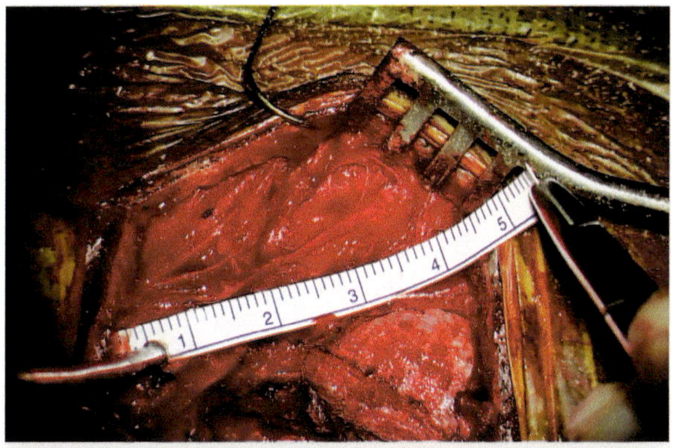


**Fig. 10.4** Dissected parietal superficial temporal artery (STA) branch, with visualization of the frontal STA branch take-off. (Used with permission from Barrow Neurological Institute, Phoenix, AZ.)

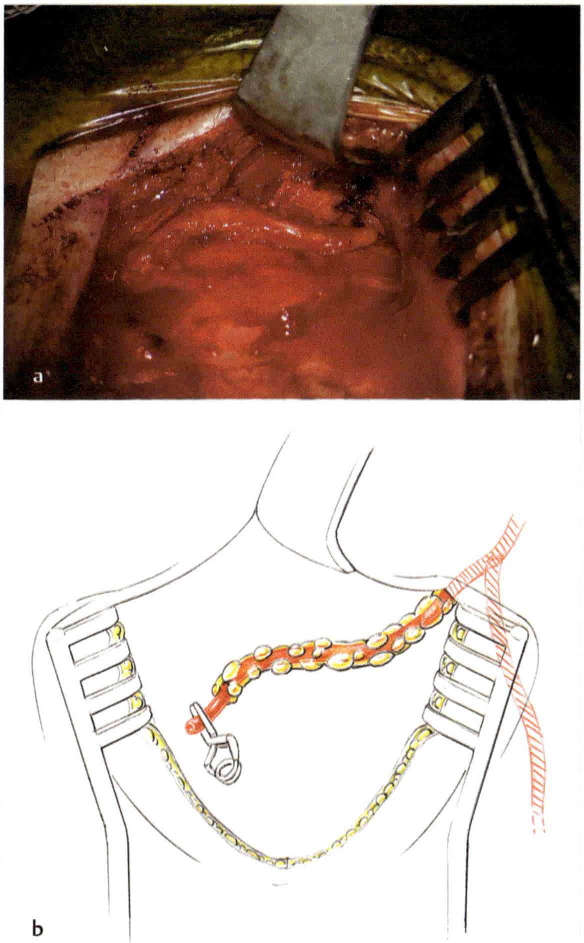


**Fig. 10.5** **(a)** Dissected frontal superficial temporal artery branch under the scalp flap. (Used with permission from Barrow Neurological Institute, Phoenix, AZ.) **(b)** An illustrated depiction of the dissected artery under the flap.

the posterior border of the scalp flap using fishhooks. The STA must remain moist and free of pressure or significant tension. The parietal STA branch remains in continuity since the decision for an EDAS has not been excluded prior to the cortical MCA evaluation.

## 10.9.2 Temporal Muscle Dissection and Craniotomy

The temporalis muscle is incised to the bone with the Bovie Force FX electrosurgery cautery unit (Covidien/ Medtronic, plc), with the incision extending from just above the zygoma to the superior temporal line. The temporalis muscle is carefully elevated anteriorly and posteriorly to expose a 5 × 5 cm area of temporal and frontal bone junction, allowing for exposure of the MCA branches above and below the sylvian fissure. The temporalis muscle is carefully retracted with the scalp using fishhooks. A matchstick drill bit is used to create a large bur hole at the root of the zygoma to allow room for the STA passage, and a second bur hole 5 to 7 cm superior to the first that allows for an EDAS, if needed (▶ Fig. 10.6). A bone flap centered 2 to 3 cm above the top of the ear to straddle the sylvian fissure is created. The STA is retracted away from the intended bone cuts for each side of the craniotomy. Careful bur holes allow for preservation of dural integrity and avoidance of damage to the middle meningeal artery (MMA) branches, which are important for collateral blood flow.

## 10.9.3 Dural Opening

The dura is opened along the course of one or two large MMA branches, leaving approximately a 5-mm strip of dura next to the MMA. Cruciate incisions of the dura

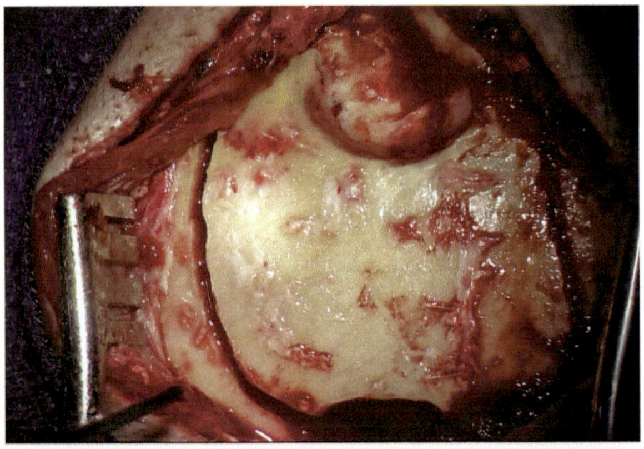

**Fig. 10.6** Bone flap with two bur holes and a carefully retracted superficial temporal artery. (Used with permission from Barrow Neurological Institute, Phoenix, AZ.)

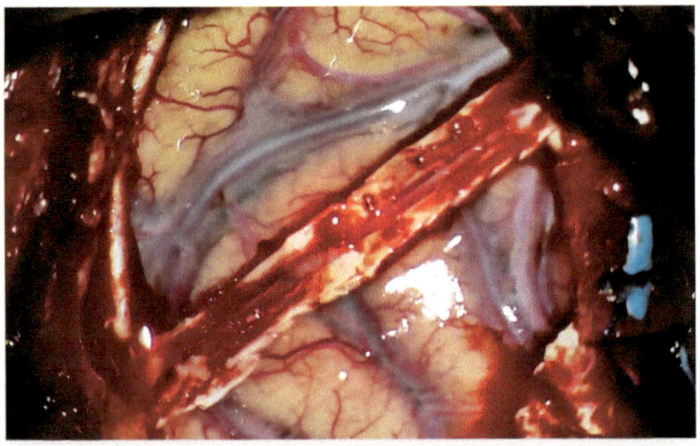

**Fig. 10.7** The dura is opened, with the middle meningeal artery preserved and the cruciate dural flaps inverted under the bone. (Used with permission from Barrow Neurological Institute, Phoenix, AZ.)

horizontal to the bone edge create triangular flaps of dura; the dura is then inverted and tucked under the bone (▶ Fig. 10.7). Preserving the MMA and the dural inversion maintains the collateral blood flow. The arachnoid membrane should be preserved, if possible, until the actual MCA dissection to minimize loss of cerebrospinal fluid, which can result in sagging of the brain.

### 10.9.4 Anastomotic Site Selection

The ideal cortical MCA recipient branches for anastomoses with the STA are 1.0 mm in diameter or larger and reside on the surface. MCA branches less than 0.7 mm in diameter are difficult to work with and provide less significant flow augmentation. Although surface MCA branches are easier to work with, dissection into a sulcus usually provides the advantage of a larger caliber vessel. For the double-barrel bypass, an MCA branch below the sylvian fissure is selected as a recipient for the frontal STA, and an MCA branch above the fissure is used for the parietal STA. Nonetheless, both anastomoses may be above or below the sylvian fissure, one anterior and one posterior if cerebral blood flow deficits support this pattern. Ideal recipient MCA branches near the bone edge can be accommodated with an additional small craniectomy. Cadaveric dissection of both the STA branches superimposed over the frontal and temporal lobes demonstrates the variety of cortical arterial branches, which can be reached by fully dissected STA branches (▶ Fig. 10.8).

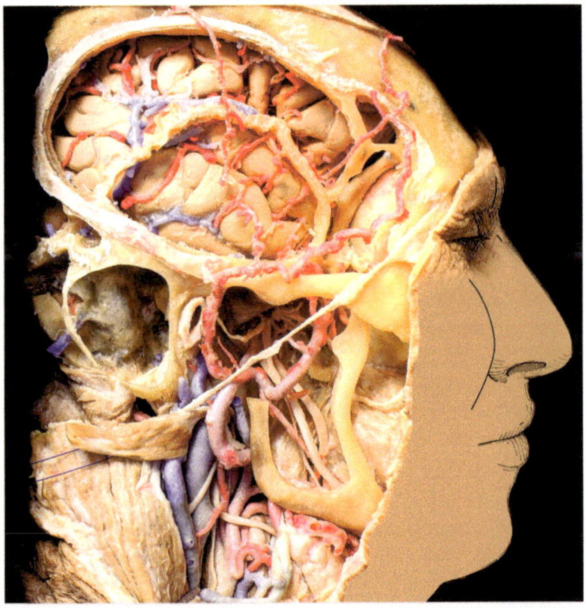

**Fig. 10.8** Cadaveric specimen (*facial features anonymized*) with dissected frontal and parietal superficial temporal artery branches superimposed as they lay naturally over the calvarium, demonstrating a broad range of potential anastomosis sites. (Used with permission from Barrow Neurological Institute, Phoenix, AZ.)

### 10.9.5 Donor STA Preparation

If possible, the frontal STA branch is prepared before opening the arachnoid membrane while the parietal STA remains intact. The frontal STA is flushed with pure heparin; a 30-degree blunt ophthalmic needle works well for flushing. The adventitia of the STA end is held by an assistant while the primary surgeon grasps the loose adventitia and dissects it sharply from the vessel to clear the distal 1 cm of the artery of adventitia. A single cut is made from the STA tip 3 mm along the barrel to create a fish-mouth opening in the vessel. A single cut avoids jagged vessel edges, and 3 mm creates a large opening

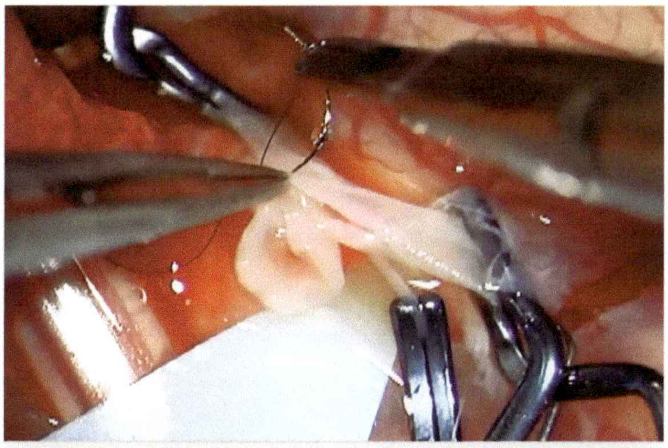

**Fig. 10.9** Superficial temporal artery (STA) fishmouthed open with microscissors 3 mm into the artery; 1 cm of the STA has been cleared of adventitia. (Used with permission from Barrow Neurological Institute, Phoenix, AZ.)

three times the diameter of the recipient artery for blood flow (▶ Fig. 10.9).

## 10.9.6 Recipient MCA Branch Preparation

The arachnoid membrane is sharply cut from a 10-mm segment of the target MCA branch; 10 mm allows extra room for the 3-mm opening in the STA donor artery and for temporary microaneurysm clips. Small perforating branches off the recipient MCA can be preserved, if they are large enough, with a temporary clip but are more commonly divided. Use of gentle bipolar cautery (settings of 25 W or less) at a safe distance (1–2 mm) from the MCA target branch helps protect the delicate lumen from injury or spasm. After the recipient branch is dissected, a colored triangular-shaped Silastic dam is placed under the artery, and 3 mm of cortical MCA is marked for the arteriotomy. A 3-French MicroVac suction catheter (PMT Corp., Chanhassen, MN) is placed under the Silastic dam to remove any pooling cerebrospinal fluid or blood (▶ Fig. 10.10**a**).

## 10.9.7 MCA Arteriotomy

The patient is placed in electroencephalographic burst suppression by anesthesia, and systolic blood pressure of 10 mm Hg above baseline is verified. Low-pressure, temporary microaneurysm clips are applied to the MCA branch to maximize the space around the planned 3-mm arteriotomy (▶ Fig. 10.10**b**). The MCA can be opened with an arachnoid knife or with the tip of a 27-gauge needle. Microscissors can then be used to extend the opening to exactly 3 mm. The vessel is flushed with pure heparin, and the edges of the opening are marked with either dye or a fresh skin marker. Adjustment of the temporary clips may be necessary if residual flow is noted, which sometimes requires a third microaneurysm clip. The assistant remains responsible for actively irrigating the lumens of both the STA and the MCA with heparinized saline.

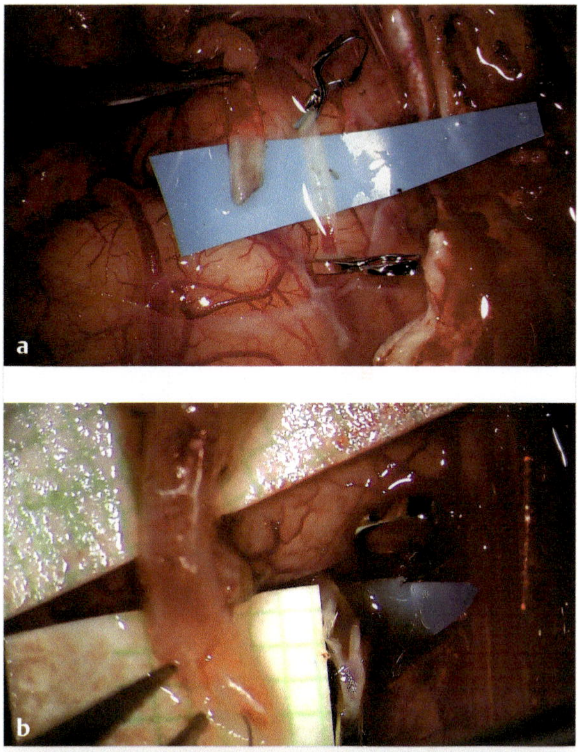

**Fig. 10.10** **(a)** Prepared superficial temporal artery branch and middle cerebral artery (MCA) branch with blue Silastic dam, microvacuum suction, and temporary clips. The microvacuum suction may also be placed in a dependent position in the craniotomy flap instead of under the MCA branch. **(b)** Arteriotomy (3 mm) into the cortical MCA branch. (Used with permission from Barrow Neurological Institute, Phoenix, AZ.)

## 10.9.8 Anastomosis

For the anastomosis, 10–0 nylon precut to 5-cm lengths is used. The arteriotomies of both the STA and MCA are placed in opposition, and the first suture passes from the adventitia of the heel of the STA to the lumen and then from the lumen of the MCA to its adventitia side, where it is secured with three knots. The second suture again starts in the adventitia side of the STA but at its toe side, passing into the lumen and then into the MCA lumen and out the adventitia. Now the STA and MCA are nicely adjacent to each other (▶ Fig. 10.11). The more difficult far limb of the anastomosis is typically done first, with three equally spaced interrupted sutures. The inside of the anastomosis is then inspected to ensure accurate suture placement. The second limb of the anastomosis is performed like the first. Although sutures can be done in

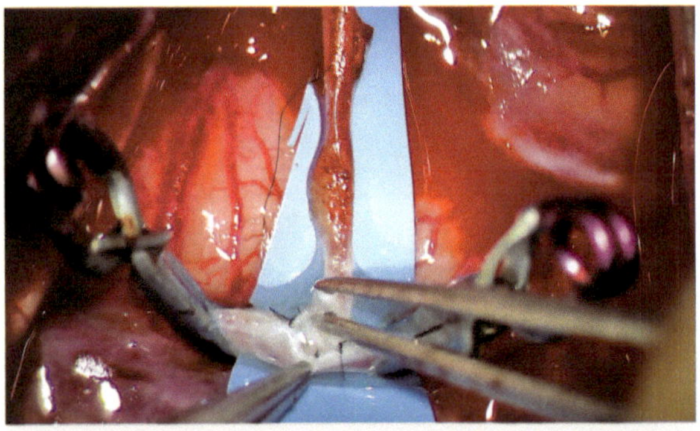

**Fig. 10.11** Bird's-eye view of the shape of the superficial temporal artery tacked down to the middle cerebral artery. The least amount of room to manipulate the suture is near the heel end. The sutures are visible within the lumen. (Used with permission from Barrow Neurological Institute, Phoenix, AZ.)

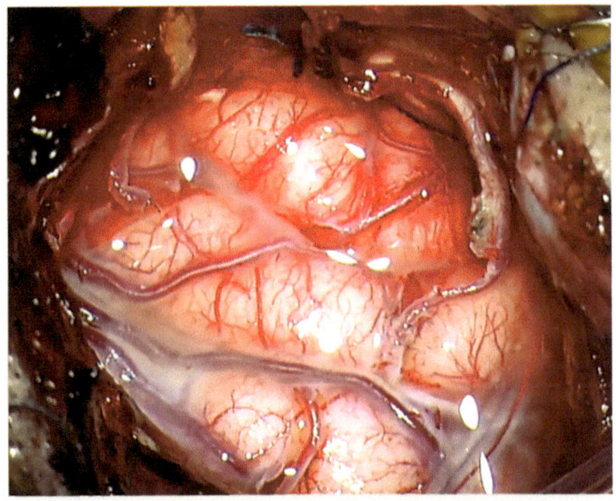

**Fig. 10.12** View of completed frontal superficial temporal artery (STA) to middle cerebral artery anastomoses with parietal STA still intact before second anastomoses. (Used with permission from Barrow Neurological Institute, Phoenix, AZ.)

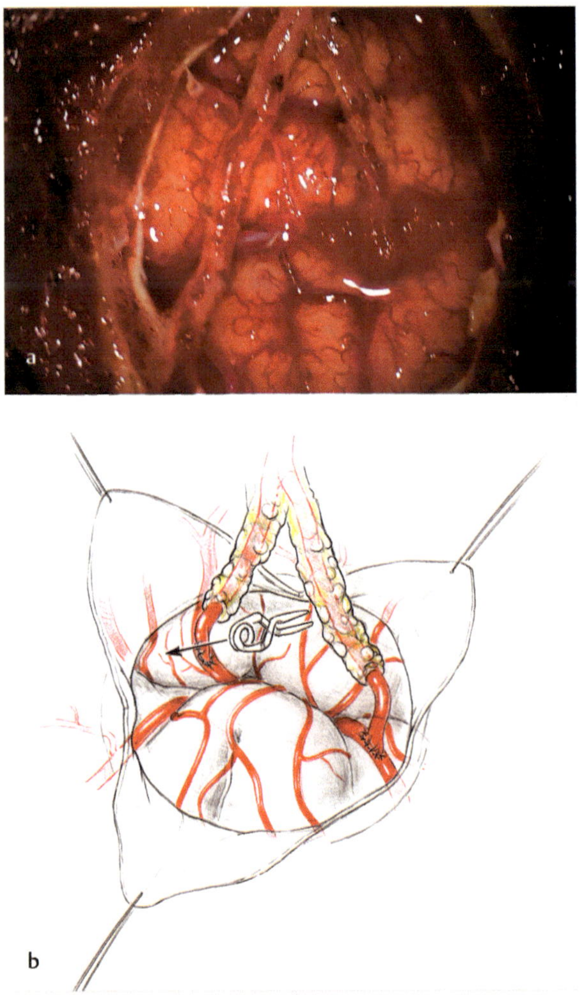

**Fig. 10.13 (a)** Final view of both frontal and parietal superficial temporal artery to middle cerebral artery anastomoses. (Used with permission from Barrow Neurological Institute, Phoenix, AZ.) **(b)** An illustrated depiction of the final view.

one pass, a separate pass for each vessel wall maximizes accuracy.

An alternative to interrupted sutures is the continuous technique, with a series of 8 to 10 loops per limb. All loops are tightened before locking down the knot to the tail of the opposing suture.

### 10.9.9 Graded Release of the Temporary Clips and Hemostasis

Release of the clip on the distal MCA, which usually has the lowest blood flow, facilitates identification of any leaking areas of the anastomosis. Single interrupted sutures can address any leaks. The use of Surgicel (Ethicon, Inc., Somerville, NJ) on the edges of the anastomosis also aids hemostasis. The proximal MCA clip is then released. Finally, the STA clip is released. The clips can be adjusted and released in such a way to allow for flushing of debris from the MCA out the parietal STA before the full release of the frontal STA (▶ Fig. 10.12). An indocyanine green (ICG) angiogram is performed to ensure adequate flow through the anastomoses.

### 10.9.10 Second Anastomoses

A second anastomotic site is chosen above the sylvian fissure posterior to the frontal STA anastomoses. If a second site is not found, then the parietal STA branch can be sutured to the pia as an EDAS procedure. The second anastomosis is performed just like the first, with preparation of the STA and then the MCA recipient artery. A temporary clip is placed on the parietal branch STA beyond the frontal branch take-off (▶ Fig. 10.13). A second ICG

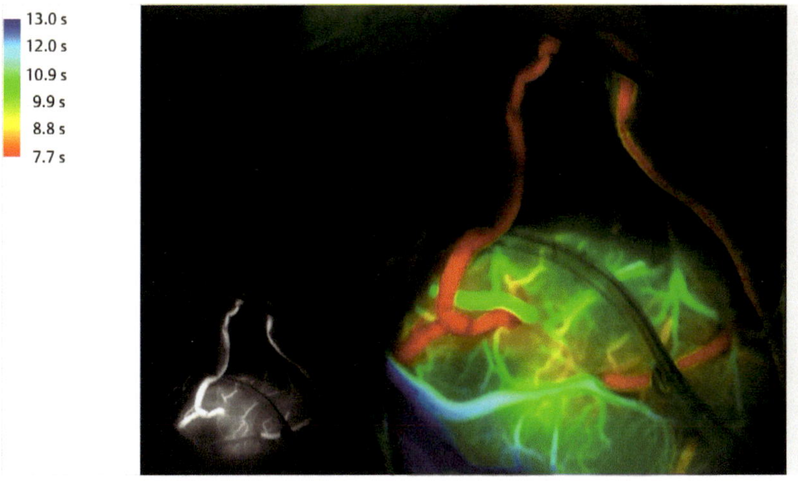


**Fig. 10.14** Indocyanine green angiogram after completion of the double-barrel bypass. (Used with permission from Barrow Neurological Institute, Phoenix, AZ.)

angiogram is performed to evaluate flow through both anastomoses (▶ Fig. 10.14).

### 10.9.11 Closure Phase

The use of Gelfoam hemostat (Pfizer, Inc., New York, NY) under the bone flap should be avoided because of the potential for impairment of collateral revascularization. The bone flap is placed back in position and secured with plates, with sufficient room for passage of the STA inferiorly and superiorly, if needed. The temporalis closure allows for gaps at the inferior and superior end, if needed. The STA must not have significant compression. The galea is closed with 2–0 Vicryl sutures (Ethicon, Inc.), and the skin is closed with staples.

### 10.9.12 Postoperative Care

We monitor patients for 48 hours postoperatively in the neurosurgical intensive care unit with critical attention to tight blood pressure control, within the range of baseline blood pressure to 30 points above baseline, usually maintaining a systolic blood pressure of 120 to 150 mm Hg. Patients continue to receive daily antiplatelet medications. Postoperative CTA is performed later on the day of surgery. A repeat noncontrast CT is obtained the following morning to assess potential hemorrhaging. Hyperventilation must be avoided to minimize hypocapnia.

We repeat the CTA and CT perfusion studies 6 months after surgery and perform a catheter cerebral angiogram yearly for 3 years. A yearly CTA is performed thereafter.

## 10.10 Difficulties Encountered

During the procedures, either the frontal or parietal STA branch may be too short to reach recipient cortical arteries. The length of available STA should be assessed before the STA branch is cut. Additional length may be gained from dissection of the proximal STA in the region of the zygoma or distally at the ends of the parietal or frontal branches.

## 10.11 Bailout, Rescue, and Salvage Maneuvers

ICG angiography is performed after each anastomosis to confirm patency.[10] If partial or total occlusion is noted at the anastomosis site, replacement of the temporary clips and removal of one or two sutures usually allows access to see the problem. Alternatively, flushing with pure heparin using a 27-gauge needle into the robust STA may clear any thrombus. This process might require a single suture to close the needle hole. If an STA branch is of poor quality, then it might be used as an onlay indirect bypass instead of for an anastomosis.

## 10.12 Tips, Pearls, and Lessons Learned

When setting up for the anastomoses, select the shorter graft for the lower division MCA bypass. After temporary clipping, ensure that there is no back-bleeding. Do not hesitate to adjust a temporary clip or add a second supporting clip to halt back-bleeding on the MCA or STA. However, avoid trapping a column of blood in the MCA or during CTA because doing so may lead to thrombosis. When performing the anastomoses, do the most difficult side first. If the recipient artery is near the bone edge, perform a small craniectomy to make the anastomoses easier. Compared to continuous suturing, interrupted sutures allow for fewer compound problems. However, interrupted sutures are more likely to leak, most commonly near the heel of the anastomosis. Placing sutures close to the heel stitch minimizes the chance of leakage. If the endothelium or the tip of the STA becomes damaged, recut the end in order to obtain a clean cut. If the MCA opening tears, the STA fish mouth may be enlarged to fit the opening.

Direct bypasses can be finicky procedures; therefore, do not rush the case. Be mindful to accurately execute the technical details of each step of the procedure. Repeating steps reduces the likelihood of success because of degradation of the arterial intima, thromboses, or fatigue. Simple technical errors can lead to bypass failure. Adherence to the procedural rules improves the likelihood of success. Placing temporary clips far enough from the anastomosis site requires some additional exposure, but the added room aids with suturing. Persistent filling of the MCA lumen due to incomplete occlusion by temporary clips impairs progress and increases the likelihood of thrombosis. Avoid the use of high bipolar cautery too close to the wall of the donor or recipient arteries. Finally, passage of the suturing needle through each arterial wall independently affords the most accurate suture placement during the anastomosis.

The importance of the surgical assistant cannot be overemphasized. Most centers involved with bypass surgery train residents or fellows who are eager for a chance to perform anastomoses. A key role for them is to keep the STA graft moist and the field free of blood by irrigating the exposed lumens with heparinized saline.

# Acknowledgment

The authors thank Dr. Kaan Yagmurlu for his skillful cadaveric skull dissection used in the photograph for ▶ Fig. 10.8.

# References

[1] Donaghy RM. Extra-intracranial blood flow diversion. Paper presented at: 36th Annual Meeting of the American Association of Neurological Surgeons; April 11, 1968, 1968; Chicago, IL

[2] Yaşargil MG, Krayenbuhl HA, Jacobson JH, II. Microneurosurgical arterial reconstruction. Surgery. 1970; 67(1):221–233

[3] Sakamoto H, Kitano S, Yasui T, et al. Direct extracranial-intracranial bypass for children with moyamoya disease. Clin Neurol Neurosurg. 1997; 99 Suppl 2:S128–S133

[4] Ishikawa T, Kamiyama H, Kuroda S, Yasuda H, Nakayama N, Takizawa K. Simultaneous superficial temporal artery to middle cerebral or anterior cerebral artery bypass with pan-synangiosis for Moyamoya disease covering both anterior and middle cerebral artery territories. Neurol Med Chir (Tokyo). 2006; 46(9):462–468

[5] Kazumata K, Ito M, Tokairin K, et al. The frequency of postoperative stroke in moyamoya disease following combined revascularization: a single-university series and systematic review. J Neurosurg. 2014; 121(2):432–440

[6] Kuroda S, Houkin K, Ishikawa T, Nakayama N, Iwasaki Y. Novel bypass surgery for moyamoya disease using pericranial flap: its impacts on cerebral hemodynamics and long-term outcome. Neurosurgery. 2010; 66(6):1093–1101, discussion 1101

[7] Duckworth EA, Rao VY, Patel AJ. Double-barrel bypass for cerebral ischemia: technique, rationale, and preliminary experience with 10 consecutive cases. Neurosurgery. 2013; 73(1) Suppl Operative: ons30–ons38, discussion ons37–ons38

[8] Wanebo JE, Zabramski JM, Spetzler RF. Superficial temporal artery-to-middle cerebral artery bypass grafting for cerebral revascularization. Neurosurgery. 2004; 55(2):395–398, discussion 398–399

[9] Amin-Hanjani S, Barker FG, II, Charbel FT, Connolly ES, Jr, Morcos JJ, Thompson BG, Cerebrovascular Section of the American Association of Neurological Surgeons, Congress of Neurological Surgeons. Extracranial-intracranial bypass for stroke—is this the end of the line or a bump in the road? Neurosurgery. 2012; 71(3):557–561

[10] Lee M, Guzman R, Bell-Stephens T, Steinberg GK. Intraoperative blood flow analysis of direct revascularization procedures in patients with moyamoya disease. J Cereb Blood Flow Metab. 2011; 31(1):262–274

# 11 Occipital Artery–Middle Cerebral Artery Bypass in Moyamoya Disease

*Ken Kazumata*

**Abstract**

The posterior cerebral artery (PCA) is involved in approximately 30% of moyamoya disease (MMD) cases. Symptomatic PCA regression following anterior revascularization was predominantly found in children and young adults. Occipital artery–middle cerebral artery (OA–MCA) bypass can be used as one of the option for revascularization in the posterior portion of the brain. OA–MCA bypass demonstrates a several advantages over conventional OA–PCA bypass. Technical points are described in this chapter.

*Keywords:* moyamoya disease, OA–PCA bypass, OA–MCA bypass, posterior cerebral artery, revascularization

## 11.1 History and Initial Description

Occlusive lesions in the posterior cerebral artery (PCA) are observed in 26 to 43% moyamoya disease (MMD) patients at the initial diagnosis, which is associated with disease advancement and poor prognosis.[1] Although majority of the patients with PCA involvement is asymptomatic, revascularization in the anterior circulation occasionally advances PCA involvement in certain patients.[2] PCA regression causes several clinical issues such as follows: (1) additional PCA lesions can cause extensive cerebral ischemia beyond the territory of the PCA, (2) ischemic injury to frontoparietal connection fibers potentially impairs cognitive function, and (3) surgical treatment involves more complex procedures. Nevertheless, revascularization in the posterior portion of the brain is generally difficult. While source for blood supply through indirect procedure is limited in the posterior portion of the head, the direct anastomosis may be less competent than the superficial temporal artery-middle cerebral artery (STA–MCA) bypass. Previous literatures describe indirect methods for revascularization in the posterior half of the brain[3,4] as well as occipital artery-posterioer cerebral artery (OA–PCA) bypass for the direct anastomosis in the posterior circulation.[5] Alterative approach such as OA–MCA bypass is described.

## 11.2 Indications

We consider that anterior revascularization as the first treatment choice at the time of diagnosis, regardless of the PCA involvement. Accordingly, patients who persistently demonstrated ischemic symptoms attributable to PCA lesions or “delayed” PCA involvement following the anterior revascularization is selected as candidates for posterior revascularization. Hemodynamic compromise is evaluated such as using single-photon emission computed tomography (SPECT) and acetazolamide test. Symptomatic occlusive lesions in PCA territories were identified by their decreased cerebrovascular reserve, an avascular area on a cerebral angiogram, or hyperintense vessels on fluid-attenuated inversion recovery (FLAIR).[6]

## 11.3 Key Principles

OA–MCA bypass procedure is not commonly used. However, it can be effective when posterior part of the brain requires additional source of blood supply. OA–MCA bypass does not require prone position and may be effective when combined with indirect procedure. Although source of indirect procedure is limited, a large craniotomy may facilitate neovascularization from the dura matter. Pericranial flap is also available.

## 11.4 SWOT Analysis

### 11.4.1 Strengths

OA–MCA bypass can effectively alleviate recurrent ischemia due to PCA involvement.[2] Furthermore, improving cerebral perfusion in the posterior portion of the brain may ultimately lead to improved revascularization in the anterior circulation territory as well.[7] Furthermore, surgical revascularization in the posterior portion of the brain may not only be effective in stroke prevention, but also potentially improve cognitive outcomes by preventing ischemic injury in fronto-parietal association fibers.[8]

### 11.4.2 Weaknesses

Patency rate might not be comparable as in the STA–MCA bypass because of its technical difficulty.

### 11.4.3 Opportunities

Symptomatic PCA lesions are the target of OA–MCA bypass. Considering the symptoms as well as the distribution of cerebral infarctions, the area susceptible to ischemia due to PCA lesions is not only confined to the visual cortex, but also extends to adjacent cortices beyond the watershed zone.

### 11.4.4 Threats

Recipient artery may not be competent as to allow direct anastomosis. Indirect procedure should always be considered as an alternative of OA–MCA bypass.

## 11.5 Contraindications

OA–MCA bypass should be avoided in patients who had demonstrated delayed wound healing in anterior revascularization, as harvesting OA could cause further damage to blood flow supply the scalp.

## 11.6 Special Considerations

In order to select optimal surgical candidates, multimodal neuroimaging studies are employed, which can ascribe ischemic symptoms to the advanced PCA lesions. However, there is a poor correlation between the PCA regression and the hemodynamic compromise, as detected by SPECT.[9] Hyperintense vessels on FLAIR (or ivy signs) may serve as a marker for critical ischemia.[10]

## 11.7 Pitfalls, Risk Assessment, and Complications

In addition to complications due to standard craniotomy, wound necrosis as well as difficulty of direct anastomosis should be mentioned for informed consent.

## 11.8 Special Instructions, Position, and Anesthesia

Patient is placed in semi-supine position with general anesthesia.

## 11.9 Patient Position with Skin Incision and Key Surgical Steps

Patient is placed in semi-supine position in revascularization via OA–MCA anastomosis. A skin incision is made along the lateral branch of the OA. The OA is then dissected from the subcutaneous tissue. The subcutaneous tissue flap is made by the periosteal and loose areolar connective tissue. The OA is anastomosed to the cortical branch of the MCA located in the parietal lobe, such as the distal segment of angular artery. The dural flaps are inverted and placed on the surface of the brain. The subcutaneous tissue flap muscle is sutured to the edge of the dura mater. (See ▸ Fig. 11.1).

## 11.10 Difficulties Encountered

It may be difficult to find competent artery for the direct anastomosis. Distal segment of angular artery may be optimal site for the anastomosis. At the distal segment of the OA, the size of the artery diminishes abruptly as the

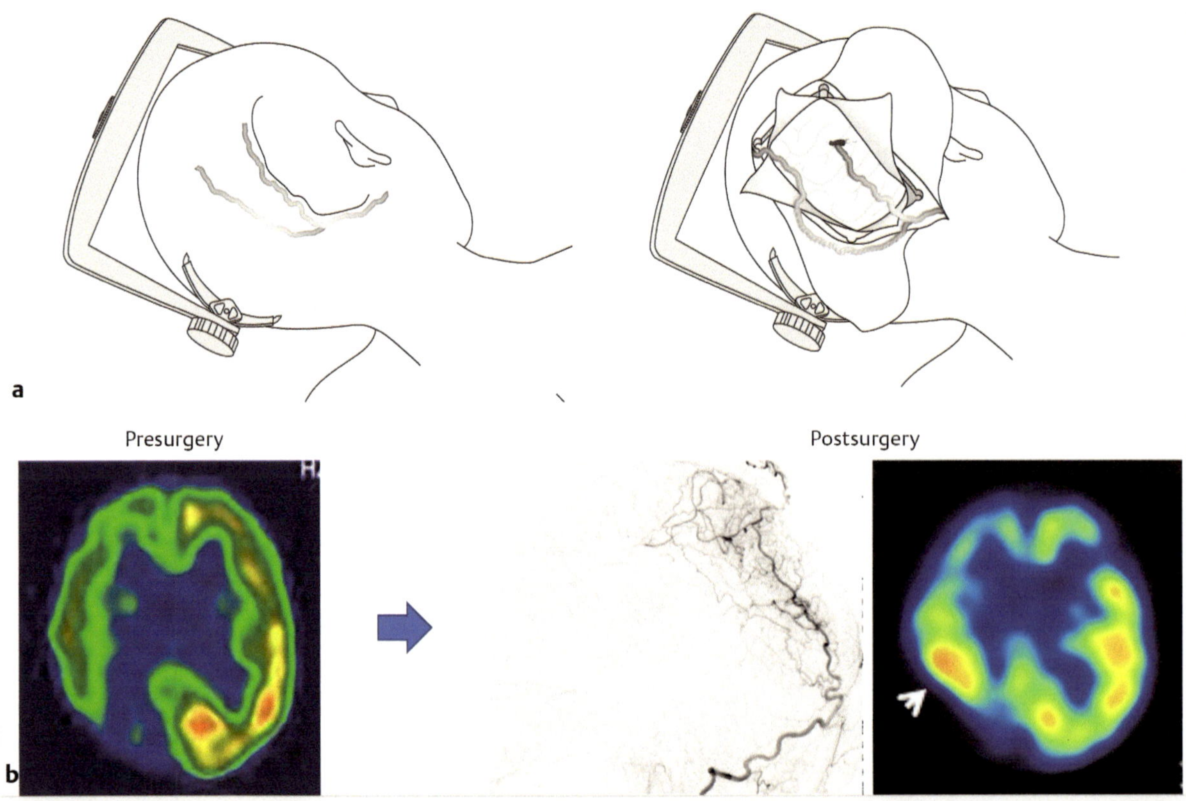


**Fig. 11.1** **(a)** Patient position and skin incision in OA–MCA bypass. **(b)** Pre- and postsurgery images.

OA runs through the subcutaneous fat layer. In addition, a relatively long pedicle necessary for reaching recipient arteries would reduce the rate of long-term patency.

## 11.11 Bailout, Rescue, and Salvage Maneuvers

It is necessary to use indirect procedure when direct anastomosis is not successful. Wide craniotomy, particularly in the anterior portion, would facilitate indirect revascularization from middle meningeal artery via the transdural anastomosis.

## 11.12 Tips, Pearls, and Lessons Learned

Anterior revascularization is the first option of the treatment, even if radiological examinations indicate additional PCA involvement. We consider that prophylactic revascularization to the PCA territory may not be necessary given that majority of the PCA fall-off after the anterior revascularization remains asymptomatic. PCA involvement can be detected either at the time of initial diagnosis or in follow-up examinations, following anterior revascularization. PCA lesions progress for several years, or even a decade, after initial revascularization.[2,5,11] Therefore, we consider that continuous scrutiny is necessary in outpatient basis in patients with a prior history of anterior revascularization.

## References


[1] Funaki T, Takahashi JC, Takagi Y, et al. Impact of posterior cerebral artery involvement on long-term clinical and social outcome of pediatric moyamoya disease. J Neurosurg Pediatr. 2013; 12(6):626–632

[2] Pandey P, Steinberg GK. Outcome of repeat revascularization surgery for moyamoya disease after an unsuccessful indirect revascularization. Clinical article. J Neurosurg. 2011; 115(2):328–336

[3] Endo M, Kawano N, Miyaska Y, Yada K. Cranial burr hole for revascularization in moyamoya disease. J Neurosurg. 1989; 71(2):180–185

[4] Mukerji N, Steinberg GK. Burr holes for moyamoya. World Neurosurg. 2014; 81(1):29–31

[5] Hayashi T, Shirane R, Tominaga T. Additional surgery for postoperative ischemic symptoms in patients with moyamoya disease: the effectiveness of occipital artery-posterior cerebral artery bypass with an indirect procedure: technical case report. Neurosurgery. 2009; 64(1): E195–E196, discussion E196

[6] Kamran S, Bates V, Bakshi R, Wright P, Kinkel W, Miletich R. Significance of hyperintense vessels on FLAIR MRI in acute stroke. Neurology. 2000; 55(2):265–269

[7] Mugikura S, Takahashi S. Letters to the Editor: posterior cerebral artery involvement and pediatric moyamoya diseaes. J Neurosurg Pediatr. 2014; 14(4):434–435

[8] Kazumata K, Tha KK, Narita H, et al. Chronic ischemia alters brain microstructural integrity and cognitive performance in adult moyamoya disease. Stroke. 2015; 46(2):354–360

[9] Lee JY, Choi YH, Cheon JE, et al. Delayed posterior circulation insufficiency in pediatric moyamoya disease. J Neurol. 2014; 261(12):2305–2313

[10] Lee KY, Latour LL, Luby M, Hsia AW, Merino JG, Warach S. Distal hyperintense vessels on FLAIR: an MRI marker for collateral circulation in acute stroke? Neurology. 2009; 72(13):1134–1139

[11] Ikeda A, Yamamoto I, Sato O, Morota N, Tsuji T, Seguchi T. Revascularization of the calcarine artery in moyamoya disease: OA-cortical PCA anastomosis—case report. Neurol Med Chir (Tokyo). 1991; 31(10):658–661

# 12 STA–ACA/MCA Double Bypasses with Long Grafts

Akitsugu Kawashima

**Abstract**
Some reports have stated that surgical treatment is needed for patients with moyamoya disease involving hypoperfusion in the anterior cerebral artery (ACA) territory. We introduced a new direct bypass technique using the long superficial temporal artery (STA) graft for such cases in 2010. Moyamoya patients who need reconstruction in the ACA territory also frequently need reconstruction in the middle cerebral artery (MCA) territory. In this chapter, we describe STA–ACA/MCA double bypasses with long grafts. This powerful revascularization technique can supply much blood flow in the greater part of the frontal lobe. It is essential to the procedure that the 10-cm-long STA graft passes intradurally under the residual bone bridge between the two separate craniotomies for the ACA and the MCA recipient arteries to prevent kinking of the long STA graft. Difficulties of this procedure are long STA graft preparation/set-up and anastomosis to the ACA cortical arteries, which are smaller in size than the MCA cortical arteries and lie in the sulcus in many cases. It is very important to prepare for the graft to avoid damage to the graft, which can include hypertextention, heat form coagulator, and insufficient dissection layer. Also, close attention should be paid to a natural STA graft course. Key to successful anastomosis is (1) having a good view of suturing, (2) avoiding suturing the contralateral wall, and (3) suturing suitable margin and interval of stitches, specifically making as small number of stitches as possible to expand the orifice.

*Keywords:* moyamoya disease, STA–MCA bypass, STA–ACA bypass, long graft, anastomosis

## 12.1 History and Initial Description

There have been some reports about surgical treatment for patients with moyamoya disease involving hypoperfusion in the anterior cerebral artery (ACA) territory. Some procedures of indirect revascularization in the ACA territory were reported to help cases of moyamoya disease to prevent ischemic stroke. However, effectiveness of indirect revascularization has some limitations, taking several months to obtain its effect and having potentially insufficient effect compared to direct bypass. Superficial temporal artery–middle cerebral artery (STA–MCA) bypass may improve ischemia in both the ACA and the MCA territories through leptomeningeal anastomosis between capillary vessels of the ACA and the MCA. However, it's unclear before operation whether blood supply in the ACA territory from STA–MCA bypass through leptomeningeal anastomosis is sufficient.

Previously, direct bypass in the ACA territory using the peripheral branch of the STA for the graft was conducted. We introduced new techniques using the long STA graft, which can allow wide blood supply from the bypass in 2010. Moyamoya patients who need reconstruction in the ACA territory also require frequently reconstruction in the MCA territory. In this chapter, we describe STA–ACA/MCA double bypasses with a long graft. This procedure has the potential for powerful revascularization that can provide blood supply in the whole frontal lobe.

## 12.2 Indications

The indication for STA–ACA/MCA bypasses with long grafts in cases of moyamoya disease are as follows: (1) hypoperfusion with poor vasoreactivity in the ACA and the MCA territories based on cerebral blood flow (CBF) study and angiographic study, and (2) ischemic symptoms including the lower extremities. A typical angiographic finding is severe internal carotid artery terminal stenosis/occlusion with poor collateral blood flow from ipsilateral posterior cerebral artery, contralateral ACA, or ipsilateral MCA.

## 12.3 Key Principle of STA–ACA/MCA Double Bypasses with Long Grafts

This procedure requires much time (about 5 hours) and takes a lot of effort, specifically a large skin incision with two separate craniotomies, long STA graft dissection, and anastomosis for small-size recipient artery. However, this procedure can achieve immediate blood supply from the bypasses in both ACA and MCA territories. Moreover, this powerful revascularization has the possibility to provide blood flow in the greater part of the frontal lobe (▶ Fig. 12.1**a, b**).

## 12.4 SWOT Analysis

### 12.4.1 Strength

- This procedure can provide immediate extensive blood supply in the whole frontal lobe in many cases.

### 12.4.2 Weaknesses

- Large skin incision and two separate craniotomies are needed in this procedure.
- Long graft dissection, usually frontal branch preparation from the galeal side, should occur, with care not to damage the graft.
- The condition of anastomosis to the ACA cortical arteries is more difficult than the condition of

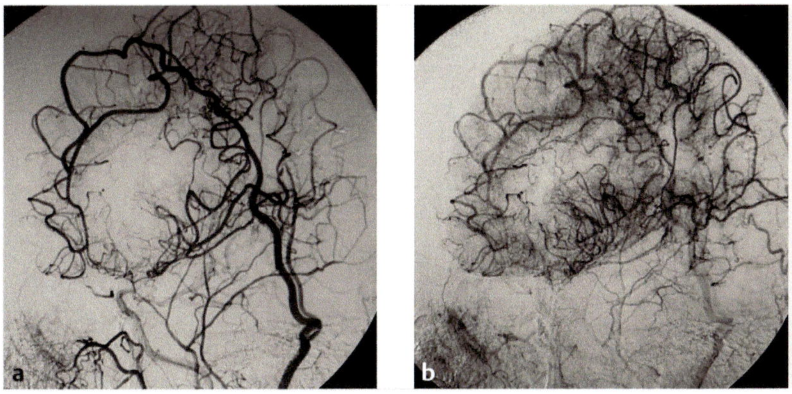


**Fig. 12.1** Postoperative right external carotid angiography **(a, b)** showing good blood supply in the whole frontal lobe from superficial temporal artery-anterior cerebral artery/middle cerebral artery double bypasses.

anastomosis to the MCA cortical arteries because size of recipient arteries in the ACA territory are smaller than in the MCA territory and recipient arteries in the ACA territory usually lie in the sulcus, thus allowing only a narrow working space.

### 12.4.3 Opportunity

- This procedure can provide extensive blood supply in the greater part of the frontal lobe in many cases, so improvement of cognitive function may be established.

### 12.4.4 Threats

- Using a long STA graft may increase the risk of graft kink/rotation and graft damage to the vessel wall of the STA. This may cause an increase in the rate of graft occlusion in long-term follow-up.
- The risk of skin trouble after operation may increase caused by the long STA dissection.

## 12.5 Contraindications

Contraindications to STA–ACA/MCA bypasses with long grafts are as follows: cases with insufficient STA development and young pediatric cases. There are probably 10 to 20% of cases where STAs are too small in size or too many in branching to be prepared as the long graft. In our experience of 62 cases, blood supply from bypasses has been commonly developing in the greater part of the frontal lobe. However, blood supply from bypasses that gradually shifted to indirect collaterals was shown particularly in pediatric cases less than 10 years old.

## 12.6 Special Considerations

To determine the suitable indication of this procedure, it is very important to evaluate preoperative angiographical findings and CBF study. To prepare the STA long graft, preoperative evaluation of the development of the STA is also needed. Taking 100 mg aspirin daily starting more than 1 week before operation is necessary to prevent intraoperative thrombosis formation at the orifice of the anastomosis. The patient should stop the use of aspirin on the day of the operation. Intravenous boluses of heparin are not needed, and aspirin is restarted 3 to 5 days after operation depending on presence of postoperative hemorrhage.

## 12.7 Pitfalls, Risk Assessment, and Complications

STA–ACA/MCA bypasses with long grafts may be challenging procedures because of the preparation of long graft of STA and the smaller size of the recipient artery with a narrow anastomosis field. However, we believe that bypass surgeons who have had certain experience with direct bypasses in cases of moyamoya disease can achieve successful bypasses in this procedure. Large skin incision and two separate craniotomies may lead to skin trouble or infection at a higher rate than the STA–MCA single bypass. In fact, rate of postoperative skin trouble and infection needing additional treatment are 0 and 1.5%, respectively, in our 68 procedures. Also, possible complications in terms of direct bypass are perioperative infarction and hyperperfusion syndrome, the same as standard direct bypass procedure.

## 12.8 Special Instructions, Position, and Anesthesia

The patient is placed in the supine position under general anesthesia. The head is elevated approximately 20 cm and fixed without pin fixation. The $PaCO_2$ should remain at 35 to 42 mm Hg during the operation. Anesthesia is maintained with Propofol venous infusion (6–10 mg/kg/h). Mannitol is not used in this operation. After the operation, the patient is kept sedated for 2 to 6 hours postoperatively and his or her blood pressure is controlled to stay between 100 and 120 mm Hg to prevent postoperative hemorrhage caused by hyperperfusion.

## 12.9 Patient Position with Skin Incision and Key Surgical Steps

The skin incision is made on the parietal branch of the STA and turned frontally to the midline (▶ Fig. 12.2**a**). One of the two STA branches undergoes about a 10-cm dissection for the STA–ACA bypass. In most patients, the frontal branch of the STA is selected, and the other branch is undergoes about a 6-cm dissection for the STA–MCA bypass. The frontal branch of the STA is dissected from the galeal side. The temporal muscle is divided, and two separate craniotomies, a frontotemporal and a medio-frontal, each 5 cm in diameter, are performed. The craniotomy for the STA–ACA bypass is made around the coronal suture (▶ Fig. 12.2**b**). *Blue line* is made on the long STA graft to avoid twisting the graft (▶ Fig. 12.2**c**).

A long STA graft is passed intradurally under the residual bone bridge between the two craniotomies to prevent kinking (▶ Fig. 12.2**d**). The recipient artery, which is a cortical branch from the ACA, is frequently located around the level of the coronal suture. However, there are some possibilities of facing difficulty in finding the proper size of the recipient artery. Some tips to detect the proper recipient artery are mentioned in Chapter 12.11. The long STA graft is anastomosed to the cortical artery of the ACA with 10–0 monofilament nylon using intermittent sutures. The short graft STA is anastomosed to the cortical artery of the MCA in the same manner (▶ Fig. 12.2**e**).

The dura is closed, the bone flaps are returned, and the temporal muscle and the skin are closed while avoiding kinking of the STA graft during these procedures.

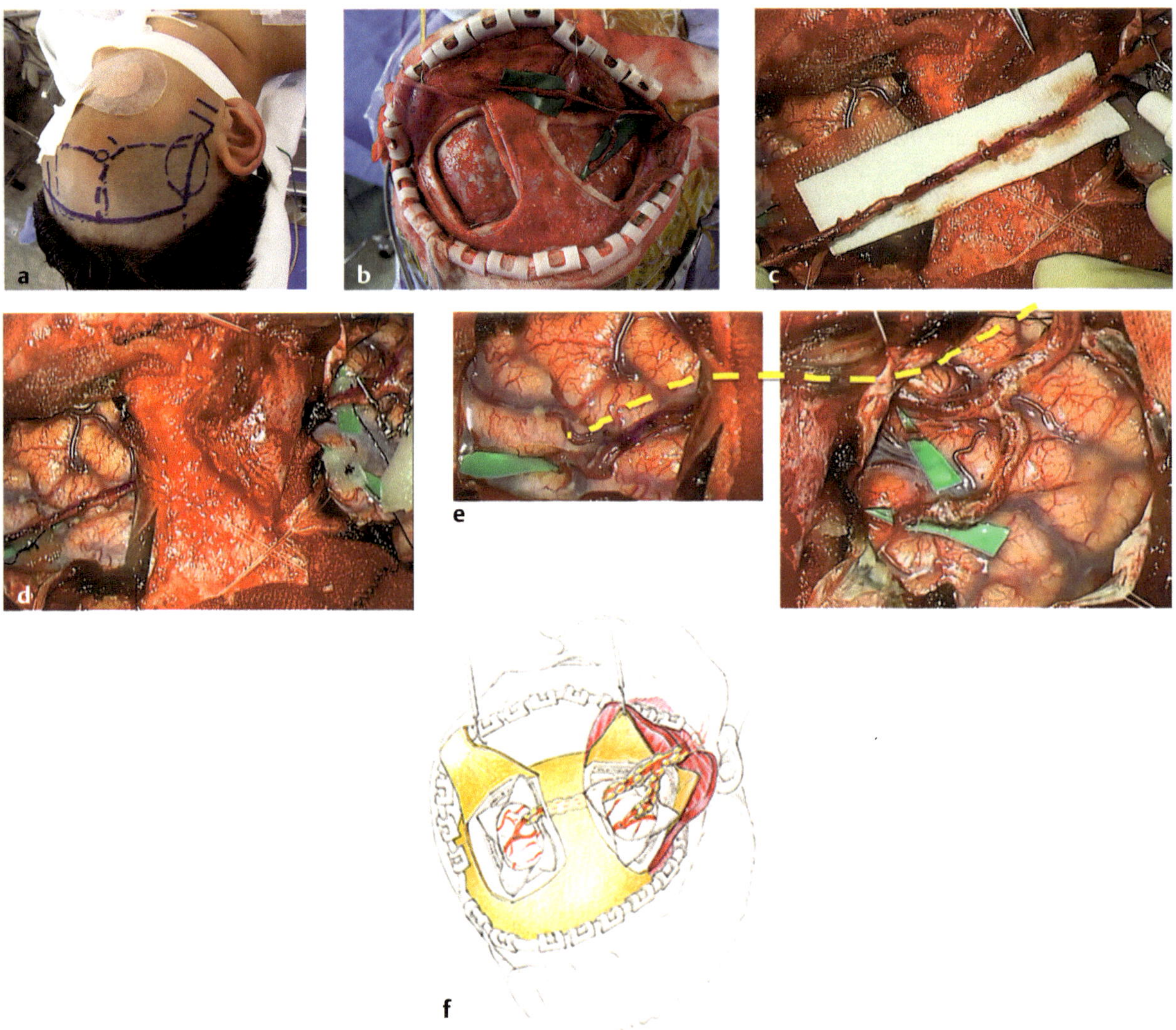

**Fig. 12.2** Skin incision **(a)** and intraoperative photograph **(b–e)**. **(a)** The posterior part of skin incision marked on the parietal branch of the superficial temporal artery (STA) and turned frontally to the midline. **(b)** Two separate craniotomies for the STA–ACA (anterior cerebral artery) bypass and STA–MCA (middle cerebral artery) bypass. Long graft for STA–ACA bypass and short graft for STA–MCA bypass were dissected. **(c)** *Blue line* on the long STA graft to avoid twisting the graft. **(d)** A long STA graft passed intradurally under the residual bone bridge between the two craniotomies to prevent kinking of the graft. **(e)** STA–ACA/MCA double bypasses with the long graft coursing naturally (*yellow dotted line*). **(f)** Established STA–ACA/MCA double bypass.

## 12.10 Difficulties Encountered

Intraoperative difficulties of STA–ACA/MCA bypasses with long grafts are divided into problems of the graft and location of the recipient arteries.

Regarding the graft, there are two difficult points. One is preparation of the graft. In many cases, the frontal branch of the STA is selected for the graft of the STA–ACA bypass. It is dissected from the galeal side as long as possible (approximately 10 cm). Especially dissection of the distal part of the frontal branch of the STA should receive close attention to prevent vessel wall damage. Careful dissection of the graft is one of the keys to achieving a good bypass. The other is prevention of kinking/rotating long graft including recipient artery around anastomosis. The long STA graft is easily kinked/rotated; however, it tends to be overlooked. The recipient artery around anastomosis is also easy to kink due to the unnatural graft course. Strongly taking care of the full-length long graft is very important.

Size of the recipient artery in the ACA territory tends to be smaller than in the MCA territory. Suitable recipient arteries of the ACA could be detected in the 5 cm in diameter craniotomy around the coronal suture as mentioned above. However, the suitable recipient artery could not be found on the brain surface in some cases. Good size of the recipient artery can be detected in the sulcus in such a case. Recipient artery in the sulcus is a tough condition for anastomosis procedures in spite of the artery having less than 1 cm of depth and being very narrow and watery.

## 12.11 Bailout, Rescue, and Salvage Maneuvers

To prevent kinking/rotating, a *blue line* is drawn on the long graft (▶ Fig. 12.2**c**) and the long STA graft is passed intradurally under the residual bone bridge between two separate craniotomies (▶ Fig. 12.2**d**).

A relatively large size cortical ACA is located in the sulcus frequently. Indocyanine green fluorescence system helps us to find suitable recipient arteries, showing dull and dark but having a large size vessel (▶ Fig. 12.3**a–c**). There are salvage maneuvers to make the more superficial and wider working space for the recipient artery in the sulcus, pulling the arachnoid at the margin of the sulcus laterally with 9–0 monofilament suturing, sheeting the suitable rubber under the recipient artery (▶ Fig. 12.4**a, b**).

We use silicone rubber stent during anastomosis to make reliable anastomosis. It helps us to get a good visualization of vessel walls to keep up the three-dimensional shape of the recipient artery after osteotomy and to avoid suturing the contralateral wall (▶ Fig. 12.5**a, b**). The silicone rubber stent is strongly effective, especially for small-sized and thin-vessel-wall recipient arteries.

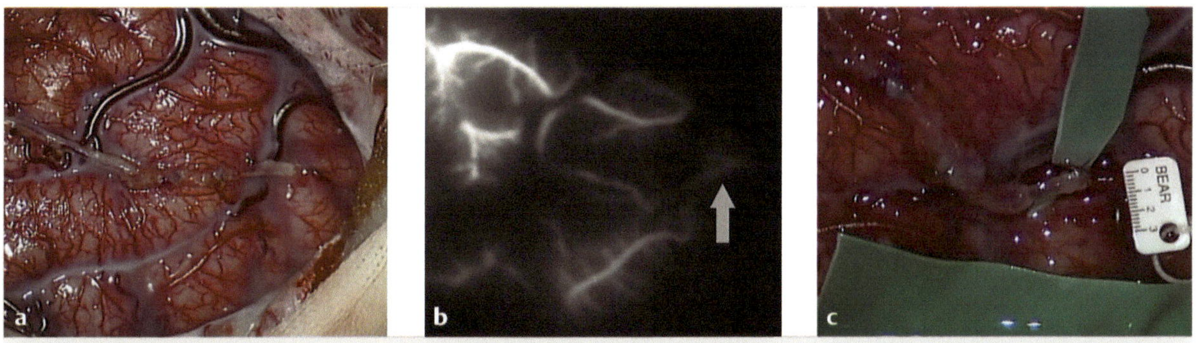


**Fig. 12.3** Intraoperative photograph. **(a, b)** Indocyanine green fluorescence system helping us to find suitable recipient arteries; showing as dull and dark but with a large size vessel (*white arrow*). **(c)** The long graft anastomosing to the anterior cerebral artery cortical artery in the sulcus.

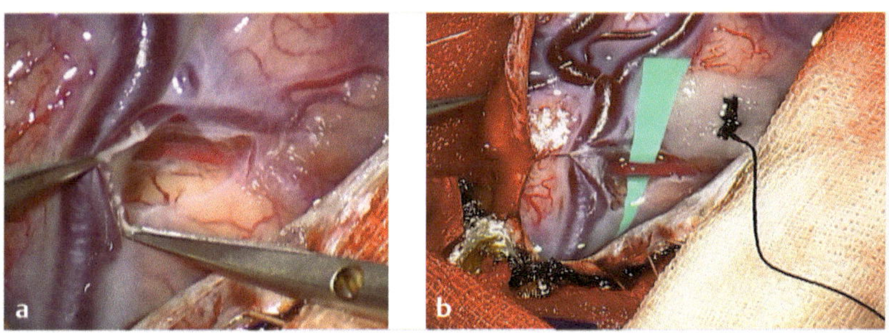


**Fig. 12.4** Intraoperative photograph. Making the more superficial and wider working space for the recipient artery in the sulcus **(a)**; pulling the arachnoid at the margin of the sulcus laterally with 9–0 monofilament suturing and sheeting the suitable rubber under the recipient artery **(b)**.

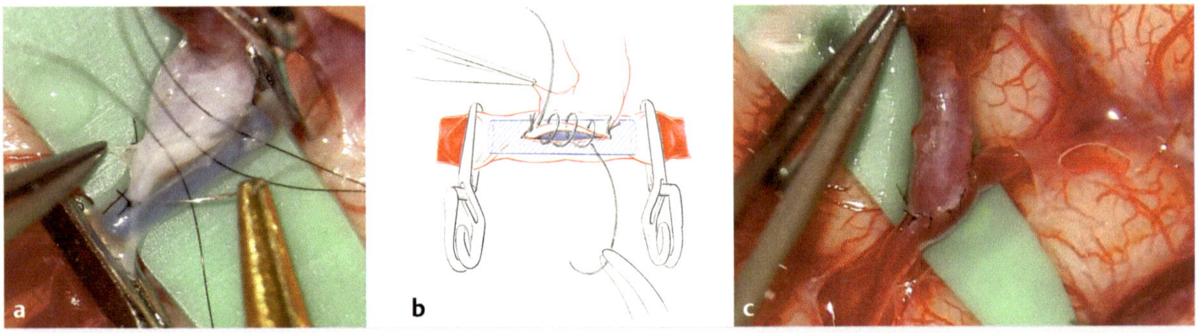


**Fig. 12.5** Intraoperative photographs and illustrative depiction of an elastic silicone rubber stent helping us to get good visualization of vessel walls to keep up the three-dimensional shape of the recipient artery after arteriotomy and to avoid suturing the contralateral wall. **(a)** Intraoperative view: note the blue silicone rubber tube in the lumen of the vessel preventing vessel wall collapse. Interrupted suturing technique where knots are made at the end, after stent removal. **(b)** Illustration highlighting usefulness of stent technique. Note this also works with continuous suturing technique where the suture line is tightened after removal of the stent. **(c)** Intraoperative view after removal of stent and finished anastomoses.

# 12.12 Tips, Pearls, and Lessons Learned

## 12.12.1 Graft Management

It's very important to prepare for the graft procedure to avoid damaging it, which could include hypertextention, transfer of overheating from the coagulator to the graft, and insufficient dissection layer. Also, the natural graft course should be paid close attention (▸ Fig. 12.2**e**).

## 12.12.2 Anastomosis

Key to successful anastomosis is (1) having a good view of the anastomotic field, (2) avoiding suturing the contralateral wall, and (3) suturing a suitable margin and interval of stitches, specifically making as small number of stitches as possible to expand the orifice (▸ Fig. 12.5**a, b**).

## 12.12.3 Training

Training is indispensable because steady hands make good anastomosis. We have trained using a silicone microtube. One handled hours of training has prepared us for the bypass surgery. One thousand hours of training has helped us to achieve a mastery skill level.

# Suggested Readings

Fujimura M, Shimizu H, Inoue T, Mugikura S, Saito A, Tominaga T. Significance of focal cerebral hyperperfusion as a cause of transient neurologic deterioration after extracranial-intracranial bypass for moyamoya disease: comparative study with non-moyamoya patients using N-isopropyl-p-[(123)I]iodoamphetamine single-photon emission computed tomography. Neurosurgery. 2011; 68(4):957–964, discussion 964–965

Iwama T, Hashimoto N, Miyake H, Yonekawa Y. Direct revascularization to the anterior cerebral artery territory in patients with moyamoya disease: report of five cases. Neurosurgery. 1998; 42(5):1157–1161, discussion 1161–1162

Karasawa J, Kikuchi H, Furuse S, Kawamura J, Sakaki T. Treatment of moyamoya disease with STA-MCA anastomosis. J Neurosurg. 1978; 49 (5):679–688

Kawashima A, Kawamata T, Yamaguchi K, Hori T, Okada Y. Successful superficial temporal artery-anterior cerebral artery direct bypass using a long graft for moyamoya disease: technical note. Neurosurgery. 2010; 67(3) Suppl Operative:ons145–ons149, discussion ons149

Khan N, Schuknecht B, Boltshauser E, et al. Moyamoya disease and moyamoya syndrome: experience in Europe; choice of revascularisation procedures. Acta Neurochir (Wien). 2003; 145(12):1061–1071, discussion 1071

Matsushima T, Inoue T, Suzuki SO, Fujii K, Fukui M, Hasuo K. Surgical treatment of moyamoya disease in pediatric patients—comparison between the results of indirect and direct revascularization procedures. Neurosurgery. 1992; 31(3):401–405

Miyamoto S, Akiyama Y, Nagata I, et al. Long-term outcome after STA-MCA anastomosis for moyamoya disease. Neurosurg Focus. 1998; 5(5):e5

Okada Y, Shima T, Yamane K, Yamanaka C, Kagawa R. Cylindrical or T-shaped silicone rubber stents for microanastomosis—technical note. Neurol Med Chir (Tokyo). 1999; 39(1):55–57, discussion 57–58

# 13 Double Anastomosis Using Only One Branch of the Superficial Temporal Artery: Single-Vessel Double Anastomosis

*Ziad A. Hage, Gregory D. Arnone, and Fady T. Charbel*

**Abstract**

Double anastomosis using only one branch of the superficial temporal artery (STA), single-vessel double anastomosis (SVDA), describes a valuable technique of direct revascularization for moyamoya disease. A proximal side-to-side anastomosis is made, followed by a distal end-to-side anastomosis with the same STA branch used on both recipient vessels. This technique may be chosen for cases in which preoperative evaluation reveals only a single robust usable STA branch on angiogram, with more than one territory requiring flow augmentation. Additionally, the decision to proceed with SVDA bypass configuration may be made based on intraoperative flow measurements of potential donor and recipient vessels, in an effort to maximize graft potential and minimize bypass failure. This chapter discusses the technique, indications, contraindications, complication avoidance, and other considerations when performing SVDA.

*Keywords:* moyamoya, direct bypass, single-vessel double anastomosis, cut-flow index, extracranial-to-intracranial bypass, superficial temporal artery bypass

## 13.1 History and Initial Description

The first description of "moyamoya" disease was by Suzuki and Takaku in 1969.[1] Three years later, professor Yasargil performed the first surgical intervention for moyamoya with a superficial temporal artery (STA) to middle cerebral artery (MCA) bypass,[2] marking the beginning of an evolution in the surgical treatment of the disease. Over the next several decades and into the 21st century, novel surgical strategies have been developed to treat moyamoya disease, and operative techniques have been continually refined. Currently, various operations for both direct and indirect bypass are described to augment blood flow to multiple vascular territories, including the anterior cerebral artery, MCA, and posterior cerebral artery territories.[3]

While double-barrel bypass techniques with both the parietal and frontal STA branches have been described,[4] the single-vessel double anastomosis (SVDA) technique is a novel strategy that involves utilizing one donor branch for both a side-to-side, and end-to-side anastomosis, provided the donor artery has sufficient flow to supply multiple bypasses. This technique can be an important addition to the bypass armamentarium in selected patients with moyamoya disease, particularly when a single anastomosis is unlikely to supply sufficient flow to multiple ischemic territories, or in cases where there is mismatch between the available flow from the donor graft exceeding the sink capacity of a single recipient bed.

## 13.2 Indications

Potential candidates for flow augmentation bypass surgery include patients with symptomatic moyamoya disease with poor cerebrovascular reserve as diagnosed on preoperative studies. We prefer to use a vasodilatory challenge paired with imaging studies to assess cerebrovascular reserve and identify areas at risk with impaired autoregulation stemming from a chronic oligemic state. Vasodilatory challenge normally causes a resultant increase in cerebral blood flow, though in instances of hemodynamic compromise, this response will be either dampened or absent in an impaired vascular territory compared to the normal circulation.[5] The studies we utilize include quantitative MRA with use of Noninvasive Optimal Vessel Analysis (NOVA) software, with a Diamox challenge, and functional MRI (regional and global blood oxygen level dependent [BOLD] imaging) with $CO_2$ challenge. Adequate donor and recipient vessels should be available as noted on digital subtraction angiography. The SVDA bypass configuration, in particular, can be selected as an option during preoperative work up if only a single robust usable STA branch is noted on the angiogram and more than one territory requires flow augmentation (such as with superior and inferior MCA division territories). On the other hand, the decision to proceed with SVDA bypass configuration may be taken intraoperatively based on flow measurements of potential donor and recipient vessels. If the cut flow (i.e., free-flowing carrying capacity) of the STA donor vessel is substantial enough to augment two vascular beds, an initial side-to-side anastomosis is performed. The cut-flow index (CFI) is then measured and calculated; if $CFI \leq 0.5$, the second anastomosis is completed in an attempt to get the CFI closer to 1, therefore maximizing the graft potential and minimizing type 2c error and bypass failure.[6,7]

## 13.3 Key Principles

Once the vascular territories in need of flow augmentation are identified based on patient symptoms (including left vs. right in bilateral disease), imaging findings, and cerebrovascular reserve testing, the skin incision and craniotomy must be carefully planned. Excessive supragaleal dissection and devascularization of the scalp can be spared if only a single branch of the STA is needed. The skin incision is tailored according to the targeted STA branch. If the parietal branch is being dissected, the skin incision will be made following its path; it can then be reflected anteriorly, distal to the superior temporal line, if a larger skin flap is needed. If the frontal branch is harvested, the incision is made to accommodate for an adequate size craniotomy while minimizing the amount of skin reflected anteriorly. The frontal STA will then be dissected from the underside of the skin flap through the galea. When performing the craniotomy and opening the dura, great care should be exercised in preserving the middle meningeal artery (MMA), as it may already provide critical extracranial-to-intracranial (EC–IC) collaterals, as often seen on preoperative angiography. Various donor/recipient vessels should be identified and different direct bypass configurations planned and selected; the surgeon should be ready to adapt and reconfigure the surgical plan based on intraoperative flow measurements. Flow-assisted surgical technique (FAST) is utilized,[7] which involves the following: performing flow measurement for the STA cut flow; calculating CFI to predict bypass patency rate[6]; optimizing type 2c error (further described in Chapter 13.4.4); optimizing CFI at 1 by performing more than one anastomosis if needed; maximizing donor capacity.

# 13.4 SWOT Analysis

## 13.4.1 Strengths

In contrast to indirect techniques, direct bypass allows for immediate flow augmentation and, in some cases, relief of symptoms. The development of adequate collaterals can take several months after indirect bypass, putting the patient at risk for repeated events in the interim. Specific to the SVDA technique, multiple anastomoses using a single donor vessel maximize its donor capacity while optimizing type 2c error (explained in Chapter 13.4.4). The technique also obviates the need to dissect a second STA branch, therefore saving time, preserving scalp blood supply for improved healing, and providing a salvage plan in case of reoperation or failure of the initial bypass.

## 13.4.2 Weaknesses

All EC–IC bypass procedures require temporary occlusion time of the recipient bed, putting patients at risk for ischemic events during the surgery; however, temporary occlusion time is required for multiple recipients in SVDA. Furthermore, any problem at the proximal anastomosis site may affect the distal anastomosis, and any potential issue affecting the donor compromises both recipients at once.

## 13.4.3 Opportunities

Techniques to reduce or eliminate temporary occlusion time will improve the safety of bypass procedures, especially when multiple bypasses are being planned as in SVDA. As such, novel suturing devices may be a target for future consideration. Additionally, the development of more advanced software that is able to accurately and quantitatively identify the amount of flow needed for augmentation in various territories with poor reserve would allow for more reliable and informed surgical planning.

## 13.4.4 Threats

Four main types of errors[7,8] are encountered with direct bypass procedures that constitute threats to the success of this surgery.

*Type 1 error*, or poor patient selection, occurs when the recipient vascular bed already has adequate collaterals (good hemodynamic reserve) and bypass is unnecessary. In these cases, often times the bypass will fail because the demand is low and there will be poor flow through the anastomosis.

*Type 2a error* refers to a problem with the donor vessel —in the case of SVDA, the STA branch. Technical issues may be secondary to vessel injury during harvesting, or thrombosis due to inadequate flushing. Of most concern in SVDA is insufficient supply of the single branch to provide adequate flow to two recipient territories, resulting in continued ischemia of both territories. Again, intraoperative flow parameters will dictate whether or not a single STA branch is sufficient.

*Type 2b error* is simply an anastomosis problem. Meticulous technique and the need for continued practice cannot be understated for bypass surgery, and increasing experience should mitigate these technical issues.

*Type 2c error* refers to recipient or distal bed problems that may limit the outflow from the bypass. Causes include atherosclerotic disease, vessel stenosis distal to the anastomosis, small recipient vessel size, and increased distal vascular bed resistance.

# 13.5 Contraindications

Contraindications to the SVDA technique encompass the usual contraindications to bypass for moyamoya in general, including preserved hemodynamic reserve, poor quality donor vessels, and poor quality recipient vessels. Inadequate vessel length or orientation may also prevent a successful SVDA. Finally, unless the cut flow from the single STA branch is sufficient to supply two separate vascular territories, an alternative technique (double barrel, for example) must be employed.

## 13.6 Special Considerations

Careful study of the preoperative angiogram will help assess the quality of donor and recipient vessels, select the adequate bypass configuration, and define the recipient territory at risk. Furthermore, it must be determined if the MMA is supplying EC–IC collaterals, in which cases one must avoid injuring the vessel during craniotomy and dural opening. Diuretics, hyperosmolar medications, and hyperventilation must not be used during the surgery because all of these techniques may compromise blood flow to an already tenuous territory during surgery and temporary occlusion time. The patient's blood pressure should be maintained at the baseline preoperative value during the surgery and especially during anesthesia induction. The pressure should be raised during temporary occlusion time and the patient should be in burst suppression. An antiplatelet agent such as aspirin (we use 325 mg) should be given the morning of surgery and continued thereafter in order to prevent thrombosis at the graft site until endothelial healing can occur. Laboratory testing for aspirin effect (platelet inhibition) may be done postoperatively to ensure therapeutic effect.

## 13.7 Pitfalls, Risk Assessment, and Complications

Several pitfalls may be encountered when performing a technically demanding surgery such as the SVDA bypass. Injuring the STA during harvest or craniotomy, failing to adequately flush the donor vessel after sectioning and clamping, failing to coagulate its side branches, or dissecting the STA wall during harvest can jeopardize the donor and consequently the success of the surgery. Moreover, inadequate craniotomy size or location may prevent exposure of adequate recipient arteries, rendering a planned bypass configuration difficult to achieve. Even worse, errant craniotomy site may lead to revascularization of the wrong territory (superior vs. inferior MCA division). Injuring the MMA during craniotomy or dural opening can eliminate important existing collaterals and further the ischemic burden. In addition, poor hemostasis prior to starting the anastomosis may cause continuous blood oozing in the field, a situation that significantly impedes efforts toward an efficient and timely bypass. Injury to a recipient vessel via coagulation or arteriotomy can thwart bypass plans and exacerbate the underlying disease. Additionally, neglecting to coagulate side branches from the recipient will cause continued bleeding despite temporary clipping. Moreover, donor–recipient mismatch can be of concern, and one must take care to bevel and fish mouth the donor when necessary. Suturing the back wall of the vessel during anastomosis is yet another cause of failure. Inadequate amount of sutures will cause an anastomosis to leak briskly. If a temporary stent is used, one must not forget to remove it prior to placing final sutures. Finally, during closure, strangulation of the STA by dura or muscle reapproximation must be avoided. In addition, meticulous skin closure is key in preventing inadvertent injury of the graft.

## 13.8 Special Instructions, Position, and Anesthesia

Bypass is performed with patients under general anesthesia with the head fixed in a Mayfield head holder. Foley catheter, arterial line, and central line are inserted prior to pinning. The head should be rotated such that the surgical field is parallel to the floor, and a shoulder roll can be helpful in certain instances where the neck is not very supple. The STA stump, bifurcation, frontal, and parietal branches should all be mapped out with a Doppler probe and adequately marked. Skin incision may vary depending on the operative plan and bypass configuration. For example, if a parietal branch is planned for an SVDA, an incision over the mapped out branch may be used (▶ Fig. 13.1). If the frontal branch is needed, a subgaleal flap can be turned anteriorly from this incision and the frontal branch can be identified from the undersurface of the flap and dissected accordingly. Burst suppression should be employed and diuretics, hyperventilation, and hypotension must be avoided at all times during surgery. The patient's blood pressure should be maintained at the baseline preoperative value during the surgery, especially during anesthesia induction. The pressure should be raised during temporary occlusion time.

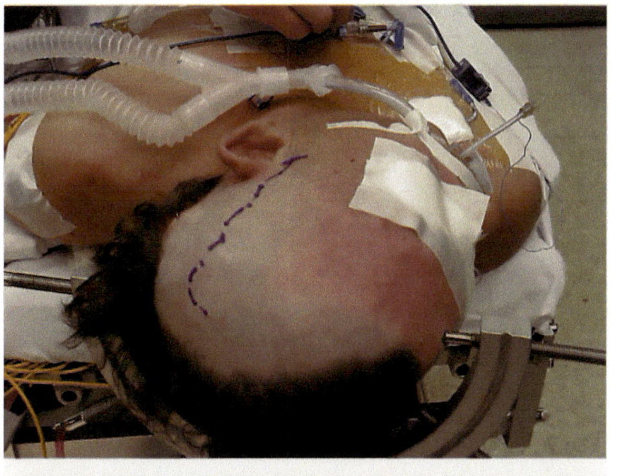

**Fig. 13.1** Patient positioning and skin marking. Note that the head is parallel to the floor, fixed in a head holder. The parietal superficial temporal artery (STA) branch has been marked out using a Doppler and the incision is directly over the path of the STA.

## 13.9 Skin Incision and Key Surgical Steps

Under microscope magnification, skin incision is made as planned, depending on the chosen STA branch that was mapped out prior to prepping and draping. The STA is dissected free of the surrounding soft tissue (▶ Fig. 13.2) and flow is measured in situ using the Charbel Micro-Flowprobe (Transonic, Ithaca, NY). Next, the STA is wrapped in a papaverine-soaked cottonoid to keep it hydrated and protected during the craniotomy, and to reduce vasospasm in the donor vessel (▶ Fig. 13.3). The microscope is removed from the field and the craniotomy is performed as planned out, depending on the location of the recipient branches and targeted revascularization. Dural tack-up sutures are placed around the craniotomy edges. The microscope is brought back into the field and the dura is carefully opened, preserving MMA branches that provide critical collaterals (▶ Fig. 13.4). After opening the dura, the STA is laid over the brain surface to plan the anastomosis sites and final position of the donor vessel (▶ Fig. 13.5). The STA is then sectioned and the cut flow is measured.[8,9] Any lower than expected flow values should prompt a search for areas of strangulation at the STA stump, as can happen with traversing veins in the soft tissue (▶ Fig. 13.6). Such vessels should be coagulated and the STA stump freed from obstruction. The STA is then flushed with heparinized saline and a temporary clip is placed on its proximal and distal ends. Next, the arachnoid is opened over the selected recipient vessels and a

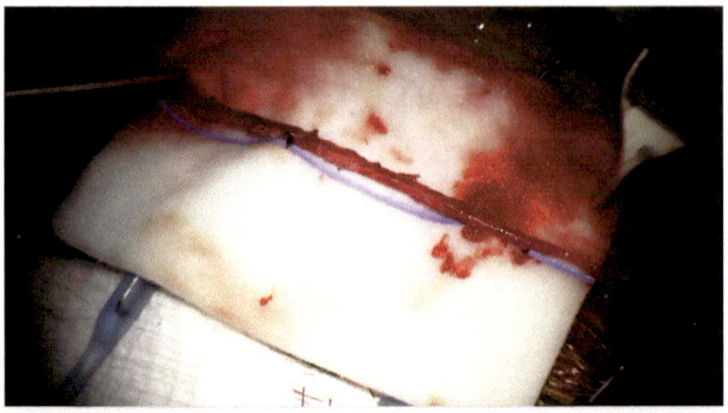

**Fig. 13.3** The superficial temporal artery, after being dissected, is wrapped in a papaverine-soaked cottonoid.

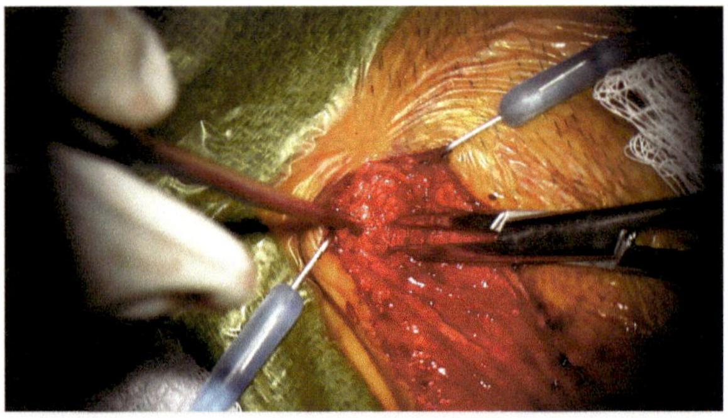

**Fig. 13.2** The superficial temporal artery (STA) dissection. Under microscope magnification, the STA is dissected in the subcutaneous layer using a curved mosquito clamp. Hooks (*in blue*) help to retract and elevate the tissue edges and facilitate dissection.

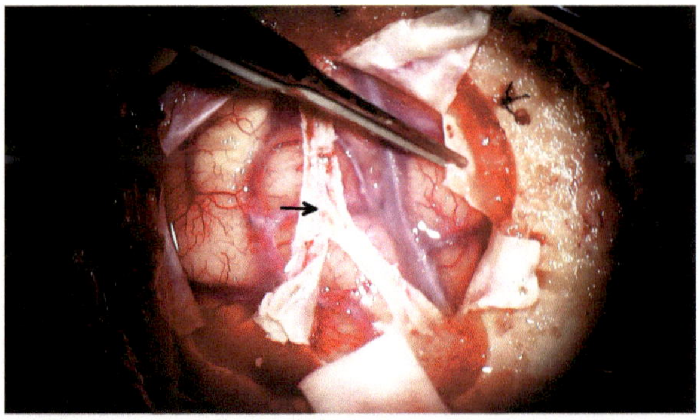

**Fig. 13.4** The dura is cut and opened in such a way to preserve the middle meningeal artery (*arrow*) and its branches.

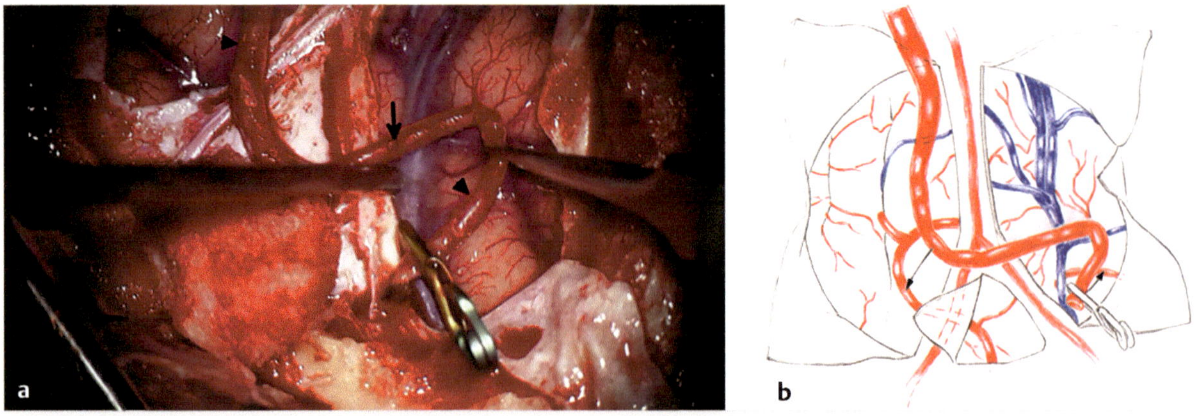



**Fig. 13.5 (a, b)** After opening the dura, the superficial temporal artery (*arrow*) is laid over the brain surface to plan anastomosis sites (*arrowheads*) and final position of the donor vessel.

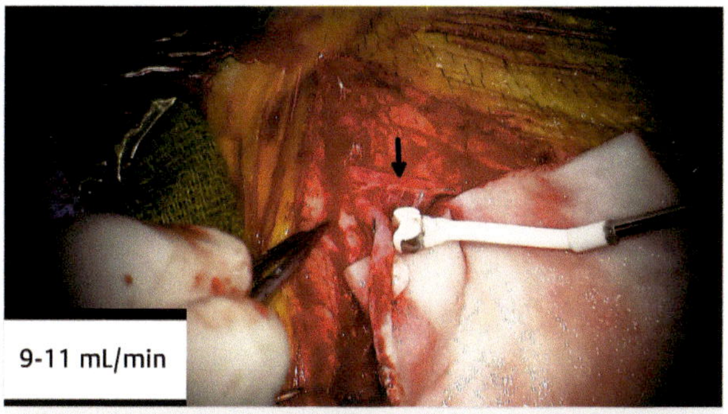


**Fig. 13.6** The cut flow is then measured in the superficial temporal artery (STA): here 11 mL/min, which is much lower than expected. Note the vein crossing over the STA (*black arrow*) and strangulating it. After coagulation and division of the vein, cut flow improved to 50 mL/min.

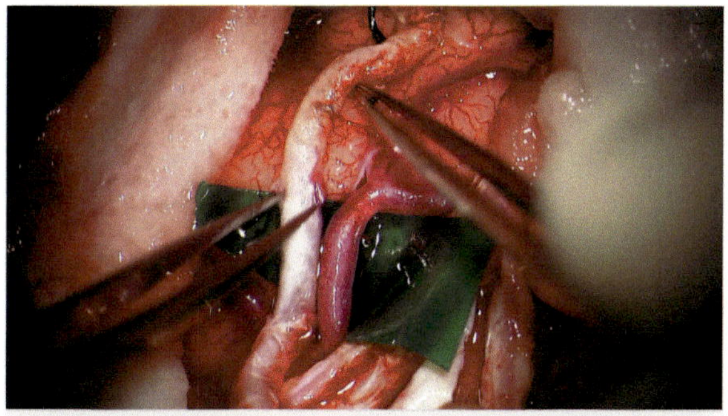

**Fig. 13.8** The superficial temporal artery is positioned in a side-to-side fashion next to the recipient in preparation for arteriotomy and anastomosis.

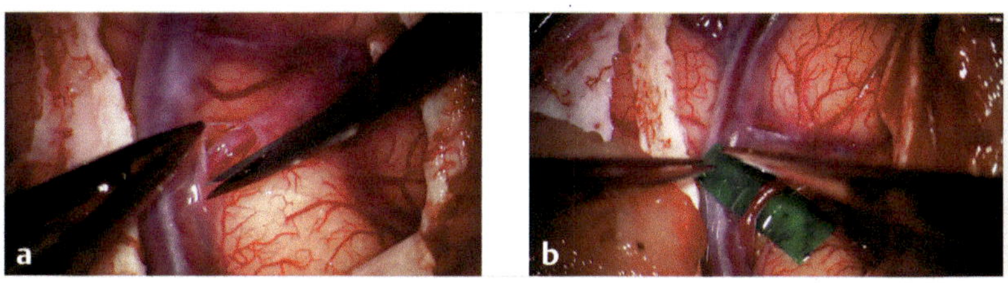

**Fig. 13.7** After arachnoidal dissection of the recipient vessel **(a)**, a rubber dam (*in green*) is placed underneath it in preparation for anastomosis **(b)**.

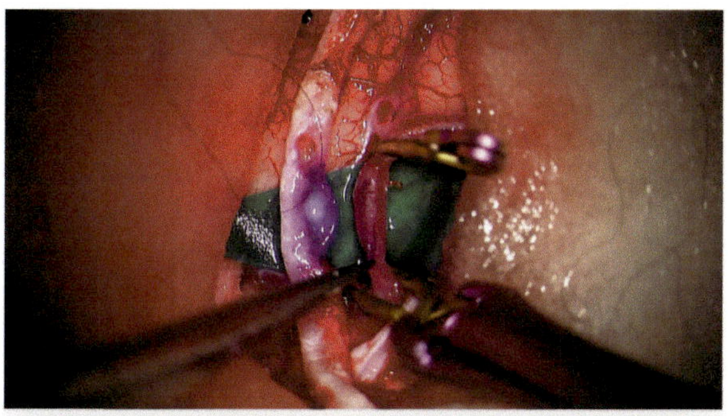

**Fig. 13.9** Arteriotomy has been performed in the superficial temporal artery (STA). A 10–0 nylon suture is first placed on one end of the STA arteriotomy, after which temporary clips are placed on the recipient vessel.

rubber dam with a small piece of gelfoam is placed under the recipient in preparation for anastomosis (▶ Fig. 13.7). The gelfoam helps in elevating the recipient vessel and surgical field during anastomosis. The second recipient vessel is also prepared as described and baseline flow measurements are taken at both recipient sites. The STA is then dissected free from its tissue cuff and positioned in a side-to-side fashion next to the recipient in preparation for arteriotomy and anastomosis (▶ Fig. 13.8). Care must be taken to position the STA while preserving its baseline anatomical configuration therefore preventing any twisting or kinking of the vessel. Arteriotomy sites are marked on donor and recipient and the first arteriotomy is performed on the STA at the proximal site where the side-to-side anastomosis will take place. The side-to-side proximal anastomosis is always performed first; if the end-to side distal anastomosis were done first, occlusion of the distal anastomosis would be necessary while performing the proximal one. This would not only put both territories at risk during temporary occlusion, but would also put the initial anastomosis at significant risk of thrombosis due to blood stasis. After placing the 10–0 nylon suture on one end of STA arteriotomy, temporary clips are placed on the recipient vessel (▶ Fig. 13.9). The arteriotomy is made on the recipient vessel to match the STA arteriotomy, and the lumen is flushed with heparinized saline. The 10–0 nylon suture is then stitched and tied to the apex of the recipient arteriotomy and the first side of the anastomosis is done in a running fashion (▶ Fig. 13.10). The stitches should remain loose until the entire length of the vessel has been sutured, and the loops of suture are then tightened sequentially. The lumen is checked making sure the back wall is not caught and the other side of the anastomosis is then completed the same way. The temporary clips are then removed from the recipient vessel and the anastomosis site is checked for hemostasis. Flow measurements are taken on the completed anastomosis. For the end-to-side anastomosis, the cut end of the STA is beveled and fish mouthed. Two 10–0 nylon sutures are then placed, one at the toe and the other at the heel of the STA (▶ Fig. 13.11).

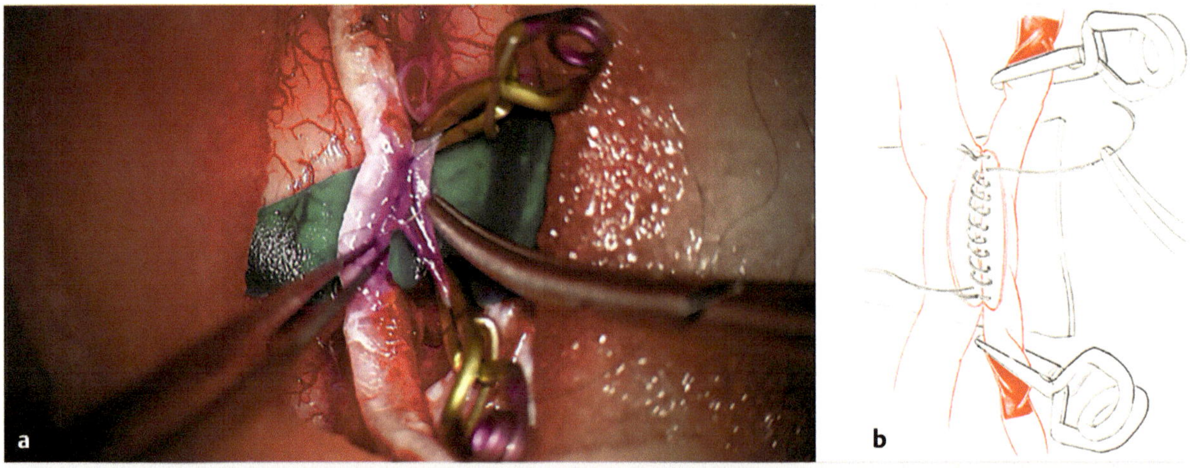

**Fig. 13.10 (a, b)** The 10–0 nylon suture is tied and the first side of the anastomosis is done in a running fashion. The lumen is checked, making sure that the back wall is not caught.

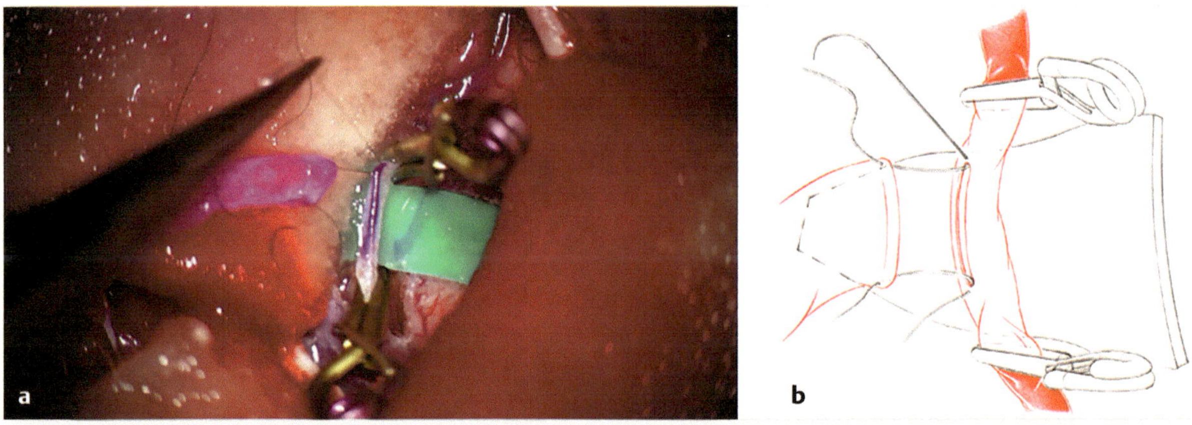

**Fig. 13.11 (a, b)** Second anastomosis. After the cut end of the superficial temporal artery (STA) is beveled and fish-mouthed, the first suture is placed and tied on the toe of the STA. The anastomosis is completed in an interrupted fashion, making sure that the needle always goes from in-to-out in the recipient to prevent wall dissection.

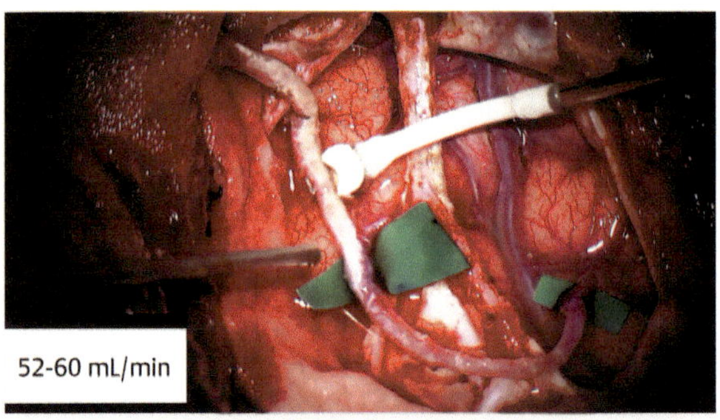


**Fig. 13.12** After completion of both anastomoses, the final bypass flow is being measured in the superficial temporal artery main stump: here around 60 mL/min.

Temporary clips are placed on the recipient vessel. Again, the arteriotomy on the recipient vessel is made to match the STA cut end, and the lumen is flushed with heparinized saline. The first suture—on the toe of the STA—is tied to one end of the recipient arteriotomy, followed by the second suture—on the heel of the STA—that is tied to the other end of the recipient arteriotomy. One side of the anastomosis is then completed in an interrupted fashion, making sure that the needle always pierces from in-to-out in the fragile recipient vessel wall to prevent arterial dissection. After completing the first side, the lumen is checked to ensure the back wall is not caught. The other side of the anastomosis is then completed in the same way. Temporary clips are removed from the recipient initially and then from the STA, and flow is reestablished. Flow measurements are again taken in the STA and both recipient vessels to assess the flow dynamics and cut flow indices (▶ Fig. 13.12). Indocyanine green fluorescence can then be performed to further confirm patency of the bypass and preserved flow in the MMA and its branches. Upon closure of dura and muscle, adequate bulk should be excised to clear the path of the STA. After each step up until skin closure, flow measurements should be obtained on the STA stump to ensure that the vessel has not been inadvertently strangulated or compromised.

Postoperatively, a CT of the head without contrast is performed to monitor for hemorrhage and a cerebral angiogram is done to assess the direct bypasses and flow-augmented territories. The patient is then observed in the intensive care unit (ICU) for a minimum of 24 to 48 hours. Systolic blood pressure is initially kept between 100 and 140 mm Hg to prevent reperfusion hemorrhage in case of prior strokes or hyperperfusion syndrome, and then liberalized from 100 to 160 mm Hg after 24 hours. Aspirin is never discontinued and levels may be monitored to ensure therapeutic antiplatelet effect. While in the ICU, hourly neurological examinations are performed until stable and then every 2 hours until the patient is transferred to the step-down unit. At that time, neurological examination is performed every 4 hours. Quantitative MRA/NOVA is performed in the postoperative period to measure bypass flow and MMA flow, establishing new baselines. After discharge from the hospital, we use functional MRI with global and regional BOLD and $CO_2$ challenge and quantitative MRA/NOVA with and without Diamox at 6 weeks and then 6 months to assess for adequacy of flow augmentation and improvement of cerebrovascular reserve. Neuropsychological testing is done preoperatively at baseline, and then at 6 months after bypass to evaluate for cognitive improvement. A follow-up cerebral angiogram is performed 1 year postoperatively to assess for any indirect bypass.

## 13.10 Difficulties Encountered

Several difficulties may be encountered during this procedure. If bypass flow is not adequate and the CFI is less than 0.5, consider the following: poor patient selection—best avoided thorough preoperative hemodynamic assessment; donor problem—avoided by careful harvest, keeping the vessel hydrated and protected in the papaverine-soaked cottonoid, flushing with heparinized saline, ensuring adequate dissection of the surrounding tissue cuff from the donor graft, and ensuring that the vessel wall is not dissected; anastomosis problem—avoided by checking the back wall during suturing or use of a stent, flushing with heparinized saline prior to completion of the bypass, ensuring a clean suture line inside the lumen, correcting any dog-ear of the vessel which may compromise the lumen and anastomosis, and ensuring good size match of donor to recipient; recipient or distal bed problem—avoided by choosing adequate vessel size, flushing with heparinized saline, and choosing an ischemic vascular bed with poor reserve.

## 13.11 Bailout, Rescue, and Salvage Maneuvers

In this technically challenging surgery, it is best to prevent an error from occurring rather than fixing it. Nonetheless, certain errors do happen occasionally. If the STA is damaged during craniotomy (caught with the drill), and the cut is distal enough, the damaged portion may be amputated to obtain a clean edge. Otherwise, the other STA branch may be harvested, mobilized, and utilized. If the bypass is not flowing after anastomosis, first check the suture line, and gently massage the vessels and the anastomosis site. If there still is paucity of flow, local thrombolytic (tissue plasminogen activator or integrillin) may be injected. Ultimately, the anastomosis may need to be opened and revised, or a new anastomosis performed on a different recipient vessel. If the bypass flow is reduced during closure of the dura or muscle layers, the closure should be reopened and revised—dura and/or muscle bulk can be excised to create enough space so that the course of the STA is unobstructed. Similarly, any strangulating craniotomy bone edge should be removed. If the bypass is punctured by a needle inadvertently, apply gentle pressure with a micro-instrument until it stops. If needed, a 10–0 suture can be placed to repair the hole.

## 13.12 Tips, Pearls, and Lessons Learned

Appropriate preoperative patient evaluation and selection cannot be understated. Exhaustive review of the preoperative angiogram, with study of MMA collaterals and planning of donor/recipient vessels and bypass configuration must be done. Donor and recipient vessels should be matched for size. Mannitol, lasix, and hyperventilation should be avoided. Anticonvulsant prophylaxis is optional but advised. Clean technique from start to end is paramount, throughout every step of the operation, from STA mapping to skin closure. The STA must be kept moist and wrapped in a papaverine-soaked cottonoid until ready for anastomosis, and must be flushed generously and repeatedly with heparinized saline. The bypass field should be elevated by placing gelfoam under the rubber dam that isolates the recipient. Do not hesitate to use a stent during anastomosis, but do not forget to remove it prior to completion! Continuously inspect the back wall of the anastomosis and the suture line prior to suturing the other side. Flow measurements during the case are critical in decision-making and evaluation. The surgeon must be prepared with troubleshooting maneuvers and alternative plans based on measurements. If leakage is observed at the anastomosis site after completion, copious irrigation is often sufficient to stop the oozing; otherwise, a stich may be added. If the bypass is not flowing well and thrombus formation is noted, local thrombolytic can be injected but one should not hesitate to reopen and revise an anastomosis. Ultimately, an anastomosis on different recipient may be performed using the same donor as salvage. Of note, in the senior author's experience, some bypasses may be visualized angiographically 1 to 2 months after appearing nonfunctional.

## References


[1] Suzuki J, Takaku A. Cerebrovascular "moyamoya" disease. Disease showing abnormal net-like vessels in base of brain. Arch Neurol. 1969; 20(3):288–299

[2] Donaghy RM. Neurologic surgery. Surg Gynecol Obstet. 1972; 134(2): 269–270

[3] Matsushima T, Inoue K, Kawashima M, Inoue T. History of the development of surgical treatments for moyamoya disease. Neurol Med Chir (Tokyo). 2012; 52(5):278–286

[4] Yoshimura S, Egashira Y, Enomoto Y, Yamada K, Yano H, Iwama T. Superficial temporal artery to middle cerebral artery double bypass via a small craniotomy: technical note. Neurol Med Chir (Tokyo). 2010; 50(10):956–959

[5] Hage ZA, Amin-Hanjani S, Charbel FT. Cerebral revascularization: state of the art. Neurosurg Q. 2013; 23(1):13–26

[6] Amin-Hanjani S, Du X, Mlinarevich N, Meglio G, Zhao M, Charbel FT. The cut flow index: an intraoperative predictor of the success of extracranial-intracranial bypass for occlusive cerebrovascular disease. Neurosurgery. 2005; 56(1) Suppl:75–85, discussion 75–85

[7] Ashley WW, Amin-Hanjani S, Alaraj A, Shin JH, Charbel FT. Flow-assisted surgical cerebral revascularization. Neurosurg Focus. 2008; 24(2):E20

[8] Amin-Hanjani S, Charbel FT. Flow-assisted surgical technique in cerebrovascular surgery. Surg Neurol. 2007; 68 Suppl 1:S4–S11

[9] Charbel FT, Meglio G, Amin-Hanjani S. Superficial temporal artery-to-middle cerebral artery bypass. Neurosurgery. 2005; 56(1) Suppl: 186–190, discussion 186–190


## Suggested Readings


Amin-Hanjani S, Singh A, Rifai H, et al. Combined direct and indirect bypass for moyamoya: quantitative assessment of direct bypass flow over time. Neurosurgery. 2013; 73(6):962–967, discussion 967–968

# Part 4

## Combined Revascularization

# 14 Combined STA–MCA Bypass and Encephalo-myo-synangiosis

*Marcus Czabanka and Peter Vajkoczy*

**Abstract**
Cerebral revascularization in moyamoya vasculopathy may be achieved by direct and indirect procedures. As both strategies are characterized by distinct advantages and disadvantages, combination strategies aim at combining the advantages of both procedures in order to achieve maximum restoration of cerebral blood flow. While direct superficial temporal artery-middle meningeal artery (STA-MMA) bypass leads to immediate supply of collateral flow, encephalo-myo-synangiosis (EMS) leads to revascularization in large area of the brain and may provide additional blood flow in the case of insufficient bypass function. In this chapter the technical aspects of combining STA-MCA (middle cerebral artery) bypass with EMS are demonstrated focusing on technical challenges and problem solving strategies.

*Keywords:* STA-MCA bypass, encephalo-myo-synangiosis, combined revascularization, moyamoya

## 14.1 History and Initial Description

In 1977 Karasawa et al published the first description of encephalo-myo-synangiosis (EMS) in moyamoya patients showing that in combination with direct superficial temporal artery-middle cerebral artery (STA-MCA) anastomosis novel collateral vessels develop on the surface of the brain supplied by the deep temporal artery that is known to deliver blood flow to the temporal muscle.[1] The introduction of this indirect revascularization procedure for moyamoya patients initiated an ongoing debate about the ideal revascularization strategy leading to the development of various combined revascularization protocols. Matsushima et al demonstrated that combined STA-MCA bypass and EMS is superior to indirect only procedures regarding development of collateral blood flow and clinical improvement of ischemic patients.[2,3] Age-dependent revascularization patterns revealed that in adult patients STA-MCA anastomosis is the main source of additional blood flow in the case of combined STA-MCA/EMS surgery, whereas in pediatric patients collateral flow via the EMS significantly improves over the course of time compensating or even replacing blood flow via the direct anastomosis.[4] Functional analysis demonstrates that in adult patients combined STA-MCA/EMS leads to a significant recovery of cerebrovascular reserve capacity while single EMS does not lead to reversal of hemodynamic compromise.[5] Therefore, combining STA-MCA anastomosis with EMS is especially beneficial in pediatric patients whereas the additional application of EMS seems of inferior importance in adult patients in the presence of a direct anastomosis.

## 14.2 Indications

Combined STA-MCA bypass and EMS is used in pediatric patients and young adults as the revascularization strategy of choice. In pediatric patients EMS has been demonstrated to lead to successful revascularization results and may represent an important additional source of collateral flow in case of small STA size and insufficient direct bypass function. In adults, EMS demonstrates less effective revascularization results and is primarily performed additionally to STA-MCA bypass in case of small or insufficient STA anatomy.

## 14.3 Key Principles

The general concept of combining STA-MCA bypass and EMS in moyamoya patients includes the idea that more blood flow is restored in a larger vascular territory of the brain via the combined strategy as compared to either single procedure. Additionally, the combination of both procedures promises maintenance of collateral flow in the case of failure of a single procedure (reciprocal compensation).Sufficient platelet antiaggregation is recommended depending on preoperative assessment of aspirin resistance using PFA-100 testing.[6] Compared to single STA-MCA bypass surgery, the size of the craniotomy is increased to the size of the temporal muscle (with the sylvian fissure as the center of craniotomy) in order to allow transposition to the brain surface. Special care has to be applied to preparation of the galea and the base of the temporal muscle in order to avoid damage to the neovascular potential of the donor tissue. This includes avoidance of compression at the base of the temporal muscle especially after bone flap reimplantation in order to avoid both compression of the donor branch of the STA and the blood supply of the temporal muscle.

## 14.4 SWOT Analysis

### 14.4.1 Strengths

STA-MCA bypass supplies direct blood flow and therefore leads to immediate hemodynamic improvement. EMS may provide additional blood flow if bypass capacity is not sufficient. In case of bypass failure EMS may compensate collateral blood flow.

### 14.4.2 Weaknesses

Combining both procedures adds surgical time and surgical risks. Especially in pediatric patients STA-MCA bypass may be difficult to achieve due to fragile and small donor and recipient vessels. Large craniotomy and muscle transposition represents a source for rebleeding from the temporal muscle and includes the risk of brain compression in case of muscle edema. Moreover, the efficacy of restoring blood flow via the EMS cannot be predicted and has been shown to be very variable.

### 14.4.3 Opportunities

The efficacy of restoring additional blood flow to the brain via the EMS may be improved by a genetic strategy.[7] Application a myoblast-mediated gene transfer of proangiogenic and porarteriogenic genes to the muscle/brain interface has been shown to improve collateral flow to the brain and to reduce the risk for ischemia.[7] Therefore, the muscle/brain interface represents a promising target for molecular biological strategies to induce arterio- and angiogenesis.

### 14.4.4 Threats

Failure of anastomosis due to fragile and thin recipient and donor vessels represent a major threat. Additional threats include risks of rehemorrhage, ischemia, or hyperperfusion syndrome. A special risk must be attributed to swelling of the temporal muscle which may induce a space occupying, compressive effect on the brain. Extremely rare are long-term complications as occlusion of the donor vessel during mouth opening resulting in transient ischemic attacks.[8]

## 14.5 Contraindications

Presence of middle meningeal artery (MMA) as part of vault moyamoya vessels or the STA as contributor of vault moyamoya vessels represent the most important contraindications. The required large dural opening imposes a significant risk for dural feeders of vault moyamoya vessels potentially leading to cerebral ischemia. As combined STA-MCA/EMS revascularization is predominantly used for pediatric patients, an insufficient caliber of the STA may be a relevant disadvantage and often represents a technical challenge for the surgeon. Nevertheless, direct anastomosis is recommended in the presence of a potentially useful donor vessel. Massive brain atrophy also represents a special contraindication as physical contact between the temporal muscle and the brain surface (brain/muscle interface) is required for successful indirect revascularization. As the temporal muscle is sutured to the dural edges, brain atrophy may increase the distance between the dura and brain surface making physical contact between muscle and brain surface impossible.

## 14.6 Special Considerations

Vascular imaging modalities represent the most important prerequisite to plan STA-MCA/EMS revascularization. Digital subtraction angiography should focus apart from the intracranial vascular status on the external carotid artery to visualize presence, size and course of the STA. Special attention has to be paid to vault moyamoya vessels, their specific contributors (i.e., occipital artery, MMA, STA, etc.) and localization. It is especially important to analyze vault moyamoya vessels in anteroposterior and lateral views in order to judge their contribution of collateral blood flow to the brain. Presence of vault moyamoya vessels fed by the MMA may either be a contraindication for this surgical strategy or it may lead to a different surgical technique for establishing EMS by opening the dura around the MMA in order to protect collateral flow via the extraintracranial anastomoses. MRI represents another important aspect not only to rule out signs of acute ischemia but also to judge brain atrophy. Major brain atrophy may represent an important obstacle making it impossible to establish a sufficient brain/muscle interface. Anticoagulation is usually established preoperatively using aspirin 100 mg orally once daily. Platelet antiaggregation is tested preoperatively using PFA-100 testing in order to rule out aspirin resistance. In the presence of aspirin resistance, the daily dose is increased to 300 mg orally, followed by PFA-100 retesting. If aspirin resistance cannot be overcome by increasing the daily dose to 300 mg, antiaggregation strategy is changed to clopidogrel 75 mg daily. In this case, surgery is then performed under clopidogrel 75 mg. It must be mentioned that other institutions deal differently with preoperative antiplatelet therapy. Some surgeons do not even perform any antiplatelet therapy before or directly after bypass surgery. Therefore, the above named antiplatelet strategy represents a recommendation in the lack of high-level evidence regarding antiplatelet therapy in moyamoya vessel patients. In the following chapters technical descriptions of each revascularization strategy include the authors' preferred antiplatelet strategy during revascularization surgery therefore a broad overview will be provided.

The anatomic specificities of the individuals STA govern the shape of the skin incision. Depending on which STA branch is used as donor vessel, a Y-shaped or a curved skin incision is used to prepare the donor vessel as well as the temporal muscle.

Special surgical care has to be applied to preparation of the temporal muscle and the galea apart from

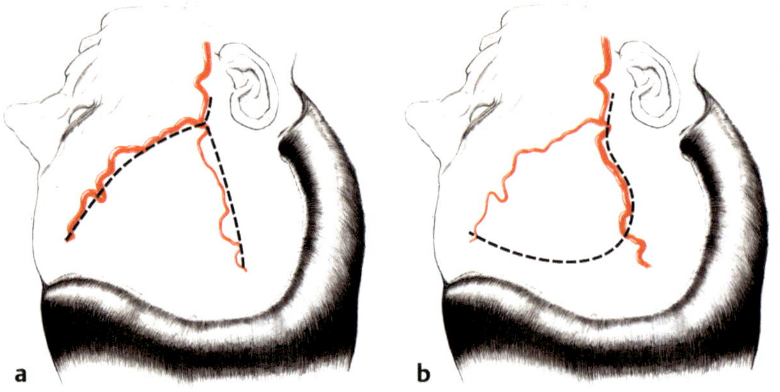

**Fig. 14.1 (a, b)** Description of skin incision strategy depending on the designated donor branch of the superficial temporal artery.

preparation of the STA, as the sacrifice of the STA and the staged preparation of the skin and temporal muscle may lead to problems with wound healing. Therefore, a clear concept for the skin incision as well as muscle preparation should be followed in order to minimize surgical trauma to these tissues (▶ Fig. 14.1). Blunt dissection of the temporal muscle from the underlying bone is performed starting from the base of the temporal muscle with stepwise dissection toward the temporal line in order to maintain structural and vascular integrity of the muscle surface. Preparation of the temporal muscle imposes an ambivalent problem as bipolar or monopolar coagulation should be avoided to protect microvascular integrity; on the other side, bleeding sources should be addressed as the surface of the temporal muscle may represent a source for postoperative hemorrhages, especially subdural hematomas. Moreover, sensitive handling of the muscle is important in order to reduce the risk for muscle edema, which may lead to compression of the cerebral surface after establishing the brain/muscle interface. As the deep temporal artery courses along the base of the temporal muscle, avoid dissection of the basal part in order to protect blood supply. The craniotomy is centered around the sylvian fissure and its individual size and shape is orientated on the shape and size of the temporal muscle before dissection is started.

## 14.7 Pitfalls, Risk Assessment, and Complications

Major pitfalls include presence of the MMA as part of vault moyamoya vessels. In these cases, opening of the dura around the MMA is performed and the temporal muscle is placed on this fenestrated transdural approach on the brain surface. Injury of the MMA during craniotomy represents a major problem for hemodynamically relevant vault moyamoya vessels as this may lead to cerebral ischemia. Establishing the craniotomy centered around the sylvian fissure usually avoids the pitfall of a nonsuitable recipient vessel on the brain surface as the perisylvian area usually represents a hotspot for sufficient recipient arteries.[9] The major risks for combined STA-MCA bypass and EMS are development of perioperative cerebral ischemia with a reported risk of 5 to 8%.[10,11] Wound healing problems occur in 2 to 6% of surgeries due to the greater wound surface generated by the combined approach compared to a targeted bypass-only approach. Hyperperfusion syndrome has been reported to range between 15 and 30% in adult moyamoya patients (lower in pediatric patients); however, most hyperperfusion syndromes present with a good prognosis.[12] Interestingly, differences are reported in hyperperfusion syndrome between Asian patient series and North American or European patient series, in which a lower incidence of hyperperfusion syndrome is reported.[10,13,14]

## 14.8 Special Instructions, Position, and Anesthesia

The patient is positioned keeping the surgical field in a horizontal plane as performed in standard STA-MCA bypass surgery. This approach includes the advantage that STA-MCA bypass may be performed in patients with unknown bypass feasibility prior to surgery. During positioning prevention of jugular venous congestion and subsequent cerebral swelling are important features that should be paid attention to as intraoperative surgical rescue maneuvers like CSF drainage to reduce brain swelling are limited in a juvenile brain with moyamoya vasculopathy. Anesthesia is usually performed following the concept of a "slack brain" in order to avoid swelling and venous congestion of the cerebral veins at the border of the durotomy. For this purpose propofol and remifentanil are key elements as they reduce cerebral metabolism and blood volume. Burst suppression on electroencephalography may be achieved by the use of barbiturates. Definitely, osmotic agents (i.e., mannitol) are administered to achieve further relaxation of the brain. Maintenance of sufficient cerebral perfusion pressure by aiming for the right mean arterial blood pressure is the second key step.

Blood pressure should be maintained at high–normal level with a mean arterial pressure targeted between 80 and 90 mm Hg at all times. A fraction of inspired oxygen of 1.0 (100%) may offer additional ischemic protection. In any case, hyperventilation should be avoided in order to prevent further reduction of the already compromised cerebral perfusion.

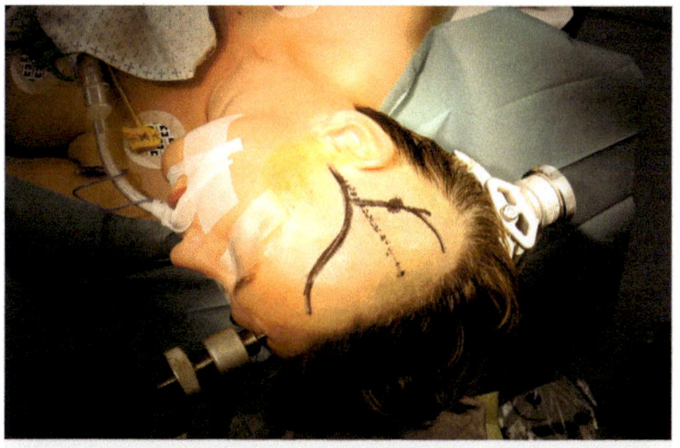

**Fig. 14.2** Head positioning and skin incision in a moyamoya patient planned for combined revascularization using superficial temporal artery-middle cerebral artery bypass and encephalo-myo-synangiosis.

## 14.9 Patient Position and Key Surgical Steps

Head is positioned in the Mayfield clamp in 90-degree rotation with the head slightly elevated above the heart level. A Y-shaped skin incision is used to dissect either the frontal or the parietal branch of the STA and to allow preparation of the temporal muscle (▶ Fig. 14.2). After skin retraction, the STA is dissected, leaving a tissue sheath around the STA to protect the vessel from manipulation and to reduce manipulation induced vasospasm (▶ Fig. 14.3). Retraction of the dissected STA branch and further skin retraction along the Y-shaped skin cut allow incision of the galea along the temporal line and the dorsal aspect of the temporal muscle (▶ Fig. 14.4). Gentle blunt preparation of the temporal muscle from proximal to distal avoiding coagulation preserves structural and vascular integrity of the temporal muscle. Avoid dissection at the base of the muscle to protect the deep temporal artery (▶ Fig. 14.5).

The size of the craniotomy is orientated on the size of the temporal muscle and it is centered around the sylvian fissure (▶ Fig. 14.6**a**). Anastomosis between the STA and a cortical perisylvian branch of the MCA is performed using a microsurgical technique (▶ Fig. 14.6**b, c**). A large dural flap is prepared and transposed upon the cortical surface

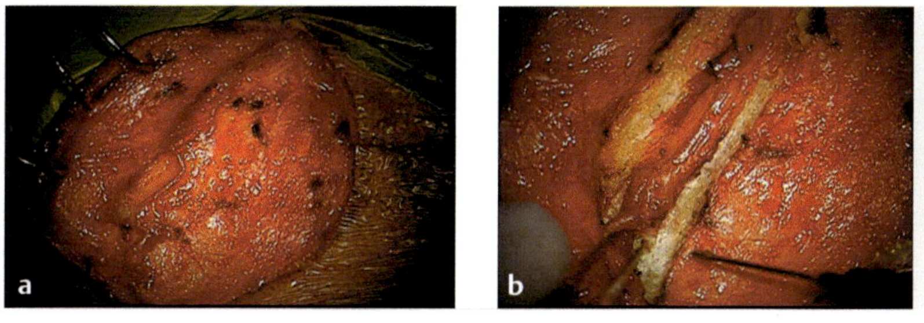

**Fig. 14.3 (a)** Identification of the frontal branch of the superficial temporal artery (STA) after skin incision. **(b)** Preparation of the STA leaving a tissue sheath around the vessel for protection purposes.

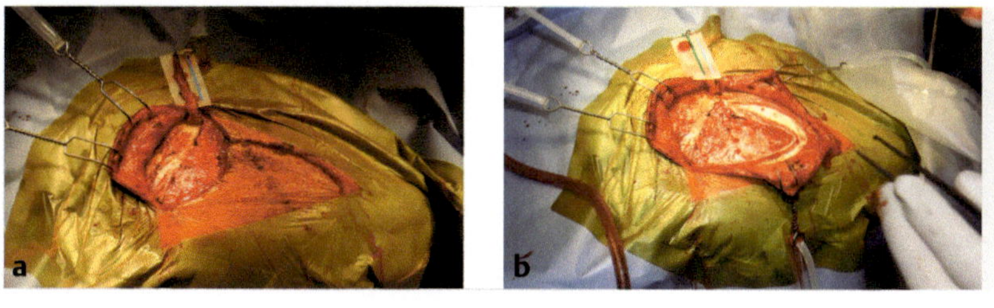

**Fig. 14.4 (a)** Skin retraction after dissection and mobilization of the frontal superficial temporal artery branch. **(b)** Skin retraction along the skin edges of the Y-shaped skin incision to allow complete exposure of the temporal muscle in order to incised the galea and mobilize the temporal muscle.

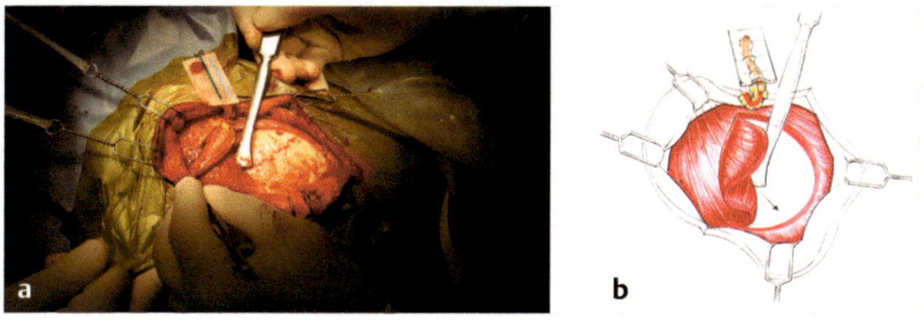

**Fig. 14.5 (a, b)** Blunt mobilization of the temporal muscle from proximal to distal in order to guarantee vascular and structural integrity of them muscle and to avoid the need for coagulation.

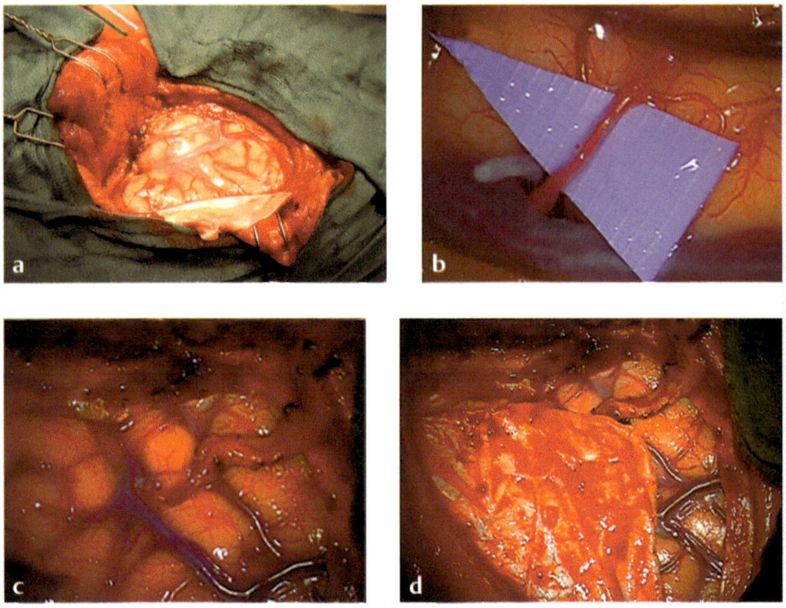

**Fig. 14.6 (a)** Visualization of the cerebral cortex after retraction for the temporal muscle and the skin edges and after opening the dura allowing clear identification of several potential recipient vessels on the cortical surface. **(b, c)** Preparation of the recipient artery in order to perform microsurgical anastomosis. **(d)** Demonstration of a dural flap which is then transposed upon the cortical surface in order to allow additional encephalo-duro-synangiosis.

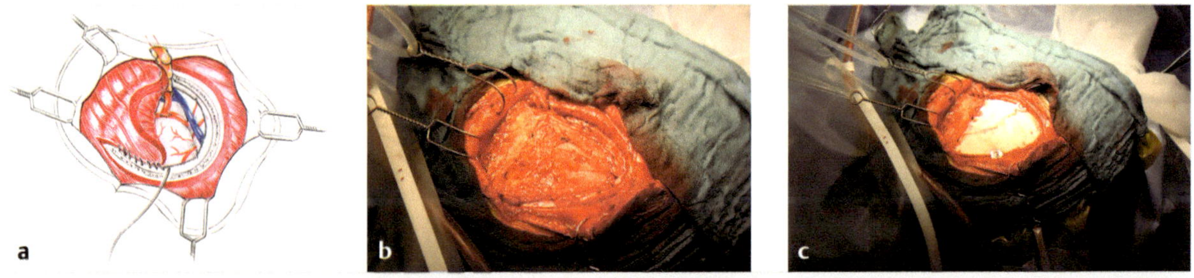

**Fig. 14.7 (a)** The temporalis muscle is sutured to the dura edge with direct contact to the cortical surface. Note that the bypass graft passes between muscle and dura edge. **(b)** Transposition of the temporal muscle upon the cortical surface; edges of the temporal muscle are sutured to the dural edges to close the epidural space and to maintain contact between the temporal muscle and the cortex avoiding slippage of the temporal muscle after wound closure. **(c)** Bone flap reimplantation; please not the osseous reduction on the base of the bone flap in order to allow enough space for the temporal muscle to transverse the skull additionally avoiding compromise to the superficial temporal artery.

to install an additional encephalo-duro-synangiosis instead of resecting the dural flap (▶ Fig. 14.6**d**).

The temporal muscle is then transposed to the cortical surface and the edges of the muscle are sutured to the dural edges (▶ Fig. 14.7**b**). Special attention has to be paid to the course of the STA donor vessel, which should not be compromised by the transposed muscle. Bone flap is reimplantated and fixed with craniofix system. Special attention has to be paid to the base of the bone flap to leave enough space for the transposed muscle flap and the STA bypass branch (▶ Fig. 14.7**c**). Avoid any compromise of either the muscle or the bypass vessel usually requiring removal of bone at the base of the bone flap.

## 14.10 Difficulties Encountered

Major difficulties include low bypass cut flow, which usually represents flow capacity of the STA. Assessment of cut flow requires measurement of blood flow in the designated bypass branch using a flow microprobe with a diameter of 1.5 mm. If cut flow is low, check for STA compression by the temporal muscle or by an accompanying vein. In the case of bypass failure after anastomosis (checked by intraoperative indocyanine green videoangiography) revision of the anastomosis should be performed. As this may be difficult in individual bases, a new anastomosis may be performed on a new recipient vessel. This rescue strategy requires sufficient length of the donor vessel and the presence of another sufficient recipient artery. If there is a lack of suitable recipient on the cortical surface, the perisylvian approach used for combined STA-MCA/EMS allows opening the sylvian fissure and preparing an M2 branch as recipient. Preparation of the temporal muscle may lead to intramuscular edema or hemorrhage which will result in a space occupying lesion if it is placed on the brain. This space occupying effect may be counteracted by leaving out the bone flap, which holds the advantage that indirect revascularization may still occur.

## 14.11 Bailout, Rescue, and Salvage Maneuvers

There are two options to deal with an insufficient bypass anastomosis. First, reopen the anastomosis and check for an intravascular thrombus occluding the anastomosis. Sometimes stitches to the posterior wall of the anastomosis become evident. In these cases redo the anstomosis. Second, cut the bypass branch, occlude the part of the branch that is left on the M4 segment of the MCA with a clip and redo the anastomosis with a new recipient. This option is only available if the donor branch provides enough length to cut it and to displace it to a novel recipient. In the case of bleeding from the temporal muscle look for careful hemostasis focusing on targeted coagulation in order to maintain vascular and structural integrity of the temporal muscle for secondary vascular sprouting to the ischmemic cerebral cortex. Applying an EMS provides the opportunity that indirect revascularization may occur in the presence of an insufficient direct anastomosis representing a rescue strategy if repetitive anastomoses fail. When massive swelling of the temporal muscle is observed during preparation, leaving out the bone flap allows for indirect decompression and may save the EMS.

## 14.12 Tips, Pearls, and Lessons learned

Skin incision was changed from a curved incision to a linear incision over the donor branch of the STA. If the frontal branch is the donor vessel of choice, a Y-shaped incision is used to allow wide access to the temporal muscle and direct preparation of the STA bypass branch with one part of the Y-shaped incision designated above the donor artery. This allows direct preparation of the donor branch without the need to prepare the donor in the skin flap after curved incision while guaranteeing good access to the temporal muscle. If the parietal branch represents the donor vessel of choice a small curved incision (as used for a small pterional approach) is performed to allow direct preparation of the parietal branch without the need to dissect the donor from the skin flap (see ▶ Fig. 14.1). Proximal to distal preparation of the temporal muscle in a blunt technique is recommended to maintain structural and vascular integrity of the temporal muscle while reducing hemorrhage from the muscle requiring coagulation. After opening the dura meticulous coagulation of dural edges is important to reduce bleeding into the operative field during the anastomosis preparation. For optimal bypass anastomosis the recipient artery is identified using intraoperative vidoeangiography assessing blood flow characteristics in the recipient prior to anastomosis. Another important aspect is to make sure that the bypass branch and the translocated temporal muscle do not interfere with each other.

## References


[1] Karasawa J, Kikuchi H, Furuse S, Sakaki T, Yoshida Y. A surgical treatment of "moyamoya" disease "encephalo-myo synangiosis". Neurol Med Chir (Tokyo). 1977; 17(1 Pt 1):29–37

[2] Matsushima T, Inoue T, Katsuta T, et al. An indirect revascularization method in the surgical treatment of moyamoya disease—various kinds of indirect procedures and a multiple combined indirect procedure. Neurol Med Chir (Tokyo). 1998; 38 Suppl:297–302

[3] Matsushima T, Inoue T, Suzuki SO, Fujii K, Fukui M, Hasuo K. Surgical treatment of moyamoya disease in pediatric patients—comparison between the results of indirect and direct revascularization procedures. Neurosurgery. 1992; 31(3):401–405

[4] Czabanka M, Vajkoczy P, Schmiedek P, Horn P. Age-dependent revascularization patterns in the treatment of moyamoya disease in a European patient population. Neurosurg Focus. 2009; 26(4):E9

[5] Czabanka M, Peña-Tapia P, Scharf J, et al. Characterization of direct and indirect cerebral revascularization for the treatment of European patients with moyamoya disease. Cerebrovasc Dis. 2011; 32(4):361–369

[6] Jussen D, Horn P, Vajkoczy P. Aspirin resistance in patients with hemodynamic cerebral ischemia undergoing extracranial-intracranial bypass surgery. Cerebrovasc Dis. 2013; 35(4):355–362

[7] Hecht N, Peña-Tapia P, Vinci M, von Degenfeld G, Woitzik J, Vajkoczy P. Myoblast-mediated gene therapy via encephalomyosynangiosis—a novel strategy for local delivery of gene products to the brain surface. J Neurosci Methods. 2011; 201(1):61–66

[8] Freyschlag CF, Seiz M, Brockmann MA, et al. Effect of mouth opening on bypass function after combined revascularization for moyamoya disease. Acta Neurochir Suppl (Wien). 2011; 112:35–38

[9] Peña-Tapia PG, Kemmling A, Czabanka M, Vajkoczy P, Schmiedek P. Identification of the optimal cortical target point for extracranial-intracranial bypass surgery in patients with hemodynamic cerebrovascular insufficiency. J Neurosurg. 2008; 108(4):655–661

[10] Guzman R, Lee M, Achrol A, et al. Clinical outcome after 450 revascularization procedures for moyamoya disease. Clinical article. J Neurosurg. 2009; 111(5):927–935

[11] Kazumata K, Ito M, Tokairin K, et al. The frequency of postoperative stroke in moyamoya disease following combined revascularization: a single-university series and systematic review. J Neurosurg. 2014; 121(2):432–440

[12] Fujimura M, Mugikura S, Kaneta T, Shimizu H, Tominaga T. Incidence and risk factors for symptomatic cerebral hyperperfusion after superficial temporal artery-middle cerebral artery anastomosis in patients with moyamoya disease. Surg Neurol. 2009; 71(4):442–447

[13] Acker G, Goerdes S, Schmiedek P, Czabanka M, Vajkoczy P. Characterization of clinical and radiological features of quasi-moyamoya disease among European Caucasians including surgical treatment and outcome. Cerebrovasc Dis. 2016; 42(5–6):464–475

[14] Acker G, Goerdes S, Schneider UC, Schmiedek P, Czabanka M, Vajkoczy P. Distinct clinical and radiographic characteristics of moyamoya disease amongst European Caucasians. Eur J Neurol. 2015; 22 (6):1012–1017

# 15 STA–MCA Bypass and EMS/EDMS

*Ken Kazumata and Kiyohiro Houkin*

**Abstract**

Moyamoya disease (MMD) primarily affects the middle and anterior cerebral arteries (MCA, ACA). The MCA as well as ACA is involved predominantly in patients with MMD. Symptomatic cases can be treated successfully by using combined (superficial temporal artery) STA–MCA anastomosis and indirect bypass procedures. Direct anastomosis can be successfully achieved in cases of infantile MMD. Combined direct/indirect bypass procedures demonstrates a several advantages over indirect procedures alone. This chapter discusses these advantages as well as technical points of the combined procedure.

*Keywords:* moyamoya disease, STA–MCA bypass, revascularization

## 15.1 History and Initial Description

Combined direct/indirect bypass for the treatment of moyamoya disease (MMD) has been utilized by the Department of Neurosurgery at Hokkaido University since 1985.[1] The procedure was developed because we had observed complications such as inconsistent and/or suboptimal growth of postoperative revascularization following indirect bypass alone, such as encephalo-duro-arterio-synangiosis (EDAS).[2] Compared with indirect procedures alone, combined superficial temporal artery–middle cerebral artery (STA–MCA) double anastomosis and indirect bypass procedures are more complex, though direct/combined bypass is more often associated with excellent revascularization than indirect bypass.[3]

## 15.2 Indications

Patients with advanced stage of MMD (Suzuki grade III or greater) who demonstrated ischemic symptoms as well as previous history of intracranial hemorrhage are considered candidates for revascularization. In ischemia, symptomatic hemispheres are treated. Asymptomatic hemispheres with hemodynamic compromise may also be treated. Revascularization surgery is performed in bilateral hemisphere of patients with prior history of intracranial hemorrhage.

## 15.3 Key Principles

Our surgical strategy is characterized by the universal application of both direct and indirect bypass regardless of the patient's age (▶ Fig. 15.1). The standard procedure consists of double STA-MCA anastomosis (▶ Fig. 15.2).

## 15.4 SWOT Analysis

### 15.4.1 Strengths

Combined direct/indirect bypass immediately increases regional cerebral blood flow (rCBF) at the site of craniotomy and prevents immediate postoperative ischemic complications.[3,4] Postoperative revascularization is more extensive following combined direct/indirect bypass than following indirect procedures alone.[6] Repeated revascularization procedures in the posterior portion of the brain are also less frequently required when compared with indirect procedures alone.

### 15.4.2 Weaknesses

This procedure can be time consuming and induce hyperperfusion and brain compression due to swelling of the temporal muscle.[5]

### 15.4.3 Opportunities

Symptomatic hemispheres (ischemic attack, stroke, and hemorrhage) are the targets of the combined direct/indirect bypass.

### 15.4.4 Threats

Bypass occlusion immediately after anastomosis is more frequent than arteriosclerotic internal carotid artery (ICA) occlusion or vascular reconstruction in aneurysmal surgery.

## 15.5 Contraindications

Patients with multiple parenchymal lesions should be treated with indirect procedures. Patients who have experienced very recent strokes or intracranial hemorrhage should be treated conservatively for the first several weeks to allow for adequate recovery from the associated brain damage. Frequent transient ischemic attacks (TIAs) represent a major risk of postoperative cerebral infarction. We try to avoid revascularization surgery during the period in which frequent TIAs are most likely to occur.

## 15.6 Special Considerations

The basic procedure consists of frontotemporal craniotomy and double STA–MCA anastomosis combined

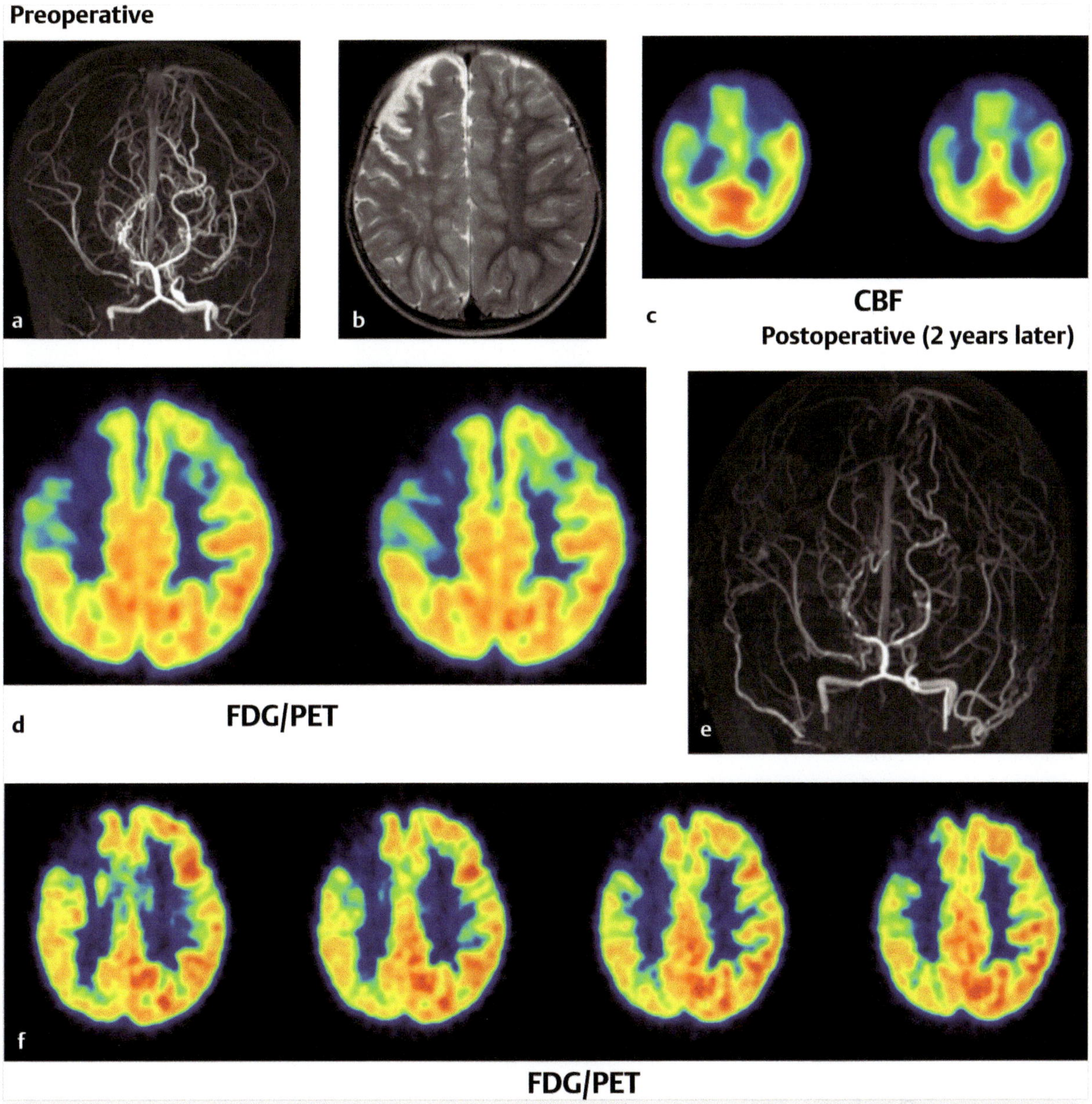


**Fig. 15.1** Combined superficial temporal artery-middle cerebral artery bypass was performed in a 3-year-old girl with right dominant arterial involvement **(a)**. T2 image suggested cerebral atrophy **(b)**, suggesting irreversible brain changes in the prefrontal regions. Cerebral blood flow was decreased beyond the area of the right frontal infarction **(c)**. Preoperative glucose metabolism (18F-FDG/PET) was also reduced adjacent to the infarction **(d)**. Nevertheless, 2 years after the successful revascularization **(e)**, an increase in glucose metabolism was observed adjacent to the right frontal infarction **(f)**.

with overlaying temporal muscle on the surface of the brain, though subsequent modifications have also been performed (▶ Fig. 15.2). For example, direct STA–ACA (anterior cerebral artery) bypass may be accomplished in addition to the standard STA–MCA bypass (▶ Fig. 15.3).[7] However, we occasionally encountered suboptimal neovascularization and skin complications using the STA–ACA/MCA bypass technique. Alternatively, indirect procedures involving the midline portion have been attempted, though the benefit of such techniques has not been clearly demonstrated with regard to postoperative stroke rates.[8] Thus, we currently utilize the conventional procedure developed in 1985.

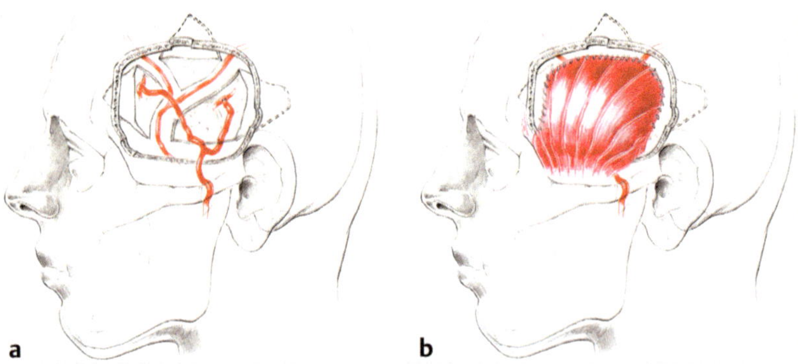


**Fig. 15.2 (a, b)** The basic procedure consists of the following three steps: (1) double superficial temporal artery–middle cerebral artery bypass, (2) preservation of the middle meningeal artery, (3) overlaying temporal muscle on the surface of the brain.

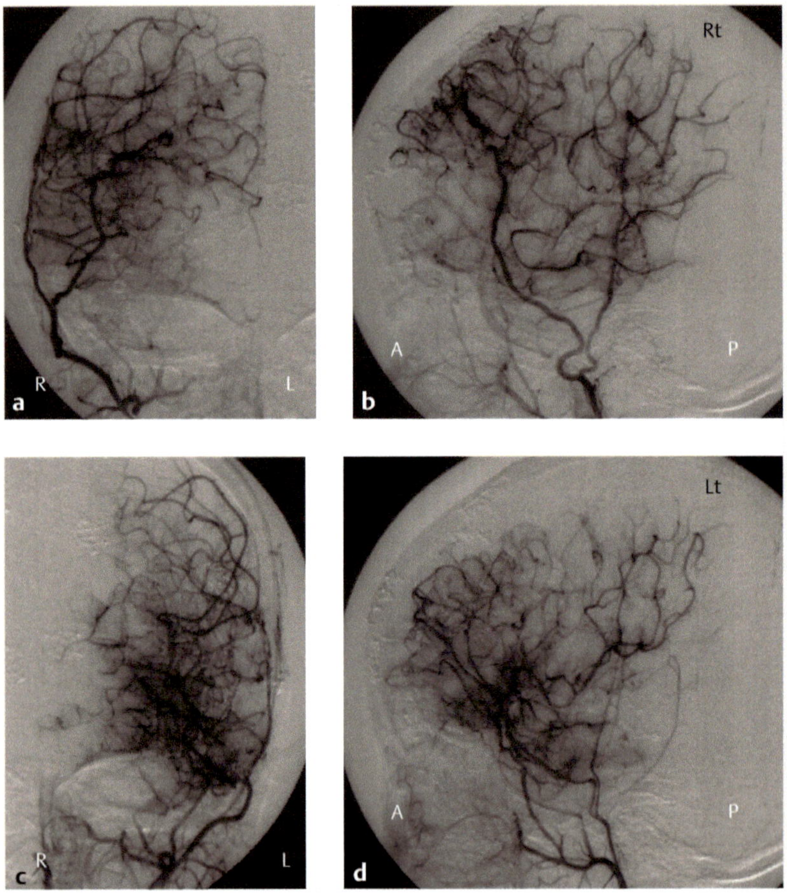


**Fig. 15.3** Postoperative angiogram after superficial temporal artery-anterior/middle cerebral artery (STA–ACA/MCA) bypass. **(a)** Right anteroposterior (AP) view; **(b)** right lateral view; **(c)** left AP view; **(d)** left lateral view. Note that the right STA–ACA supplies the right superior frontal gyrus.

## 15.7 Pitfalls, Risk Assessment, and Complications

Perioperative stroke event should be informed. We observed perioperative stroke events more frequently in adults compared with pediatric patients (adults: 7.9% of surgeries; pediatric patients: 1.7% of surgeries).[3] Overall, postoperative complications (stroke events) were observed in 4.7% of surgeries. A low-lying frontal branch of the STA leads to increases in the rate of postoperative facial palsy. Deformity of forehead is also observed due to the use of temporal muscle for indirect anastomosis. Postoperative hyperperfusion induces neurological symptoms such as headache, seizure, speech dysfunction, and numbness in mouth as well as in upper extremity. It can cause intracerebral hemorrhage.

## 15.8 Special Instructions, Position, and Anesthesia

Patients should be placed in supine position under general anesthesia. We instruct patients to discontinue antiplatelet and/or anticoagulant use prior to surgery. No

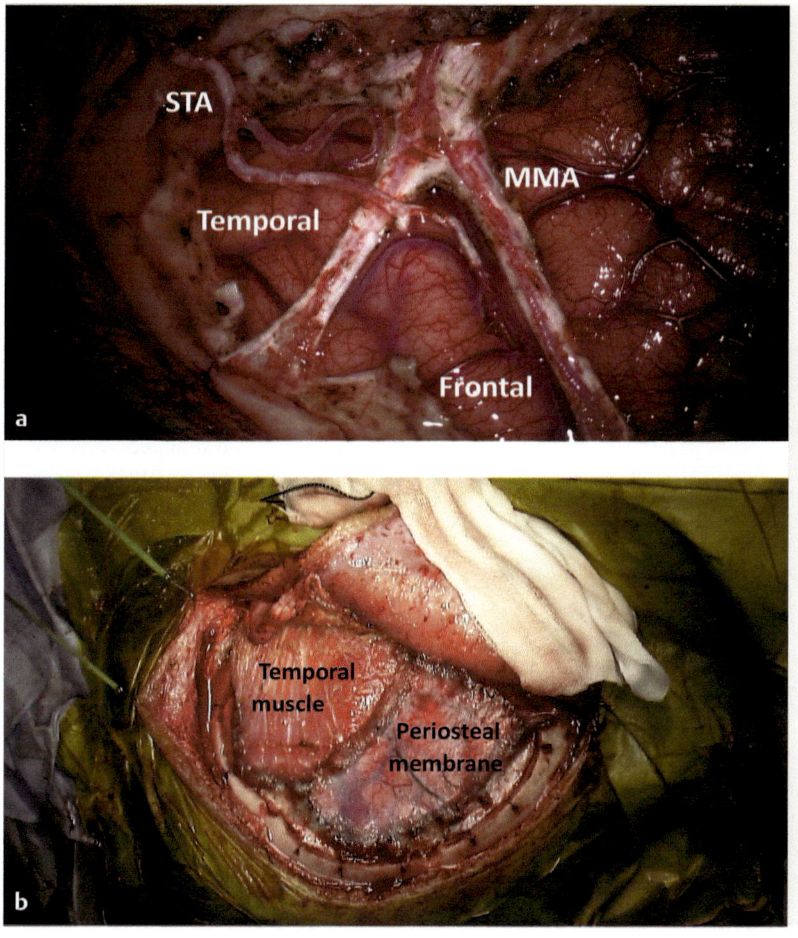


**Fig. 15.4 (a, b)** The technique of encephalo-duro-arterio-myo-synangiosis (EDMAS).

standard regimen has been established with regard to postoperative use of antiplatelet agents.

## 15.9 Patient Position with Skin Incision and Key Surgical Steps

Patients are placed in supine position. An incision line is drawn on the skin directly above the parietal branch of the STA, and a microscope is used for subsequent dissection of the STA. This maneuver likely decreases the rate of skin complications. After extensive frontotemporal craniotomy, the dura is opened while preserving the middle meningeal artery (MMA). Both the parietal branch and the frontal branch of the STA are anastomosed to the cortical branch of the MCA. The dural flap is inverted and placed on the surface of the brain to increase collateral formation (See ▶ Fig. 15.4). The temporal muscle is placed on the surface of the brain and sutured to the edge of the dura, completing encephalo-duro-arterio-myo-synangiosis (EDMAS).[1,9]

## 15.10 Difficulties Encountered

Frequently, bypass thrombosis occurs.

## 15.11 Bailout, Rescue, and Salvage Maneuvers

To avoid bypass occlusion and an STA pedicle, single anastomosis can be performed with the parietal branch of the STA left intact and laid over the surface of the brain (arterial synangiosis). While some surgeons may not perform indirect procedures in adult patients, we always perform the indirect procedure in addition to the direct procedure. The additional benefit of the indirect procedure has been investigated and reported elsewhere.[10]

The MMA should be preserved due to its significant contribution to postoperative neovascularization (▶ Fig. 15.5). Normocapnia and normotension should be maintained throughout the surgery.

## 15.12 Tips, Pearls, and Lessons Learned

In the immediate postoperative period, rCBF increases predominantly in the basal ganglia, which is followed by

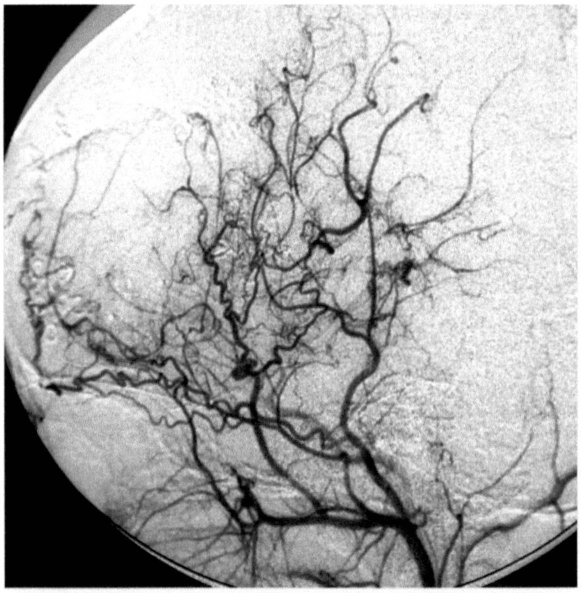

Fig. 15.5 Typical postoperative angiogram (lateral view of carotid angiogram) after combined superficial temporal artery-middle cerebral artery bypass. The deep temporal artery is also involved in neovascularization in the frontal lobe.

a gradual increase in lateral prefrontal hyperperfusion.[4] Immediate postoperative increases rCBF in subcortical structures are potentially associated with intracerebral hemorrhage following surgery. Prefrontal hyperperfusion is associated with transient neurological deterioration. Regional CBF is assessed using 123I-IMP/SPECT on postoperative day 1 and day 7. Systolic blood pressure is controlled below 140 mm Hg via continuous intravenous administration of $Ca^{2+}$ antagonists, if necessary. In general, hyperperfusion is a self-limiting process, though transient neurological deficits may occur during the first 2 weeks. Necrosis along with skin incision may also be observed. Therefore, the surgical site should be monitored for proper healing after discharge from the hospital. Bypass patency can be evaluated via magnetic resonance angiography (▶ Fig. 15.6). Immediate postoperative posterior cerebral artery (PCA) regression is observed in approximately 10% of patients (▶ Fig. 15.7).

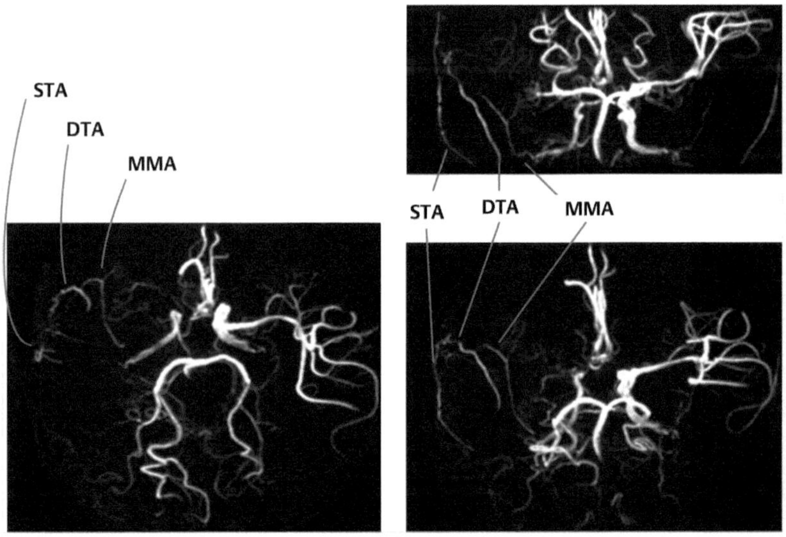


Fig. 15.6 Postoperative monitoring can be performed using magnetic resonance angiography. There are three routes of collateral supply from the external carotid system after the combined direct and indirect bypass: superficial temporal artery, deep temporal artery, and middle meningeal artery.

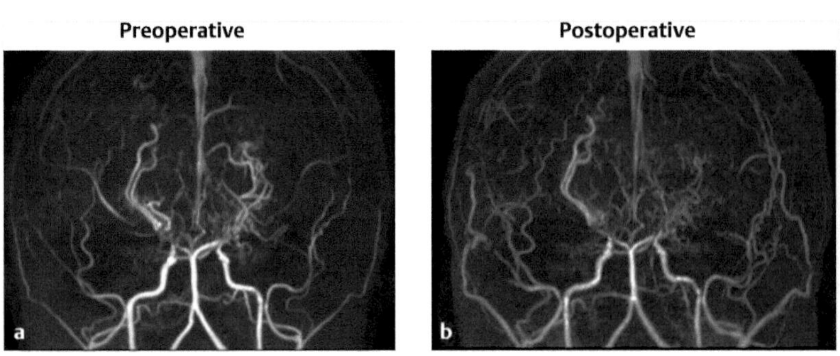


Fig. 15.7 Left posterior cerebral artery regression was observed following combined superficial temporal artery-middle cerebral artery. **(a)** Presurgery; **(b)** postrevascularization surgery.

# References


[1] Houkin K, Kamiyama H, Takahashi A, Kuroda S, Abe H. Combined revascularization surgery for childhood moyamoya disease: STA-MCA and encephalo-duro-arterio-myo-synangiosis. Childs Nerv Syst. 1997; 13(1):24–29

[2] Matsushima T, Fujiwara S, Nagata S, et al. Surgical treatment for paediatric patients with moyamoya disease by indirect revascularization procedures (EDAS, EMS, EMAS). Acta Neurochir (Wien). 1989; 98 (3–4):135–140

[3] Kazumata K, Ito M, Tokairin K, et al. The frequency of postoperative stroke in moyamoya disease following combined revascularization: a single-university series and systematic review. J Neurosurg. 2014; 121(2):432–440

[4] Kazumata K, Tha KK, Uchino H, et al. Topographic changes in cerebral blood flow and reduced white matter integrity in the first 2 weeks following revascularization surgery in adult moyamoya disease. J Neurosurg. 2017; 127(2):260–269

[5] Uchino H, Kuroda S, Hirata K, Shiga T, Houkin K, Tamaki N. Predictors and clinical features of postoperative hyperperfusion after surgical revascularization for moyamoya disease: a serial single photon emission CT/positron emission tomography study. Stroke. 2012; 43 (10):2610–2616

[6] Bang JS, Kwon OK, Kim JE, et al. Quantitative angiographic comparison with the OSIRIS program between the direct and indirect revascularization modalities in adult moyamoya disease. Neurosurgery. 2012; 70(3):625–632, discussion 632–633

[7] Ishikawa T, Kamiyama H, Kuroda S, Yasuda H, Nakayama N, Takizawa K. Simultaneous superficial temporal artery to middle cerebral or anterior cerebral artery bypass with pan-synangiosis for moyamoya disease covering both anterior and middle cerebral artery territories. Neurol Med Chir (Tokyo). 2006; 46(9):462–468

[8] Kuroda S, Houkin K, Ishikawa T, Nakayama N, Iwasaki Y. Novel bypass surgery for moyamoya disease using pericranial flap: its impacts on cerebral hemodynamics and long-term outcome. Neurosurgery. 2010; 66(6):1093–1101, discussion 1101

[9] Kuroda S, Houkin K. Bypass surgery for moyamoya disease: concept and essence of sugical techniques. Neurol Med Chir (Tokyo). 2012; 52 (5):287–294

[10] Uchino H, Kim JH, Fujima N, et al. Synergistic interactions between direct and indirect bypasses in combined procedures: the significance of indirect bypasses in moyamoya disease. Neurosurgery. 2016

# 16 Combined Direct (STA–MCA) and Indirect (EDAS) EC–IC Bypass

*Erez Nossek, Annick Kronenburg, and David J. Langer*

**Abstract**

We espouse utilization of both the frontal and parietal branches of the superficial temporal artery (STA) when anatomically appropriate to treat symptomatic moyamoya disease (MMD) and syndrome (MMS). The frontal branch is used as the direct donor by performing an anastomosis with a cortical middle cerebral artery (MCA) artery, while the parietal branch is combined with dural reflections to create a large surface area of vascularized tissue for indirect revascularization. Patients are treated when they present with clear symptoms of ischemia or hemorrhage. Ischemic patients are exclusively treated when hemispheric blood flow testing demonstrates clear hypoperfusion. Asymptomatic hemispheres are only considered for treatment following successful treatment of a symptomatic contralateral hemisphere. MMD and MMS represent an uncommon but increasingly recognized cause of stroke in young and middle-aged adults in North America. Excellent outcome of treatment can be achieved by carefully selecting patients and maintaining a technical proficiency in the creation of both direct STA–MCA as well as indirect grafts for cerebral revascularization.

*Keywords:* moyamoya vasculopathy, cerebral revascularization, stroke, bypass

## 16.1 History and Initial Description

Extracranial–intracranial (EC–IC) bypass for the treatment of the symptomatic hypoperfused hemisphere in intracranial steno-occlusive diseases, secondary to atherosclerotic disease or moyamoya vasculopathy (MMV), is currently the treatment of choice.[1,2] The use of a combined direct superficial temporal artery to middle cerebral artery (STA–MCA) and indirect encephalo-duro-arterio-synangiosis (EDAS), by performing an STA onlay with flipped dural flaps, is advocated as an optimal treatment option as it allows immediate augmentation of blood flow in the postoperative period, while providing the brain to acquire additional indirect flow in the long term.[3] Dual placement of direct and indirect bypasses within the same hemisphere has been demonstrated by formal diagnostic angiogram, regardless of patients' age and the hemodynamic status, to be of benefit with the indirect graft serving as an adjunct to a direct bypass in order to maximize revascularization.[3] Quantitative magnetic resonance imaging (QMRI) studies have shown a reciprocal relationship between the direct and the indirect bypasses after combined bypass surgery, thus providing complementary revascularization.[4]

The STA is the terminal branch of the external carotid artery (ECA). It supplies the anterolateral part of the scalp. This artery usually (in 71.4–95.7% of the vessels) bifurcates *above* the level of the superior margin of the zygomatic arch. The mean inner diameter of the STA at the level of the zygomatic arch is approximately 2.2 to 2.7 ± 0.5 mm.[5,6] The STA commonly bifurcates into an anterior frontal branch that courses anterosuperiorly and a posterior parietal branch that courses posterosuperiorly. The vessel however can be highly irregular in its anatomy and therefore its course must be studied angiographically preoperatively to insure adequate mapping of its trajectory (▸ Fig. 16.1). The inner diameter of the frontal and parietal branches is approximately 1.4 to 2.1 and 1.4 to 1.8 at 7 cm respectively, distal to the zygomatic arch.[6,7]

## 16.2 Indications

The operative benefits of combined cerebral revascularization have been previously demonstrated with combined

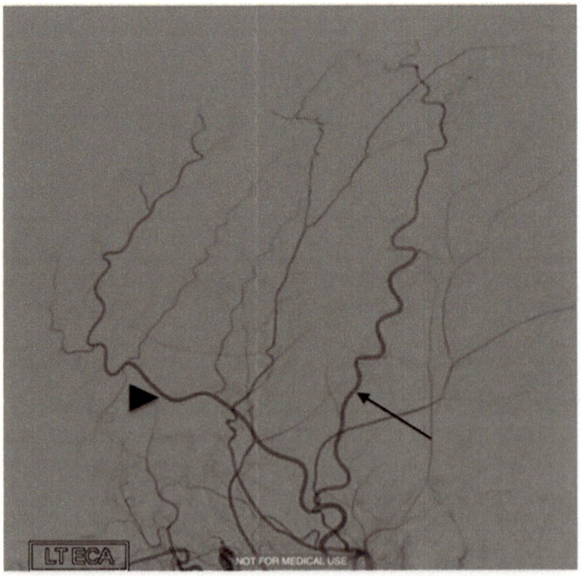


**Fig. 16.1** Preoperative diagnostic angiography. External carotid artery (ECA) injection, lateral projection, demonstrating the STAfb (*arrowhead*) and STApb (*arrow*).

hemispheric revascularization shown to decrease rates of both ischemic and hemorrhagic stroke.[8,9] Increased attention has also been directed at cognitive function, an important determinant of the quality of life, in patients with MMD. Cognition in MMD has been shown to be affected,[10] possibly due to occult strokes, although it has also been shown in patients without stroke.[11] Definitive benefits on cognition following revascularization have yet to be fully characterized. A recent systematic review concluded that combined cerebral revascularization was superior in producing favorable long-term clinical outcome.[12] However, combining both techniques at the same procedure may be challenging and its nuances are critical for a good surgical and long-term outcome. In our previously published case series of patients treated with neurosurgical revascularization, the number of peri- and postoperative complications was acceptable, supporting evidence for the safety of these procedures in selected groups of patients.[13] To favor optimal cerebral revascularization of the affected hemisphere, combined direct and indirect bypass therapy should become a standard treatment modality among vascular neurosurgeons when treating symptomatic MMV. Although little is known about the optimal timing of surgical intervention, we prefer not to perform revascularization surgery in the acute phase, which is in accordance with common practice.[14] Patients presenting with hemorrhage are initially managed conservatively, with surgical consideration and radiographic workup performed following at least 2 to 3 months after recovery. Patients with transient ischemic attacks or those with small watershed ischemic infarction can be treated earlier following their full workup. Patients with larger recent infarctions are treated in more of a delayed fashion but usually within a month of their stroke, depending upon their neurological condition. We consider treating asymptomatic hemispheres in patients with bilateral MMV who have been revascularized on their symptomatic side, when there is evidence of hypoperfusion on cerebral hemodynamic studies.

## 16.3 Key Principles

The bypass procedure consists of (1) distal to proximal donor vessel preparation of the frontal STA branch (STAfb) for direct and the parietal STA branch (STApb) for indirect revascularization, followed by (2) a craniotomy in the region of interest (preferably a hypoperfused area as demonstrated on hemodynamic studies), (3) performing the anastomosis with a cortical M4 branch and verifying patency, (4) performing the EDAS, and (5) meticulous wound closure.

## 16.4 SWOT Analysis

- **Strength:** Bypass surgery is the only surgical therapy for MMD and MMS that carries a low complication risk and favorable clinical outcome.
- **Weakness:** Extensive surgical experience in bypass surgery and familiarity with the clinical key aspects of moyamoya are mandatory for successful treatment.
- **Opportunity:** Due to a low caseload, this surgical therapy is only performed in a few centers worldwide, which is creating an inadequate number of experienced treating facilities.
- **Threat:** Since the footprint of endovascular therapy is growing, fewer neurosurgeons are trained in microvascular surgery.

## 16.5 Contraindications

Surgery in patients who carry a high general anesthesia risk should be extensively studied and great care taken should be taken before recommending operative intervention. Asymptomatic moyamoya patients without hemodynamic compromise should not be operated on, but should be monitored over time instead. Bypass surgery in large infarcted areas should be avoided since it carries a great risk of intracerebral hemorrhage.

## 16.6 Special Considerations

### 16.6.1 Preoperative Considerations

MMV management requires a comprehensive workup including a directed medical history of the patient and physical examination. We study patients with MRI, quantitative magnetic resonance angiography (QMRA) by using noninvasive optimal vessel analysis software (NOVA; VasSol, River Forest, Chicago, IL) to assess cerebral blood flow, and single-photon emission computed tomography (CT) with and without acetazolamide to assess cerebral perfusion and vascular reserve. Conventional digital subtraction angiography (DSA) is utilized primarily in patients where treatment is being contemplated. A six-vessel DSA is performed as close to the planned surgical date as possible, since vascular anatomy can change over time in this dynamic disease. Preoperative angiographic assessment includes assessment of the specific course of the STA branches (▶ Fig. 16.1) in order to evaluate and support successful harvesting of the donor artery. We discuss each pertinent finding with the patient and family and review the procedure step by step with our neurovascular team. We review the plan starting from hospital admission and continuing through preoperative preparation, the procedure itself, and the postoperative period. We believe that the well-educated patient familiar with all periprocedural details will achieve a better overall experience and outcome.

### 16.6.2 Postoperative Considerations

The first 24 hours postoperatively patients are admitted to an intensive care unit and special attention is paid to

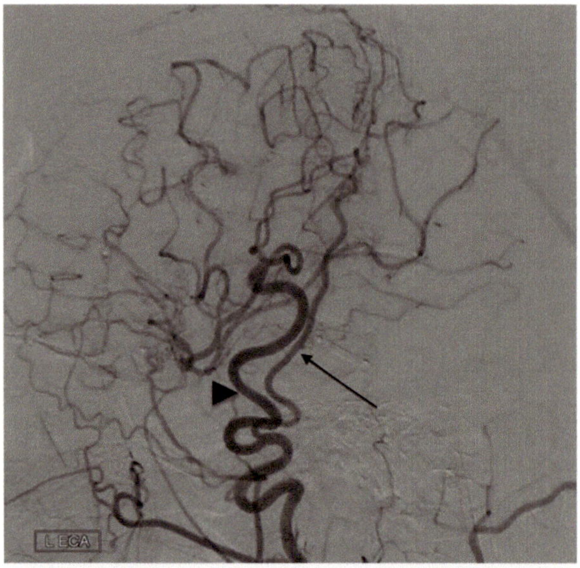


**Fig. 16.2** A 24-month follow-up, subtracted external carotid artery (ECA) angiography demonstrating the STApb (*arrow*) passing through the craniotomy site and the STAfb (*arrowhead*) with robust flow into the distal middle cerebral artery (MCA) branches.

maintain normotension to ensure the patency of the bypass and to prevent hyperperfusion syndrome, which may cause temporary neurological deficits. A postoperative conventional CT angiography or DSA is performed to confirm bypass patency. In the illustrative case presented here, the postoperative angiogram at 6 months shows a robust flow through the both the STAfb direct bypass in to the MCA branches and the STApb continues to flow distal to the craniotomy site. We also perform QMRA in the immediate postoperative period. We continue to follow the patient both clinically and by QMRA at 3 months and DSA at 6 months follow-up (▶ Fig. 16.2). The indirect graft is assessed and a contralateral "indirect only" surgery is considered on the asymptomatic hemisphere if robust collateral flow from the EDAS is seen on angiography. We maintain the patient on aspirin 81 mg per day unless there is a medical contraindication. Patients who have presented with hemorrhage have their aspirin stopped 3 months postoperatively.

## 16.7 Pitfalls, Risk Assessment, and Complications

An important complication of the procedure is graft thrombosis. Special attention must be paid to ensure anastomosis patency intraoperatively and postoperative secondary measures to prevent graft occlusion, such as maintaining normotension, normovolemia, and the administration of antiplatelet therapy (aspirin) is of importance. Bypass surgery should not be performed in large infarcted areas, since it carries the risk of intracerebral hemorrhage in damaged brain tissue. Wound healing problems and (low-grade) infections may occur at a higher rate due to diminished blood supply of the skin. With the careful selection of patients, morbidity and mortality rates in our and other centers[12,13,15] have been acceptable and outweigh the possible complications of the procedure, especially since bypass surgery remains the only proven therapy for these patients.

## 16.8 Special Instructions, Position, and Anesthesia

Aspirin (325 mg) is administered the night before the procedure. In the perioperative period moyamoya patients are at risk of developing ischemia in a hypoperfused hemisphere during general anesthesia. This is of particular concern in patients with bilateral MMV. The following four principles are followed by an experienced neuroanesthesia team: normotension, normovolemia, normoventilation, and normothermia. Hyperventilation (causing cerebral vasoconstriction) and fluctuating blood pressures, which may cause watershed infarction, need to be avoided. Furthermore, hemoglobin and hematocrit levels need to be within the baseline levels. Mannitol and diuretic therapy should be avoided.

## 16.9 Patient Position with Skin Incision and Key Surgical Steps

### 16.9.1 Description of the Technique

We place the patient in supine position in a Sugita head frame with the head rotated contralateral to the treatment side without flexion or extension. The pinning of the calvarium should be done 7 cm posterior to the marked STApb in order to allow incision without any limitations, and especially for posterior retraction of the skin flap (▶ Fig. 16.3). Following pinning, a hand-held Doppler is used to mark the course of both the anterior frontal branch of the STAfb and the STApb (▶ Fig. 16.4). These branches are marked from their proximal bifurcation at the level of the tragus. The STApb is mapped distally up to 2 cm above the superior temporal line, and the STAfb distally up to the level of the frontal process of the zygomatic bone ("Key Hole") at the anterior, superior margin of the temporal muscle.

Donor vessel dissection is performed under the microscope or exoscope. We start with the STApb dissection from distal to proximal in order to avoid proximal damage to the vessel. By using a blunt malleable brain retractor that is inserted into the subgaleal plane directly over the STA to dissect the STApb, it allows us to create a linear

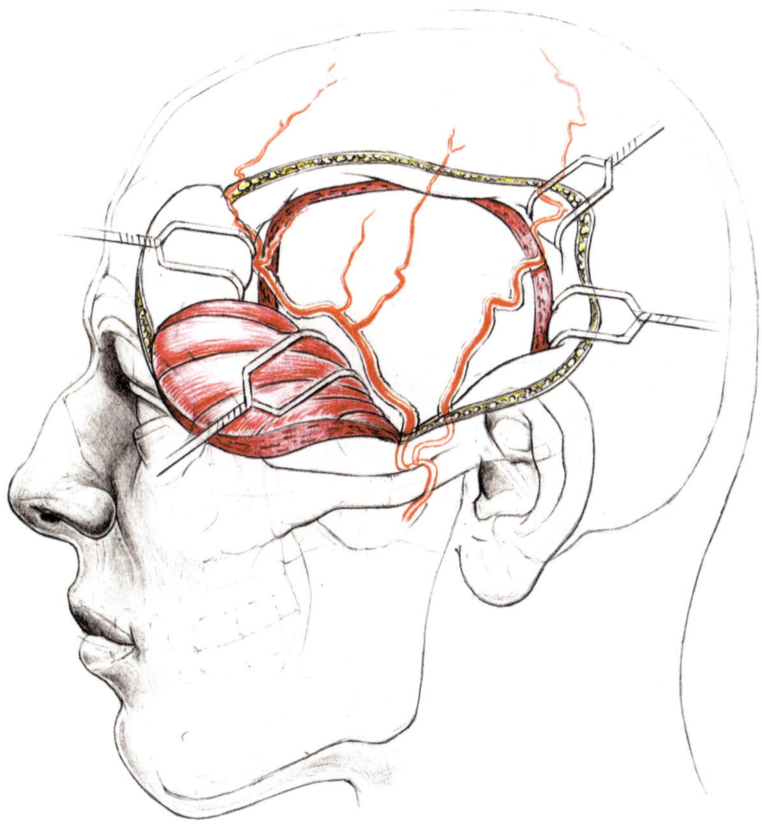

**Fig. 16.3** The temporalis muscle is "tunneled" anteriorly under the STAfb. Inset: Contemplated skin incision and location of the STAfb and STApb. The ascending limb of the skin incision is done over the ultrasound-based marking of the STAfb. (Note the posterior retraction of the skin in order to allow for a free onlay indirect bypass.)

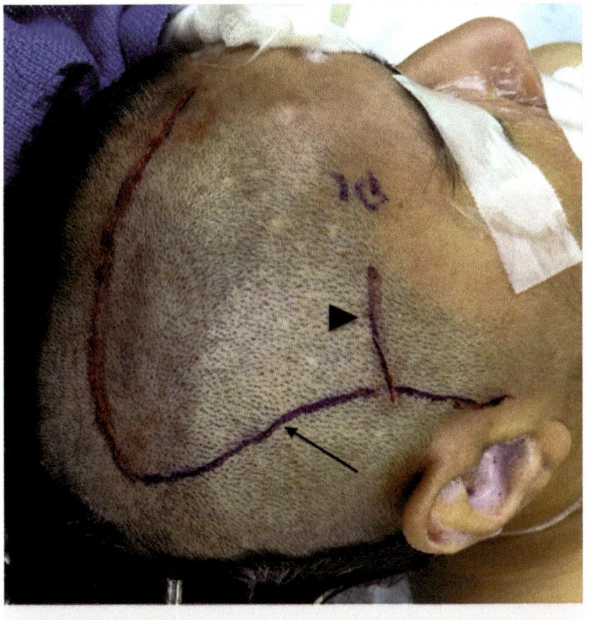

**Fig. 16.4** Preoperative ultrasound-based marking of the STAfb (*arrowhead*) and STApb (*arrow*).

incision and concurrent protection of the STA in its bed.[16] As we progress with the dissection, we place fish hooks over the skin flap anteriorly and posteriorly to allow for easier retraction and safer vessel dissection. We leave a periadventitial cuff along the vessels in order to avoid spasm of the vessel. We follow the vessel proximally to identify the bifurcation of the STA. At this level, veins may be adherent to the STA, which should not be mistaken for the STAfb and subsequently followed instead of the actual branch. We recommend a total length of 10 to 12 cm to be dissected to achieve good dissection of the vessel in order to prevent tension of the artery when covering the brain beneath the bone flap. The caliber of the STAfb is preferably at least 0.8 mm. Great care needs to be taken as the dissection extends to the origin of the STAfb proximally. The surface skin marking of the STAfb can serve as a target to identify the frontal branch origination point. At this point we continue the distal skin incision where we turn it anteriorly toward the mid pupillary line, an imaginary line extending from the pupil to the mid frontal region. The proximal part of the anterior limb of the skin incision should be carried with great attention not to damage the distal STApb (▶ Fig. 16.5).

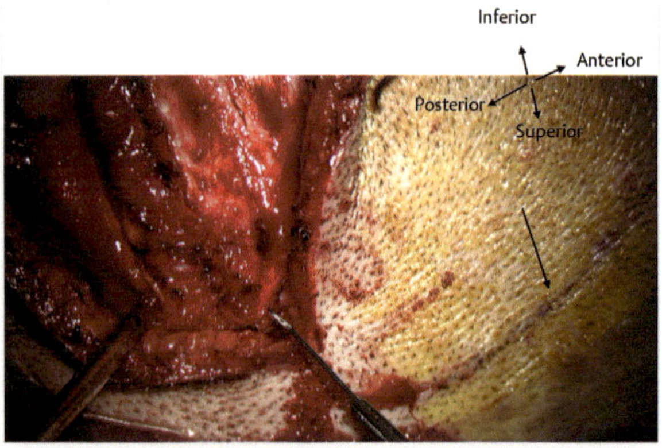


**Fig. 16.5** Skin incision anterior to the distal segment of the STApb to connect with the frontal limb of the incision (*arrow*).

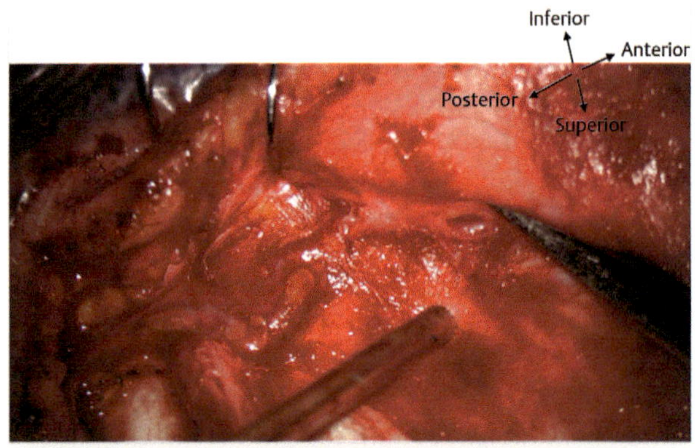


**Fig. 16.6** Dissection of the STAfb from proximal toward its distal segment. The dissection of the vessel is done within the subcutaneous tissue of the frontal skin flap.

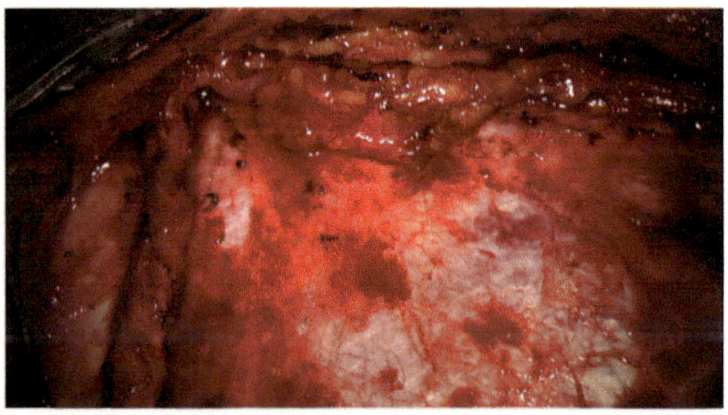

**Fig. 16.7** The two branches of the superficial temporal artery (STA) lay over the temporalis fascia.

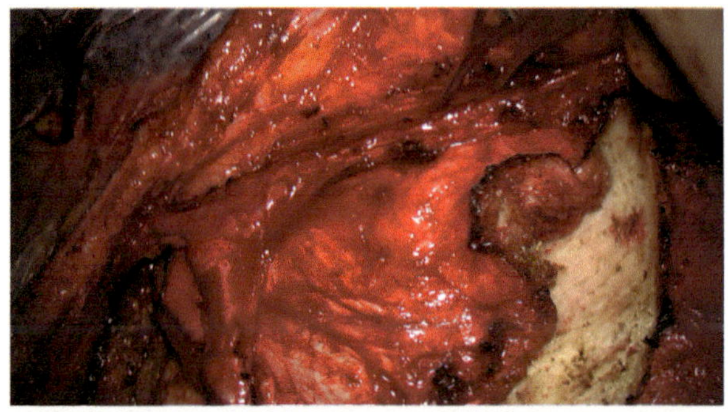

**Fig. 16.8** Subperiosteal detachment of the temporalis muscle.

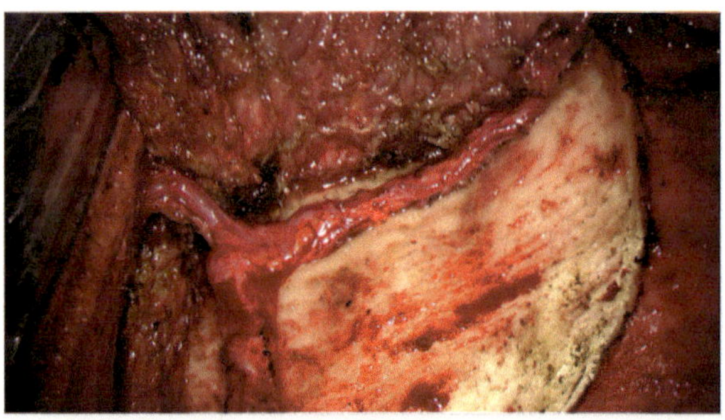

**Fig. 16.9** The temporalis muscle is "tunneled" anteriorly under the STAfb.

We elevate the skin flap anteriorly and dissect the STAfb from proximal toward its distal segment (▶ Fig. 16.6). The dissection of the vessel is done within the subcutaneous tissue of the frontal skin flap utilizing tenotomy scissors and microforceps under the operating microscope. We dissect the STAfb distally beyond the level of the pterion and keyhole, where it lays over bone, at the superior edge of the temporal muscle (▶ Fig. 16.7).

We retract the skin flap using fish hooks posteriorly, thus exposing the posterior part of the temporal muscle. The posterior cut of the temporal muscle is done at least 2 cm posterior to the STApb, and the muscle flap is elevated anteriorly under the two dissected vessels that are left in situ until the brain is exposed (▶ Fig. 16.8). By tunneling the muscle beneath the frontal branch, the vessel is brought into the field prior to the craniotomy and does not have to be reaccessed during the course of the surgery as would be the case when rereflecting the temporal muscle (▶ Fig. 16.9). The STAfb is marked in order to prevent twisted donor vessel (▶ Fig. 16.10).

Two burr holes under the trajectory of STApb are created: one temporal and one parietal. These holes become the entry and exit points for the EDAS, and need to be in line with the anatomic course of the vessel. The craniotomy is performed through the burr hole to elevate a free round bone flap with diameter of approximately 4 cm (▶ Fig. 16.11). Care must be taken not to damage the middle meningeal artery when serving an intracranial dural collateral during the craniotomy. The craniotome is used only in trajectories away from the vessels. The dura is then opened in a curved fashion and a flap is elevated anteriorly tunneled under the STAfb (▶ Fig. 16.12).

The donor STAfb is then addressed. Preferably, a cortical M4 branch is chosen as a recipient for the direct bypass (▶ Fig. 16.13). We measure the length of the vessel to verify that the transposition will reach the anastomosis site without tension by using a silk suture as measurement (▶ Fig. 16.14, ▶ Fig. 16.15). The vessel is temporarily clipped as proximal as possible. The distal STAfb is cut and vessel fully heparinized. Coloring of the distal vessel with ink often helps to identify loose adventitial tissue that should be removed. The distal vessel is then fishmouthed. We measure the cut flow in the STAfb using the Charbel flow probe (Transonic Systems Inc. Ithaca, NY). The distal aspect of the STAfb utilized for the direct graft must be cleaned thoroughly by dissecting all distal periadventitial tissue over a length of 1.0 to 1.5 cm. We then proceed with the direct bypass as described in Chapter 2 (▶ Fig. 16.16, ▶ Fig. 16.17, ▶ Fig. 16.18, ▶ Fig. 16.19, ▶ Fig. 16.20). We use 10–0 nylon with a BV 75-3 needle from Ethicon Surgical. We verify flow by using micro-Doppler (Mizuho Inc. Tokyo, Japan), measure cut flow index utilizing the Charbel flow probe and patency by using indocyanine green videoangiography.

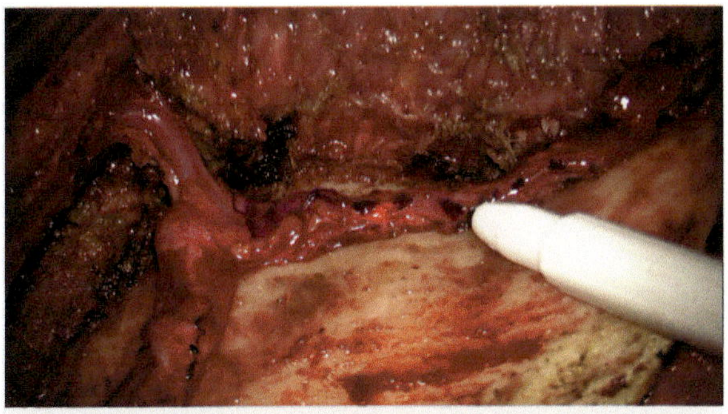

**Fig. 16.10** The STAfb is marked in order to prevent twisted donor vessel.

With the bypass completed, we proceed with the EDAS: the STApb is laid over the cortex. Several openings of the arachnoid are created underlying the STApb in order to enhance spontaneous vascularization. The STApb cuff is sutured to the pia or dural edge with a 9–0 Ethilon nylon monofilament needle (BV130-5) to achieve fixation of the vessel over the cortex (2–3 sutures). This graft must be tension free and the vessel must lay loosely and with adequate contact to the brain surface. We then divide the dural flap into two flaps based on anterior pedicle to facilitate their flipping with their periosteal layer over the cortex (▶ Fig. 16.21, ▶ Fig. 16.22).

We prepare the bone flap with enlargement of the burr hole sites to allow for the EDAS and direct graft vessels to enter and exit under the bone without compression or kinking. The temporalis muscle is closed with 2–0 vicryl. Very often the muscle itself is partially incised with a monopolar to avoid muscular compression of the two grafts. A submuscular drain is placed. The closure of the skin is performed with great attention especially at the penetrating site of the donor vessels under the bone flap. The skin is closed in layers with the subgaleal layer closed with 2–0 vicryl and the skin closed with a nylon stitch. We usually do no not use a subgaleal suture over the proximal STA, but prefer continuous nylon sutures of the skin. Care must be taken not to strangle the skin edges as the flap is at risk for wound healing problems due to reduced blood supply to the skin of the STA.

## 16.10 Difficulties Encountered

- Dissection of the STA branches may be difficult since small veins may cross the course of the arteries.

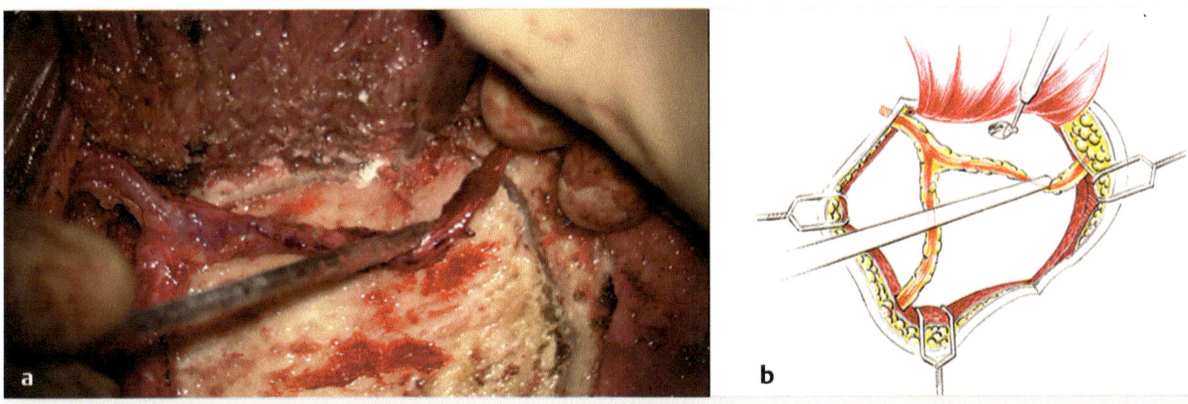

**Fig. 16.11 (a, b)** The craniotomy is done through the burr hole to elevate a free round bone flap with diameter of 4 cm. Care must be taken not to damage the vessels during the craniotomy.

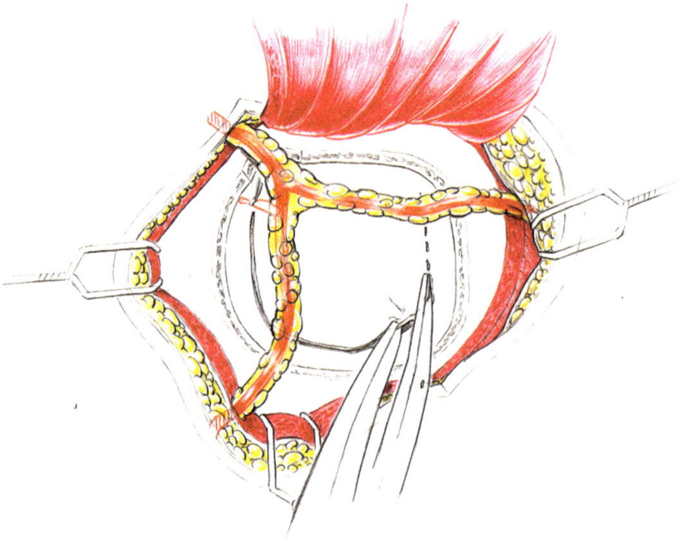

**Fig. 16.12** Opening of the dura: the indirect STApb is laid over the exposed brain. The STApb is traveling from the temporal burr hole toward the parietal burr hole. Inset: Contemplated burr holes under the trajectory of the STApb.

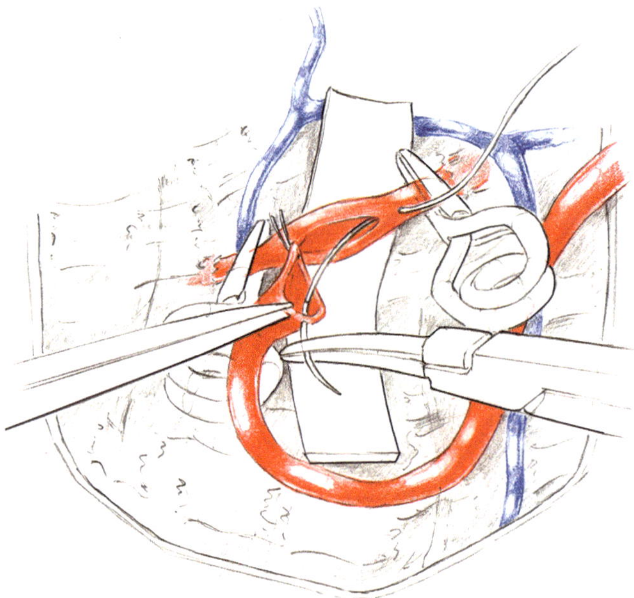

**Fig. 16.13** The anastomosis site is chosen on a cortical M4 segment anteriorly to the STApb.

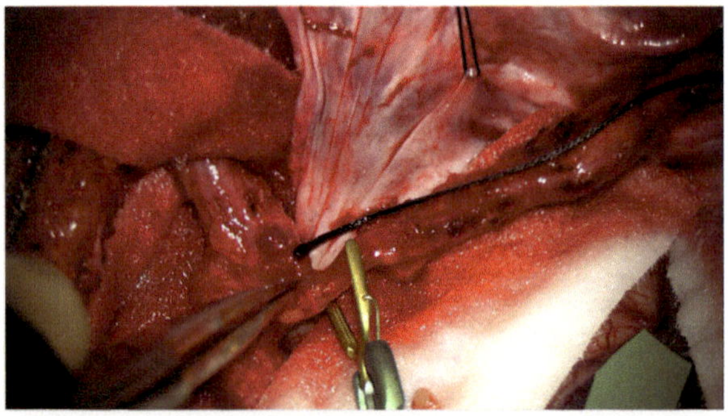

**Fig. 16.14** We measure the length of the vessel to verify that the transposition will reach the anastomosis site without tension utilizing a silk suture.

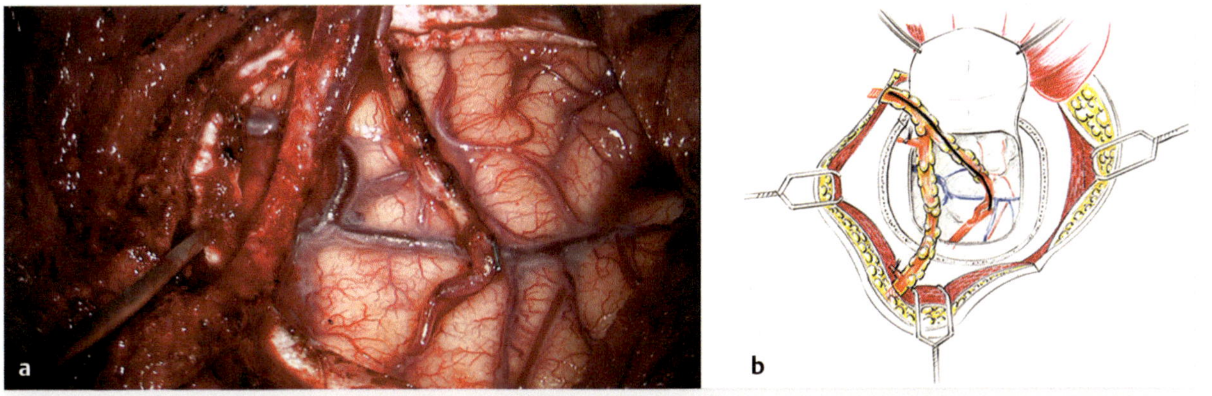

Fig. 16.15 (a, b) The indirect graft is freed so that it will rest on the cortical surface without tension. We verify that the direct graft, when transposed, will reach the anastomosis site without tension as well.

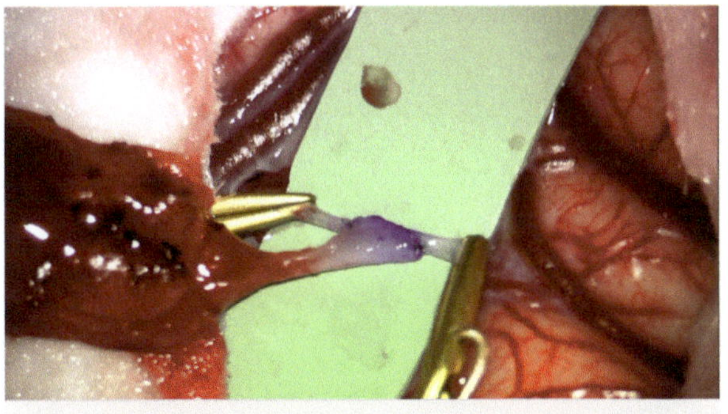

Fig. 16.16 The M4 recipient is temporarily occluded, incised, and locally heparinized. We then begin the anastomosis with apical sutures.

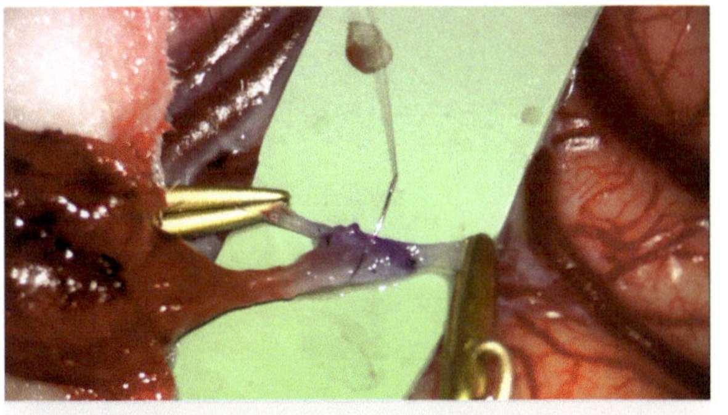

Fig. 16.17 A back wall retention stitch is placed and left untied to tent the back wall away from the front wall.

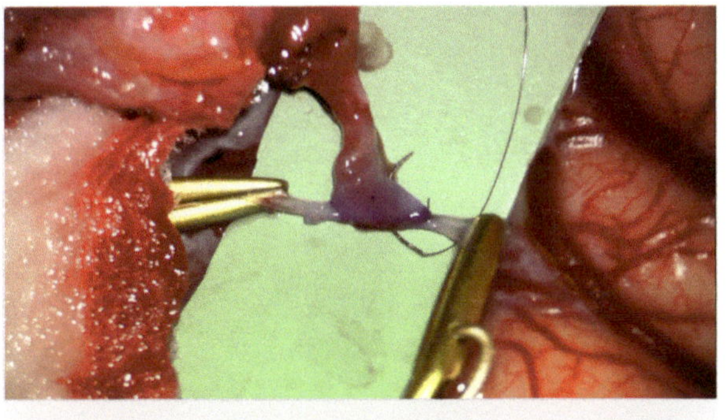

Fig. 16.18 The anastomosis site is flipped to begin with the anterior wall. Note the retention untied stitch on the back wall.

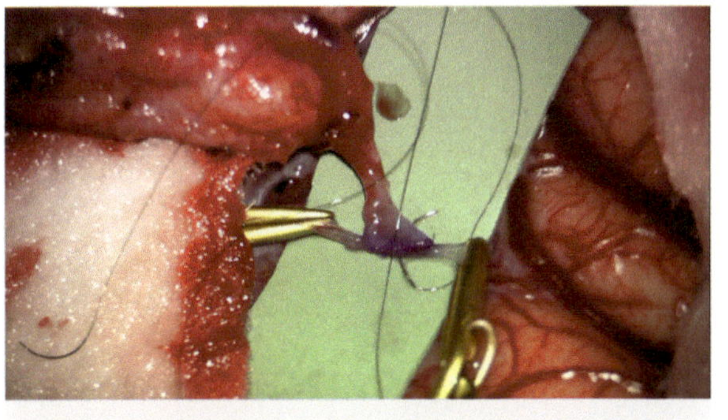

Fig. 16.19 The anastomosis site is flipped and the first stitch on anterior wall is placed.

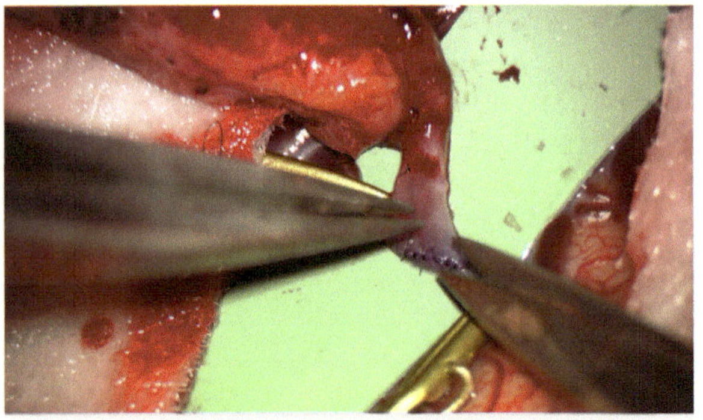

**Fig. 16.20** Final appearance of front wall anastomosis. We prefer an interrupted technique; however, a continuous suturing technique can be utilized as well.

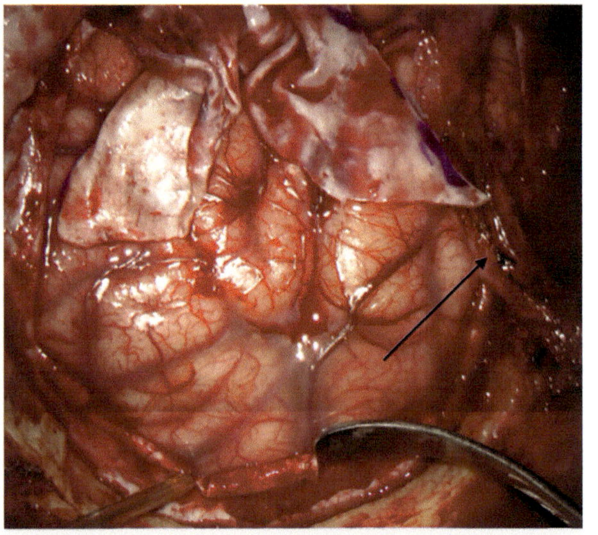

**Fig. 16.22** Intraoperative image of the final result of combined direct/indirect bypass, with STApb onlay bypass (*arrow*), STAfb direct bypass and encephalo-duro-arterio-synangiosis, with flipped dural flaps.

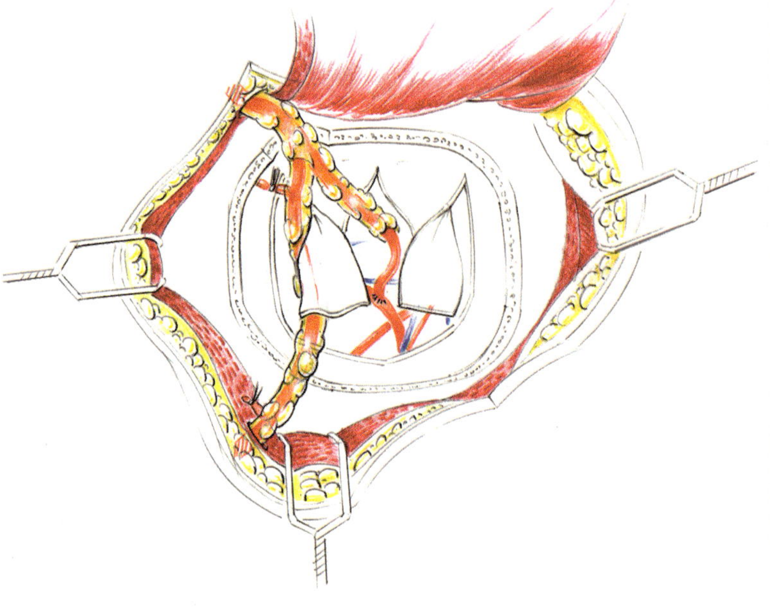

**Fig. 16.21** Final result of combined direct/indirect bypass, with STApb onlay bypass, STAfb direct bypass and encephalo-duro-arterio-synangiosis, with flipped dural flaps.

- The middle meningeal artery can be damaged during craniotomy (which may serve as an indirect transdural collateral).
- If the donor graft is not of adequate length, tension on the anastomosis may make the bypass impossible.
- Donor vessel spasm can occur. Generous use of papaverine-soaked Gelfoam and cottonoids may be of benefit.
- Opening of the arachnoid while performing the EDAS may cause small cortical bleedings from the typical cortical moyamoya vessels resulting in microinfarcts.
- Whenever the bone flap is not fitted to allow the graft vessels to enter and exit under the bone, the arteries may be compressed and occlude.
- During skin closure sutures may entangle or perforate the grafts possibly rendering them useless.

## 16.11 Bailout, Rescue, and Salvage Maneuvers

In case the STAfb is extensively damaged during the dissection, it may be considered to use the STApb for the direct procedure. Preoperatively the flow and patency of the anastomosis is verified. Whenever the graft is not patent, it has to be reopened to ensure that sutures are not misplaced and/or to inspect if blood clots are occluding the graft. To prevent puncturing of the direct graft during skin closure, a small surgical spatula can be placed covering and protecting the graft while suturing the cutaneous layer of the skin.

## 16.12 Tips, Pearls, and Lessons Learned

- Gain experience in a laboratory facilitating the training in microsurgical and anastomosis procedures.
- Besides mastering the technical skills, it is of importance to familiarize with all aspects of this rare disease to optimize clinical outcome in this group of patients.
- The right indication and patient selection has as much if not more to do with the success of the procedure than the physical performance of the surgery. “Far more patients suffer form poor indication rather than poor operation.”

## References

[1] Esposito G, Amin-Hanjani S, Regli L. Role of and indications for bypass surgery after carotid occlusion surgery study (COSS)? Stroke. 2016; 47(1):282–290

[2] Kuroda S, Houkin K. Moyamoya disease: current concepts and future perspectives. Lancet Neurol. 2008; 7(11):1056–1066

[3] Uchino H, Kim J-H, Fujima N, et al. Synergistic interactions between direct and indirect bypasses in combined procedures: the significance of indirect bypasses in moyamoya disease. Neurosurgery. 2017; 80(2):201–209

[4] Amin-Hanjani S, Singh A, Rifai H, et al. Combined direct and indirect bypass for moyamoya: quantitative assessment of direct bypass flow over time. Neurosurgery. 2013; 73(6):962–967, discussion 967–968

[5] Marano SR, Fischer DW, Gaines C, Sonntag VK. Anatomical study of the superficial temporal artery. Neurosurgery. 1985; 16(6):786–790

[6] Pinar YA, Govsa F. Anatomy of the superficial temporal artery and its branches: its importance for surgery. Surg Radiol Anat. 2006; 28(3): 248–253

[7] Kim BS, Jung YJ, Chang CH, Choi BY. The anatomy of the superficial temporal artery in adult Koreans using three-dimensional computed tomographic angiogram: clinical research. J Cerebrovasc Endovasc Neurosurg. 2013; 15(3):145–151

[8] Jiang H, Ni W, Xu B, et al. Outcome in adult patients with hemorrhagic moyamoya disease after combined extracranial-intracranial bypass. J Neurosurg. 2014; 121(5):1048–1055

[9] Kazumata K, Ito M, Tokairin K, et al. The frequency of postoperative stroke in moyamoya disease following combined revascularization: a single-university series and systematic review. J Neurosurg. 2014; 121(2):432–440

[10] Kronenburg A, van den Berg E, van Schooneveld M, et al. Cognitive functions in children and adults with moyamoya vasculopathy: a systematic review and meta-analysis. J Stroke. 2018; 20(3): 332–341

[11] Karzmark P, Zeifert PD, Bell-Stephens TE, Steinberg GK, Dorfman LJ. Neurocognitive impairment in adults with moyamoya disease without stroke. Neurosurgery. 2012; 70(3):634–638

[12] Sun H, Wilson C, Ozpinar A, et al. perioperative complications and long-term outcomes after bypasses in adults with moyamoya disease: a systematic review and meta-analysis. World Neurosurg. 2016; 92: 179–188

[13] White TG, O'Donnell D, Rosenthal J, et al. Trends in cerebral revascularization in the era of pipeline and carotid occlusion surgery study. World Neurosurg. 2016; 91:285–296

[14] Kronenburg A, Braun KPJ, van der Zwan A, Klijn CJM. Recent advances in moyamoya disease: pathophysiology and treatment. Curr Neurol Neurosci Rep. 2014; 14(1):423

[15] Guzman R, Lee M, Achrol A, et al. Clinical outcome after 450 revascularization procedures for moyamoya disease. Clinical article. J Neurosurg. 2009; 111(5):927–935

[16] Schirmer CM, David CA. Superficial temporal artery dissection: a technical note. Neurosurgery. 2013; 72(1) Suppl Operative:6–8, discussion 8

# 17 STA–MCA Anastomosis and EDMAPS

*Satoshi Kuroda*

**Abstract**

Superficial temporal artery to middle cerebral artery (STA–MCA) anastomosis and encephalo-duro-myo-arterio-pericranial synangiosis (EDMAPS) is one of the combined bypasses for moyamoya disease. The novel indirect bypass, EDMAPS enables us to most widely cover the frontal lobe by using the vascularized frontal pericranium. This technique can provide collateral blood flow to almost the entire territory of the internal carotid artery, including the anterior cerebral artery. Thus, STA–MCA anastomosis and EDMAPS may be named as an "ultimate" bypass for moyamoya disease. In this chapter, the author introduces the concept, surgical technique, and pitfalls of STA–MCA anastomosis and EDMAPS for moyamoya disease.

*Keywords:* moyamoya disease, STA–MCA anastomosis, EDMAPS, ultimate bypass

## 17.1 History and Initial Description

### 17.1.1 STA–MCA Anastomosis and EDMAPS as an "Ultimate" Bypass

▶ Fig. 17.1 shows the historical flow of bypass surgery for moyamoya disease at Hokkaido University Hospital. Nakagawa et al established encephalo-myo-arterio-synangiosis (EMAS) in the early 1980s. The temporal muscle and superficial temporal artery (STA) were used as the donor for indirect bypass.[1] However, the incidence of perioperative ischemic complications was not low.[2] Subsequent studies also showed that cerebral hemodynamics was impaired in the frontal lobe even several years after surgery.[3] At that time, STA–MCA (middle cerebral artery) single or double anastomosis was routinely performed, and craniotomy was extended to the frontal area in order to further supply collateral blood to the frontal lobe in the late 1980s. The temporal muscle, STA, and dura mater were utilized as the donor for indirect bypass, called as encephalo-duro-myo-arterio-synangiosis (EDAMS). As a result, the incidence of perioperative ischemic stroke markedly decreased probably because of immediate improvement of blood flow after direct bypass.[2,4] Postoperative blood flow studies revealed significant improvement of cerebral hemodynamics in the frontal lobe after STA–MCA anastomosis and EDAMS. Intellectual outcome significantly improved in pediatric patients.[5] However, about 10% of pediatric patients still experienced paraplegic transient ischemic attack (TIA) even after surgery probably because the temporal muscle, a main donor tissue for indirect bypass, covers mainly the MCA territory. Hemorrhagic stroke also recurred in about 20% of adult patients even after STA–MCA anastomosis and EDAMS.[6]

Based on these historical observations, Kuroda et al performed STA–MCA single or double anastomosis and extended craniotomy to the medial frontal area to further improve cerebral hemodynamics in the anterior cerebral artery (ACA) territory in the late 1990s. The frontal pericranial flap was used to widely cover the medial frontal lobe in addition to the temporal muscle, STA, and dura mater. A pericranial flap has been widely used to reconstruct the anterior cranial fossa because of its simplicity, reliability, and low morbidity. As reported by Yoshioka and Rhoton, the frontal pericranium receives blood flow mainly from the supraorbital and supratrochlear arteries arising from the ophthalmic artery.[7] The indirect bypass procedure was named as encephalo-duro-myo-arterio-pericranial synangiosis (EDMAPS). As a result, no pediatric patients have experienced paraplegic TIA after surgery. Clinical results strongly suggest that the incidence of recurrent hemorrhagic stroke is much lower than before.[8] Now, we are routinely performing STA–MCA anastomosis and EDMAPS for patients with moyamoya disease. Very recently, we evaluated cumulative incidence of late morbidity/mortality among 93 patients who underwent STA–MCA anastomosis and EDMAPS and were followed up for longer than 5 years post-surgery (mean, 10.5 ± 4.4 years). As per results, 92 of 93 patients were free from any stroke or death, but one recurred hemorrhagic stroke during follow-up periods (0.10% per patient-year, submitted data). Therefore, we believe that STA–MCA anastomosis and EDMAPS would be the best choice to prevent further cerebrovascular events for longer than 10 years by widely providing surgical collaterals to both MCA and ACA territories. In this chapter, therefore, the author describes the concept, surgical procedures, pitfalls, risk, and perioperative managements of STA–MCA anastomosis and EDMAPS.

## 17.2 Indications and Contraindications

Direct bypass procedures can quickly improve cerebral hemodynamics after surgery, and thus can significantly lower the incidence of perioperative ischemic events, including TIA and ischemic stroke.[1] Furthermore, TIA and/or headache attack quickly decreases in frequency or disappears during follow-up periods after direct bypass procedure. These clinical results of direct bypass are supported by immediate blood flow improvement just after surgery.[2,3] The procedures can flexibly be modified as

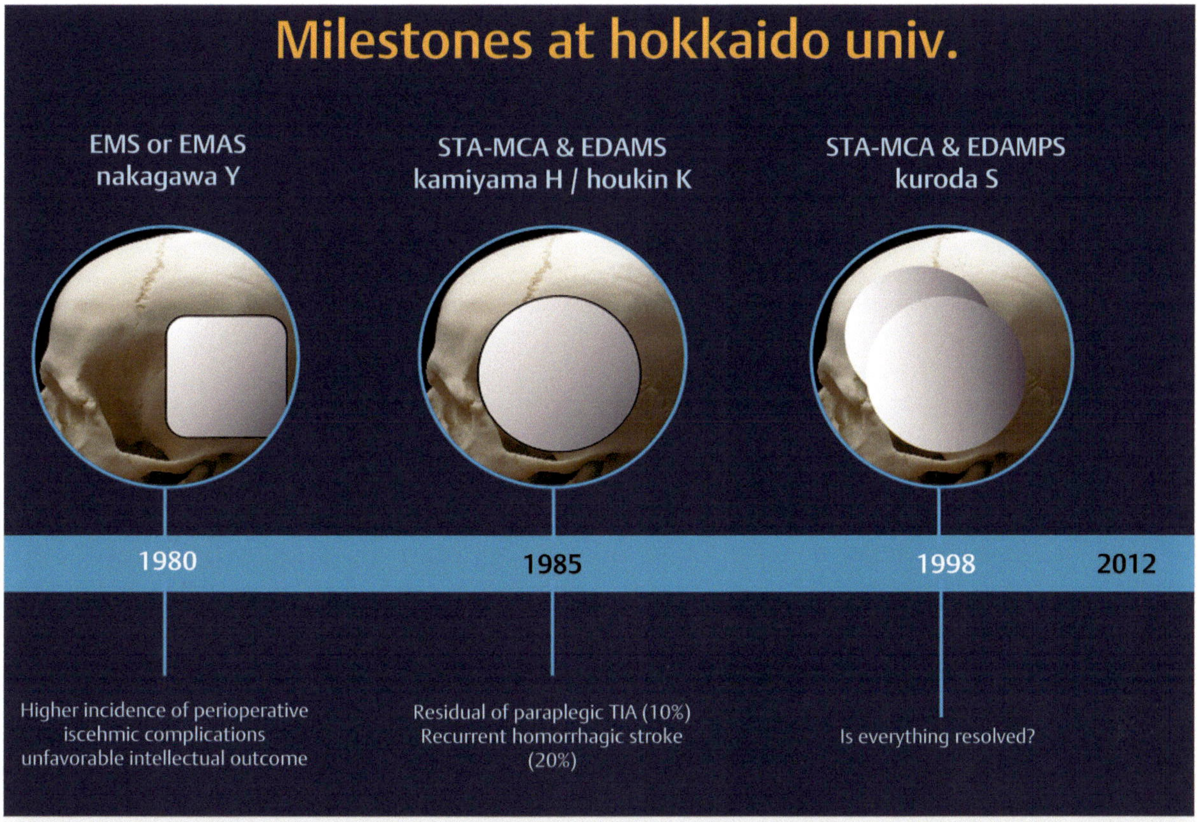


**Fig. 17.1** Milestones of bypass surgery for moyamoya disease at Hokkaido University Hospital.

STA–anterior cerebral artery (ACA) or STA–posterior cerebral artery (PCA) anastomosis according to patients' condition, such as dense ischemia in the territory of the ACA or PCA.[4] However, surgical procedure for direct bypass requires skillful technique and thus a certain surgical training, because the recipients have a small caliber (0.5–1.0 mm in diameter) and more importantly a very thin wall in a majority of patients with moyamoya disease. In addition, it should be reminded that direct bypass procedure would carry the risk for postoperative hyperperfusion, which sometime causes severe neurological sequelae and/or mortality unless appropriate managements are indicated (see ▶ Fig. 17.1).[5] On the other hand, indirect bypass procedures are technically simple and easy, because the vascularized donor tissues are only put onto the surface of the brain. Surprisingly, an aggressive neovascularization occurs between the donor tissues and the brain and start to provide collateral blood flow to the ischemic brain in moyamoya disease. However, indirect bypass may increase the incidence of perioperative TIA and/or ischemic stroke especially in patients with dense ischemia before surgery, because the neovascularization requires 3 to 4 months to establish collateral blood flow.[2,6] It is well known that surgical collaterals develop in almost all pediatric patients, although previous reports have shown that efficient surgical collaterals develop through indirect bypass in about 50 to 70% of adult patients with moyamoya disease.[7] Furthermore, surgeons should be aware that the extent of craniotomy largely determined the extent of surgical collaterals through indirect bypass. As aforementioned, it is well known that cerebral ischemia is most dense in the frontal lobe, thus craniotomy for indirect bypass should widely be extended to the frontal area.

**Table 17.1** Indirect bypass versus direct bypass

| | Advantage | Disadvantage |
|---|---|---|
| Indirect bypass | • Simple and easy | • Surgical collaterals develop 2 to 3 months postsurgery<br>• Higher incidence of perioperative ischemic stroke<br>• Effective in only 50% of adults |
| Direct bypass | • CBF improves just after surgery<br>• Lower incidence of perioperative ischemic stroke<br>• TIA quickly disappears | • Surgical training needed<br>• Possibility of hyperperfusion |

Combination of direct and indirect bypass may be the best choice for moyamoya disease because an immediate supply of collateral blood flow can compensate for the shortcoming of indirect bypass. Indirect bypass often functions as a major source of surgical collaterals in a certain subgroup of patients even after combined bypass procedure in a majority of pediatric patients and a certain subgroup of adult patients. Thus, reciprocal STA regression occurs in about 30% of the hemispheres during the transition from the postoperative acute phase to the chronic phase during indirect bypass development.[7]

## 17.2.1 Asymptomatic Moyamoya Disease

Recent studies have shown that the prevalence of asymptomatic moyamoya disease is much higher than considered before. Based on the exhaustive survey in Hokkaido Island, Japan, about 20% of patients with newly diagnosed moyamoya disease were asymptomatic.[9] Although the natural course of asymptomatic moyamoya disease is not fully understood, previous nation-wide observational study in Japan revealed that the annual risk of any cerebrovascular events and stroke was 5.7 and 3.2%, respectively. Disturbed cerebral hemodynamics at initial diagnosis was significantly linked to ischemic episodes. Disease progression during follow-up periods also highly caused ischemic cerebrovascular episodes. However, the cohort of this study was small ($n = 34$).[10] Therefore, the Research Committee on Moyamoya Disease in Japan started a prospective multicenter, nation-wide observational study, called as Asymptomatic Moyamoya Registry (AMORE) in January 2012 to further clarify the epidemiology, pathophysiology, and prognosis in asymptomatic moyamoya disease. As a result, a total of 109 subjects were enrolled during 4 years, and they were carefully followed-up for 5 years. Therefore, the author believes that no bypass surgery should be indicated for asymptomatic moyamoya disease at least until AMORE study reaches any conclusion in 2020.[11]

## 17.2.2 Ischemic-Tpe Moyamoya Disease

There are no effective medical therapies to reduce or prevent further TIA and/or ischemic stroke in moyamoya disease. Importantly, the physicians should be aware that headache attack is closely related to cerebral ischemia and should be recognized as one symptom of TIA in pediatric moyamoya disease. Most of "symptomatic" hemispheres have disturbed cerebral hemodynamics in the territory of internal carotid artery (ICA) due to the reduction of cerebral perfusion pressure (CPP), which is characterized by the most severe ischemia in the frontal lobes. In addition, the involvement of the posterior cerebral artery (PCA) may often impair cerebral hemodynamics in the occipital lobe.

When determining the indication of bypass surgery for moyamoya disease, it is quite valuable to assess the CPP by measuring cerebral blood flow (CBF) before and after intravenous injection of acetazolamide using single photon emission computed tomography (SPECT), positron emission tomography (PET), or cold xenon CT. Reduced reactivity to acetazolamide would be a key finding to identify the reduced CPP in the involved hemispheres. Therefore, STA–MCA anastomosis and EDMAPS should be indicated to the "symptomatic" hemispheres of both pediatric and adult patients who experienced TIA and/or ischemic stroke.[8]

## 17.2.3 Hemorrhagic-Type Moyamoya Disease

For a long time, it remained to be debated whether surgical revascularization would reduce the incidence of recurrent hemorrhagic stroke in adult patients with moyamoya disease. Recently, however, Japan Adult Moyamoya (JAM) Trial Group has shown that direct or combined bypass could significantly reduce it in adult patients who developed hemorrhagic stroke due to bilateral-type moyamoya disease within 6 months after the onset.[12]

# 17.3 Key Principles

STA–MCA anastomosis combined with EDMAPS can quickly improve cerebral hemodynamics through direct bypass procedure and can widely improve it through indirect bypass that entirely covers the involved hemisphere by using the whole vascularized donor tissues around the head, including the artery, dura, muscle and pericranium. Our 20-year experience has proved that this procedure can markedly reduce any further stroke for up to 20 years after surgery.

# 17.4 SWOT Analysis

- **Strengths:** STA-MCA anastomosis combined with EDMAPS quickly improves cerebral hemodynamics through direct bypass procedure and widely improves it through indirect bypass that entirely covers the involved hemisphere by using the whole vascularized donor tissues around the head, including the artery, dura, muscle and pericranium. In addition, this procedure can markedly reduce any further stroke for up to 20 years after surgery.
- **Weakness:** Only well-trained or experienced surgeons are allowed to perform this procedure in order to minimize the incidence of surgical and/or perioperative complications.
- **Opportunities and Threats:** Refer to the detailed description under Chapter 17.2.

## 17.5 Special Considerations

As described in Chapter 3, CBF measurement is essential to determine the surgical design, including the extent of craniotomy and the recipient. Especially, craniotomy and dural opening should be planned to cover the frontal lobe as widely as possible, because the frontal lobe is severely exposed to cerebral ischemia in moyamoya disease. Indeed, intellectual outcome is significantly poor in pediatric patients who underwent surgical revascularization through a small craniotomy that does not cover the frontal lobe.

It is still determined whether the antiplatelets or anticoagulants would be useful to reduce the frequency of ischemic attacks or the incidence of perioperative complications, including ischemic stroke and graft occlusion. However, the author never uses either of them because TIA and ischemic stroke occur due to hemodynamic compromise, but not artery-to-artery embolism. Furthermore, adult patients are at high risk for hemorrhagic stroke before and even after surgical revascularization.

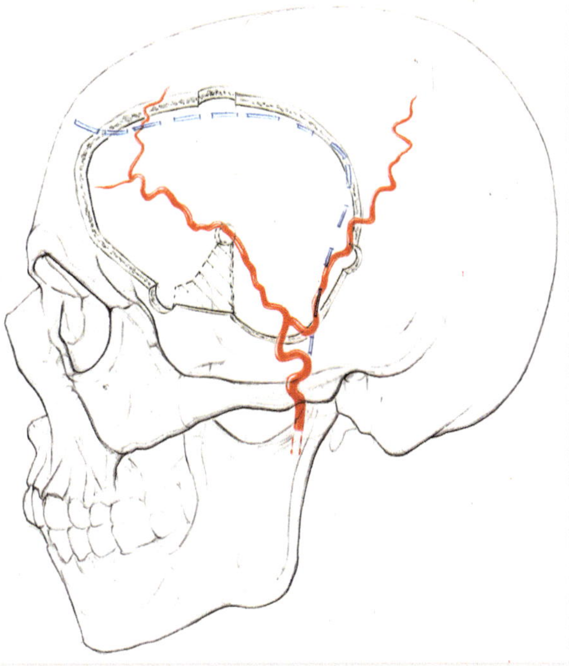

**Fig. 17.2** Design of skin incision (*blue interrupted line*) and craniotomy for STA–MCA anastomosis and EDMAPS.

## 17.6 Pitfalls, Risk Assessment, and Complications

As reported previously, STA–MCA anastomosis and EDMAPS may carry perioperative complications with 3-month morbidity of 4.3%. No mortality is recorded in our institute.[8] Therefore, the author informs the patients and their family that surgical risk of STA–MCA anastomosis and EDMAPS is around 5% according to his 20-year experience, but may be higher in patients with frequent ischemia attach and/or dense ischemia.

## 17.7 Special Instructions and Anesthesia

All patients should receive intravenous drip (500 to 1,000 mL) overnight before surgery to avoid ischemic complications during and after surgery. After induction of general anesthesia, $PaCO_2$ is strictly maintained around 40 mm Hg.[8]

## 17.8 Patient Position with Skin Incision and Key Surgical Steps

### 17.8.1 Skin Incision and Donor Tissue Preparation

Refer to ▶ Fig. 17.2 for a design of skin incision. The patients are placed in the supine position and their head is fixed with a three-point fixation device. The course of the STA is identified with a Doppler ultrasound probe. The skin incision is then made along the course of the parietal branch of the STA (▶ Fig. 17.3, ▶ Fig. 17.4). The parietal branch of the STA was dissected from the surrounding tissues, being kept patent at the point where the STA crosses the skin incision, so that the patency can be preserved just before STA–MCA anastomosis. After the scalp flap was reflected laterally, the frontal branch of the STA was also dissected under a surgical microscope (▶ Fig. 17.5). The vascularized frontal pericranial flap, consisting of the cranium periosteum and the overlying loose areolar layer, is created for subsequent encephalo-pericranio-synangiosis (▶ Fig. 17.6). Then, the temporal muscle was dissected as widely as possible and was made as a vascularized flap for encephalo-myo-synangiosis (EMS). Careful dissection is essential to preserve the arterial and venous pedicles of the muscular and pericranial flaps (▶ Fig. 17.6).

### 17.8.2 Craniotomy and Dural Opening

A frontotemporal craniotomy extending into the frontal area is made, preserving the middle meningeal artery (MMA). The size of craniotomy should be extended to the frontal area as widely as possible (▶ Fig. 17.7). The dura is incised and rolled back, preserving the main branches of the MMA. Thorough hemostasis is essential for direct STA–MCA anastomosis (▶ Fig. 17.7).

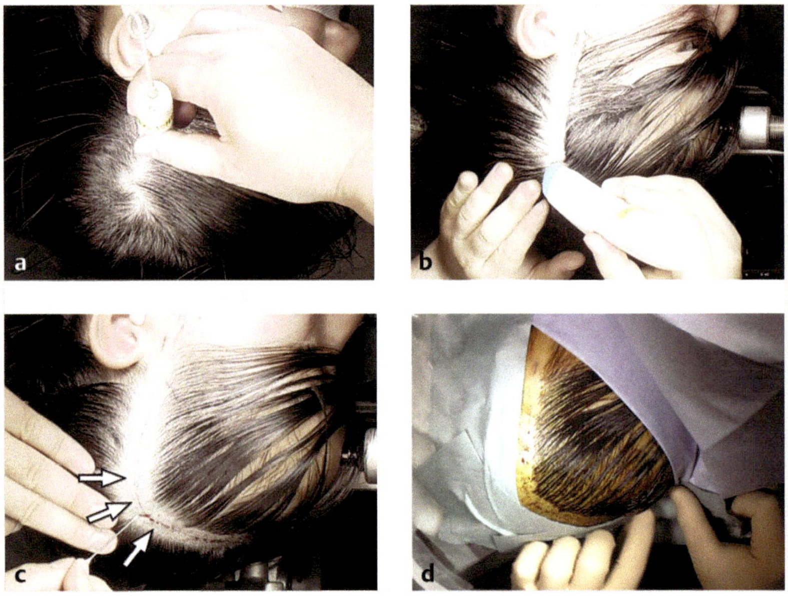

**Fig. 17.3** The first step of STA–MCA anastomosis and EDMAPS for moyamoya disease. **(a)** Doppler ultrasound probe is useful to trace the course of the parietal branch of the STA. **(b)** Partial shaving is performed along the course of the parietal branch of the STA. **(c)** The curvature of skin incision should be designed at an obtuse angle to avoid the delayed wound healing (*arrows*). **(d)** The draping.

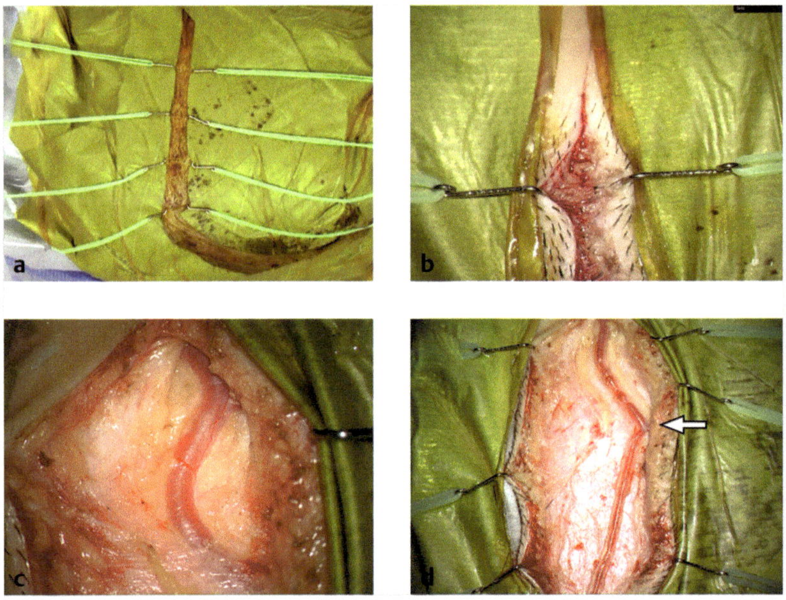

**Fig. 17.4** The second step of STA–MCA anastomosis and EDMAPS for moyamoya disease. **(a)** Only the shaved scalp is exposed. **(b)** Skin incision under surgical microscope. **(c)** The parietal branch of the STA is exposed and dissected from the surrounding galeal tissue. **(d)** The main trunk and the parietal branch of the STA are completely dissected. *Arrow* shows the origin of the frontal branch of the STA.

## 17.8.3 Direct STA–MCA Anastomosis

STA–MCA single or double anastomosis is performed in an end-to-side fashion with 10- or 11–0 nylon threads. The author prefers 11–0 nylon threads for pediatric patients younger than 10 years and 10–0 nylon threads for adolescent and adult patients. The frontal branches of the MCA should be selected as the first recipients of anastomoses in every case, because cerebral hemodynamics is impaired especially in the frontal lobe in moyamoya disease. The second recipient should be the cortical branch of the MCA that is feeding the temporal lobe. The diameter of the recipients ranges from 0.5 to 1.1 mm. The wall of the recipients is also very thin. The blue dye is put onto the surface of cut ends of the donor and recipient to visualize them clearly. A green silicon sheet is inserted beneath the recipient for the same purpose. Usually, 12 to 14 sutures would be enough to complete STA–MCA anastomosis. The clamping time of recipient is approximately 20 to 30 minutes (▸ Fig. 17.8). Indocyanine green (ICG) videoangiography is quite useful to confirm the patency of STA–MCA anastomosis and also the MMA (▸ Fig. 17.9).

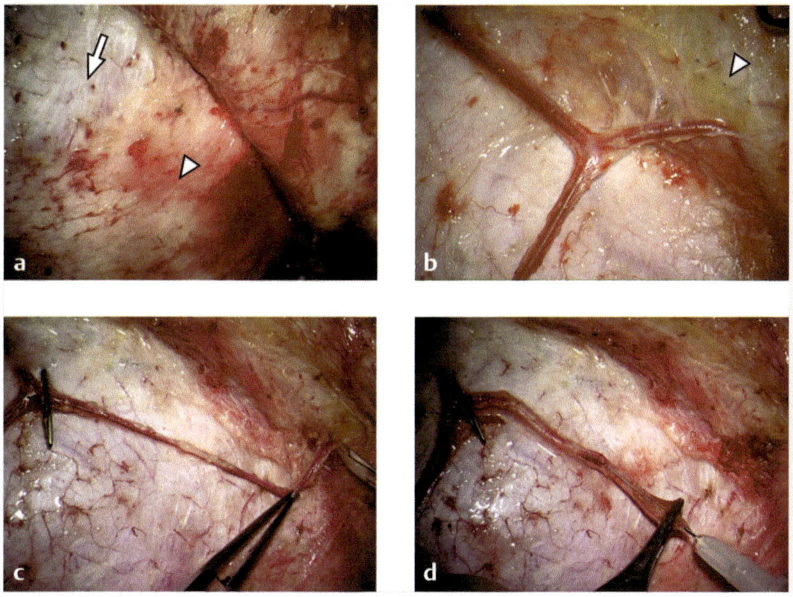

**Fig. 17.5** The third step of STA–MCA anastomosis and EDMAPS for moyamoya disease. **(a)** The skin incision is extended to the forehead, and the scalp flap is made so that the temporal muscle (*arrow*) and frontal pericranium can be identified (*arrowhead*). **(b)** The frontal branch of the STA is dissected from the surrounding galeal tissue. Note that the "track" of the fat tissue after the dissection of the frontal branch of the STA (*arrowhead*). **(c)** The frontal branch of STA is clamped and cut. **(d)** Heparinized saline is filled within the frontal branch of the STA to avoid thrombosis within it.

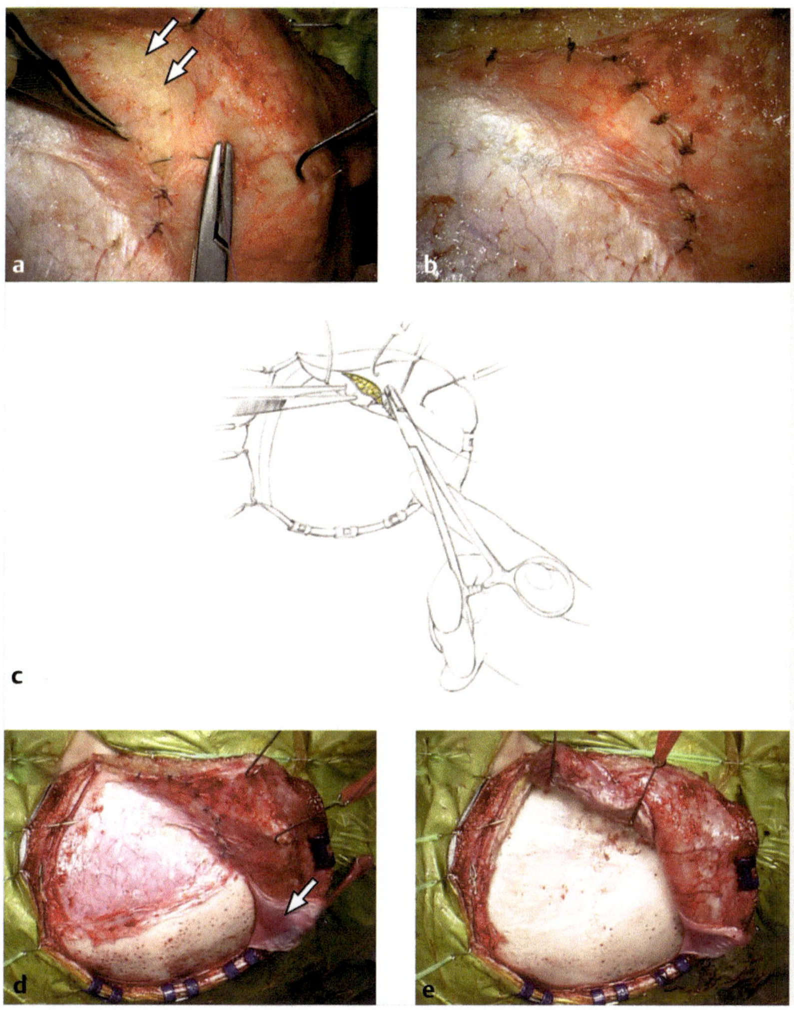

**Fig. 17.6** The fourth step of STA–MCA anastomosis and EDMAPS for moyamoya disease. **(a)** The "track" of the fat tissue is repaired by suturing the galeal tissue (*arrows*). **(b)** The "track" is completely repaired. **(c, d)** The frontal pericranium (*arrow*) is dissected from the skull. **(e)** The temporal muscle is dissected from the skull.

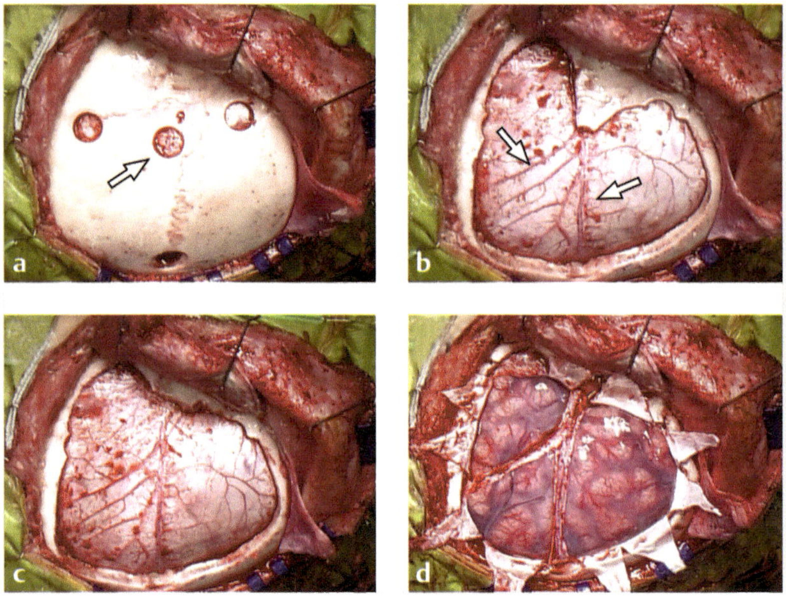

**Fig. 17.7** The fifth step of STA–MCA anastomosis and EDMAPS for moyamoya disease. **(a)** A total of five burr holes were made. The burr hole at the center is made to dissect the MMA during craniotomy (*arrow*). **(b)** A heart-shaped frontotemporal craniotomy is made by leaving the lesser wing of the sphenoid to preserve the MMA. Note two main branches of the MMA (*arrows*). **(c)** The lesser wing of the sphenoid should carefully be removed with a rongeur or high-speed drill. **(d)** The dura mater is opened by leaving the main branches of the MMA intact. Note the dural pedicles like a flower for subsequent indirect bypass, encephalo-duro-synangiosis (EDS).

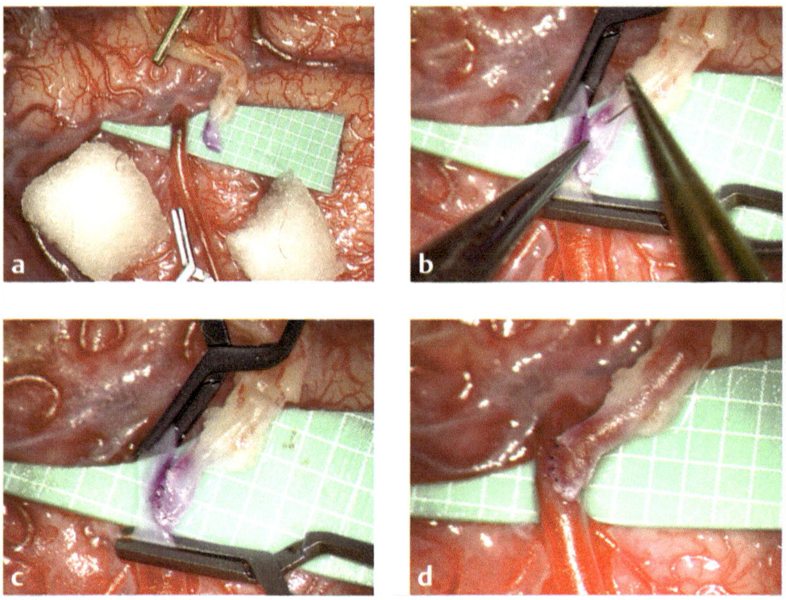

**Fig. 17.8** The sixth step of STA–MCA anastomosis and EDMAPS for moyamoya disease. **(a–d)** STA–MCA anastomosis is performed in an end-to-side fashion with 10–0 or 11–0 nylon threads.

### 17.8.4 Indirect Bypass and Cranioplasty

The dural flaps are turned into the epiarachnoid space for the development of surgical collaterals between the outer surface of the dura and the brain (encephalo-duro-synangiosis [EDS]). Then, the dural opening through frontotemporal craniotomy is covered with both the temporal muscle and pericranial flap (▶ Fig. 17.9). Cranioplasty is performed as usual. Titanium plates are usually employed for cranioplasty, but the author prefers the absorbable plates for pediatric patients younger than 10 years not to disturb the normal growth of their skull. The wound is closed in a layer-by-layer fashion. Total operation time ranges from 5 to 6 hours. Blood transfusion is usually unnecessary.

## 17.9 Difficulties Encountered

### 17.9.1 Preservation of Scalp Blood Flow

It is quite important to avoid the delayed wound healing after surgical revascularization for moyamoya disease. The

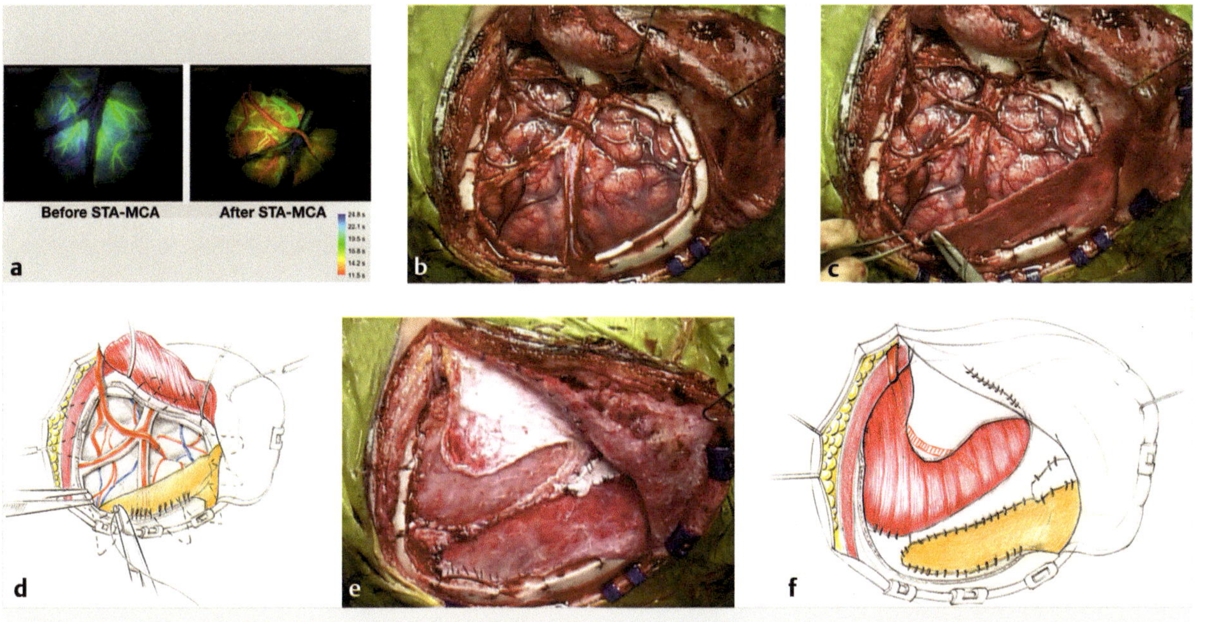


**Fig. 17.9** The final step of STA–MCA anastomosis and EDMAPS for moyamoya disease. **(a)** ICG videoangiography is useful to confirm the patency of STA–MCA anastomosis and also the MMA. **(b)** The dural pedicles are inserted into the epiarachnoid space so that their outer surface can be contacted with the brain surface. **(c, d)** The frontal lobe is covered with the frontal pericranial flap by suturing it to the dura mater. **(e, f)** Finally, the dural opening is closed with the temporal muscle.

delay of wound healing may prolong a hospital stay and furthermore require surgical repair. The author has modified surgical technique to avoid this problem for these 20 years. First, the curvature of skin incision should be designed at an obtuse angle so that the blood flow would be maintained at the top of curvature (▶ Fig. 17.3**d**). Second, the STA branches should be carefully dissected from the surrounding galeal tissue under the surgical microscope. The dissected STA should be "naked," because the surrounding galeal tissue is quite important for wound healing and should be left to the scalp (▶ Fig. 17.4**c, d**). Third, the galeal "track" after dissecting the frontal branch of the STA should always be repaired by suturing the galeal tissue so that the scalp blood flow would be recovered earlier after surgery (▶ Fig. 17.6**a, b**). The small amounts of time and effort contribute to the preservation of scalp blood flow, thus supporting wound healing.[13]

## 17.9.2 Preservation of the MMA during Craniotomy

The MMA is known to function as important collaterals to the ACA territory, but often courses within the lesser wing of the sphenoid bone. Therefore, usual fashioned craniotomy easily injures the MMA. Therefore, the author has evaluated the surgical anatomy around the lessor wing of the sphenoid and developed a novel technique to preserve it during craniotomy. Briefly, the anatomical relationship between the anterior branch of the MMA and the lesser wing of the sphenoid bone can be classified into three types: bridge, monorail, and tunnel types. In the bridge type (18.5%), the anterior branch of the MMA runs within the shallow groove in the medial surface of bone, which looks like a bridge over a river. In the monorail type (37.0%), the anterior branch of the MMA runs within the deep groove in the medial surface of bone, which looks like a monorail vehicle over a rail. In the tunnel type (44.5%), the anterior branch of the MMA is completely enclosed within the bony canal in the lesser wing of the sphenoid bone, which looks like a tunnel. Patients' age is closely related to the anatomical relationship between the anterior branch of the MMA and the lesser wing of the sphenoid wing. The bridge-type MMA can frequently be observed in younger patients.

During large frontotemporal craniotomy, a total of five burr holes are made. The burr hole at the center of craniotomy site is made rostral to the pterion to preserve the anterior branch of the MMA, because it is known to pierce the bony tunnel of the middle meningeal groove just beneath the junction of the sphenoparietal, sphenosquamosal, and squamosal sutures (▶ Fig. 17.7**a**). A heart-shaped craniotomy is performed, preserving the lesser wing of the sphenoid bone. Then, the lesser wing is resected carefully preserving the anterior branch of the MMA, using a rongeur or high-speed drill. Careful resection of the lesser wing with a rongeur can preserve the bridge- and monorail-type MMA (100 and 71.4%, respectively). However, drilling out of the lesser wing under a surgical microscope is essential to preserve the tunnel-type MMA (▶ Fig. 17.10).

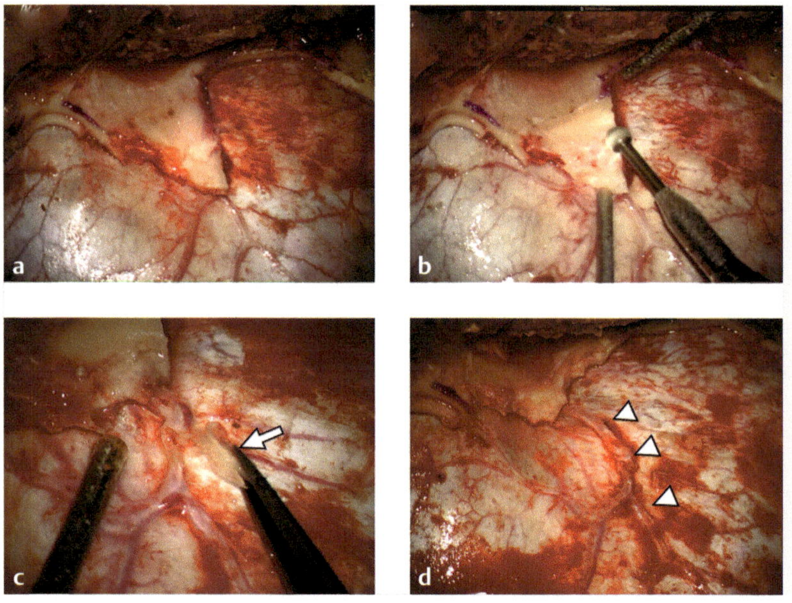


**Fig. 17.10** Preservation of the MMA during craniotomy. **(a)** The lesser wing of the sphenoid is left intact during craniotomy to avoid the injury of the MMA. **(b)** A high-speed drill is quite useful when the MMA courses within the bony tunnel. **(c)** Careful drilling and dissection enables us to remove the sphenoid bone around the MMA (*arrow*). **(d)** Finally, the MMA can be preserved completely (*arrowheads*).

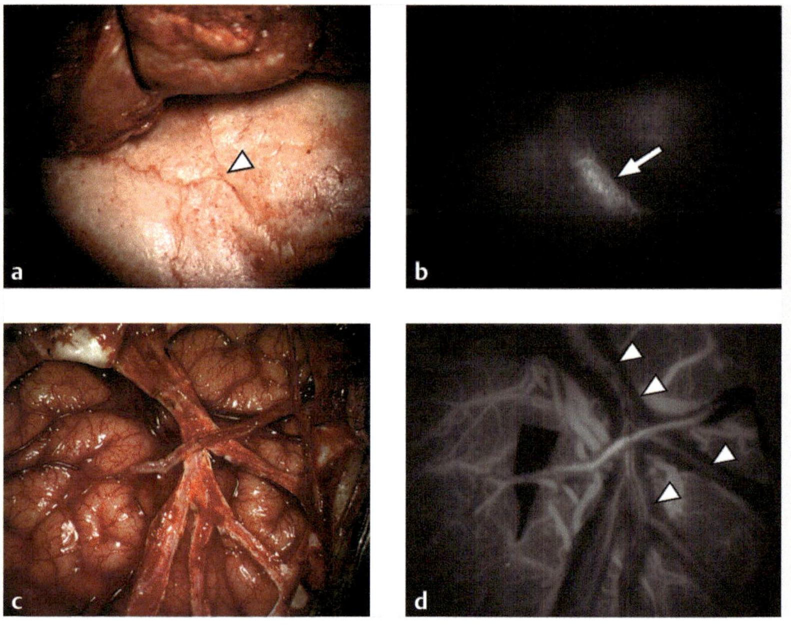


**Fig. 17.11** ICG videoangiography to preserve the MMA during craniotomy. **(a)** Intraoperative photograph of the pterion (*arrowhead*). **(b)** ICG videoangiography can visualize the MMA through the skull. **(c)** Intraoperative photograph of the preserved MMA and STA–MCA anastomosis. **(d)** ICG videoangiography can visualize the patency of STA–MCA anastomosis and also the patency of the main branches of the MMA (*arrowheads*).

Before surgery, the anatomical relationship between the anterior branch of MMA and the lesser wing of the sphenoid bone can precisely be analyzed on the raw images of time-of-flight (TOF) MR angiography. Plain CT scans are also useful to visualize the bony groove or tunnel around the pterion in all patients.[14]

### 17.9.3 ICG Videoangiography before Craniotomy

Using ICG videoangiography, the author has visualized the course of the MMA before craniotomy to further advance the methodology to preserve the MMA during craniotomy. Precise analysis has revealed that ICG videoangiography could clearly visualize the anterior branch of the MMA in 10 (37%) of 27 sides. The patients with the "visible" MMA are significantly younger than those without. ICG videoangiography can visualize it through the cranium when the diameter of the MMA is more than 1.3 mm and the sphenoid bone thickness over the MMA is less than 3.0 mm. The MMA can be preserved during craniotomy in all "visible" MMA, but not in 4 (23.5%) of the 17 "invisible" MMA. Therefore, ICG videoangiography can visualize the anterior branch of the MMA before craniotomy in about one-third of patients with the large-diameter MMA (> 1.3 mm) and thin sphenoid bone (< 3.0 mm). ICG videoangiography would be a safe and valuable technique to preserve it during craniotomy for moyamoya disease in them (▶ Fig. 17.11).[15]

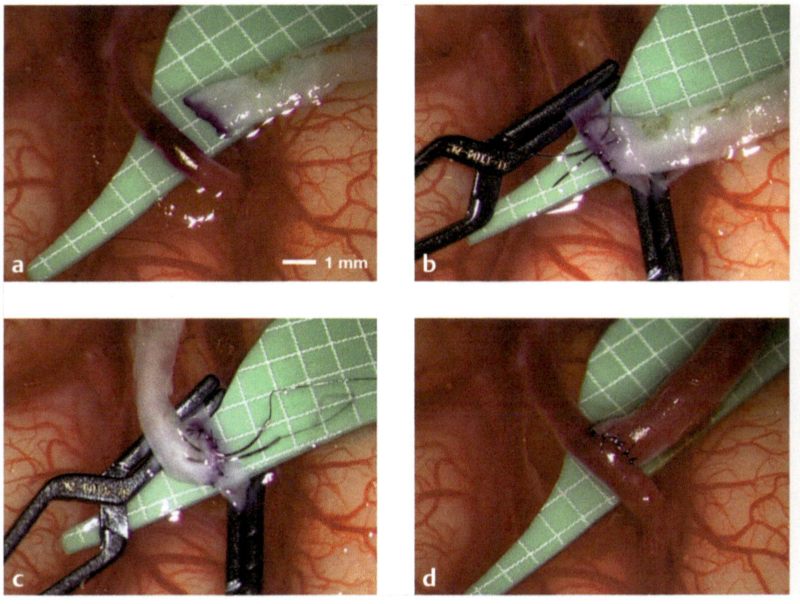


**Fig. 17.12 (a–d)** A "marking pin" technique for STA–MCA anastomosis.

### 17.9.4 STA–MCA Anastomosis

The recipients are known to have a very small caliber and a very thin wall in moyamoya disease. Therefore, accurate suturing is essential to yield a good patency of direct bypass. For this purpose, a marking pin technique is quite useful. Thus, each needle should be left keeping the surface of both cut ends in good position until the next needle is placed, like a pin fastens pieces of cloth together when sewing (▶ Fig. 17.12).

## 17.10 Bailout, Rescue, and Salvage Maneuvers

The surgeons should postpone direct STA–MCA anastomosis when the diameter of all recipients is too small (<0.5 mm). The surgeons should carefully observe the patency of direct STA–MCA anastomosis because the incidence of its thrombotic occlusion is higher than usual STA–MCA anastomosis for patients with atherosclerotic carotid occlusion. In such a case, the surgeons should open the anastomosed site by removing several stitches, remove the thrombus, and reanastomose it.

## References

[1] Nakagawa Y, Abe H, Sawamura Y, Kamiyama H, Gotoh S, Kashiwaba T. Revascularization surgery for moyamoya disease. Neurol Res. 1988; 10(1):32–39

[2] Ishikawa T, Houkin K, Kamiyama H, Abe H. Effects of surgical revascularization on outcome of patients with pediatric moyamoya disease. Stroke. 1997; 28(6):1170–1173

[3] Kuroda S, Houkin K, Ishikawa T, et al. Determinants of intellectual outcome after surgical revascularization in pediatric moyamoya disease: a multivariate analysis. Childs Nerv Syst. 2004; 20(5):302–308

[4] Houkin K, Ishikawa T, Yoshimoto T, Abe H. Direct and indirect revascularization for moyamoya disease surgical techniques and peri-operative complications. Clin Neurol Neurosurg. 1997; 99 Suppl 2:S142–S145

[5] Kuroda S, Kamiyama H, Abe H, et al. Cerebral blood flow in children with spontaneous occlusion of the circle of Willis (moyamoya disease): comparison with healthy children and evaluation of annual changes. Neurol Med Chir (Tokyo). 1993; 33(7):434–438

[6] Houkin K, Kamiyama H, Abe H, Takahashi A, Kuroda S. Surgical therapy for adult moyamoya disease. Can surgical revascularization prevent the recurrence of intracerebral hemorrhage? Stroke. 1996; 27 (8):1342–1346

[7] Yoshioka N, Rhoton AL, Jr. Vascular anatomy of the anteriorly based pericranial flap. Neurosurgery. 2005; 57(1) Suppl:11–16, discussion 11–16

[8] Kuroda S, Houkin K, Ishikawa T, Nakayama N, Iwasaki Y. Novel bypass surgery for moyamoya disease using pericranial flap: its impacts on cerebral hemodynamics and long-term outcome. Neurosurgery. 2010; 66(6):1093–1101, discussion 1101

[9] Baba T, Houkin K, Kuroda S. Novel epidemiological features of moyamoya disease. J Neurol Neurosurg Psychiatry. 2008; 79(8): 900–904

[10] Kuroda S, Hashimoto N, Yoshimoto T, Iwasaki Y, Research Committee on Moyamoya Disease in Japan. Radiological findings, clinical course, and outcome in asymptomatic moyamoya disease: results of multicenter survey in Japan. Stroke. 2007; 38(5):1430–1435

[11] Kuroda S, Group AS, AMORE Study Group. Asymptomatic moyamoya disease: literature review and ongoing AMORE study. Neurol Med Chir (Tokyo). 2015; 55(3):194–198

[12] Miyamoto S, Yoshimoto T, Hashimoto N, et al. JAM Trial Investigators. Effects of extracranial-intracranial bypass for patients with hemorrhagic moyamoya disease: results of the Japan Adult Moyamoya Trial. Stroke. 2014; 45(5):1415–1421

[13] Kuroda S, Houkin K. Bypass surgery for moyamoya disease: concept and essence of surgical techniques. Neurol Med Chir (Tokyo). 2012; 52(5):287–294

[14] Hori S, Kashiwazaki D, Akioka N, et al. Surgical anatomy and preservation of the middle meningeal artery during bypass surgery for moyamoya disease. Acta Neurochir (Wien). 2015; 157(1):29–36

[15] Tanabe N, Yamamoto S, Kashiwazaki D, et al. Indocyanine green visualization of middle meningeal artery before craniotomy during surgical revascularization for moyamoya disease. Acta Neurochir (Wien). 2017; 159(3):567–575

# 18 STA–MCA Bypass and Encephalo-duro-arterio-synangiosis

*Sepideh Amin-Hanjani*

**Abstract**

Although many procedures have been described for surgical revascularization in moyamoya disease, the combined direct and indirect bypass procedure of superficial temporal artery (STA) to middle cerebral artery (MCA) bypass with encephalo-duro-arterio-synangiosis (EDAS) is a staple among these. The operation provides complementary benefits of immediate revascularization through direct bypass, as well as longer term collateral formation through indirect EDAS. The procedure is indicated for patients with symptomatic moyamoya with adequate donor and recipient vessels. The key elements and surgical steps of this operation are outlined in this chapter and include harvesting and preparation of the frontal and parietal branch of the STA, craniotomy with cruciate dural opening sparing major branches of the middle meningeal artery, selection and preparation of the recipient cortical MCA branch, performance of direct STA–MCA anastomosis, and technique for encephalo-duro and encephalo-arterio-synangiosis. The use of intraoperative blood flow measurements in performing direct bypass is also described: measurement of the STA cut flow prior to anastomosis and bypass flow following anastomosis allows determination of the bypass cut flow index (i.e., bypass flow/cut flow), which serves as a useful indicator of bypass function. Important elements of perioperative management are also reviewed including preoperative hydration, avoidance of hypotension and hypocarbia intraoperatively, and careful blood pressure control postoperatively.

*Keywords:* blood flow, bypass, middle cerebral artery, moyamoya, superficial temporal artery, surgery

## 18.1 History and Initial Description

The general approach of performing combined direct and indirect revascularization evolved from observations of moyamoya disease (MMD) cases in the 1980s where indirect procedures, especially encephalo-duro-arterio-synangiosis (EDAS) alone, failed to provide sufficient collaterals.[1–3] Descriptions of combining direct superficial temporal artery (STA)–middle cerebral artery (MCA) bypass with various indirect procedures including EDAS, encephalo-myo-synangiosis (EMS), and encephalo-duro-arterio-myo-synangiosis (EDAMS) emerged in subsequent years, and demonstrated superior results in terms of revascularization.[4,5] The STA–MCA bypass with EDAS is one of the simple and elegant options for performing combined direct and indirect revascularization.

## 18.2 Indications

STA–MCA with EDAS can be considered the standard operation for treatment of MMD in adults. The procedure is indicated in these patients, if the following criteria are present:

1. Symptomatic patient, that is, patients presenting with stroke (hemorrhagic or ischemic), transient ischemic attack, or progressive cognitive decline.
2. Evidence of hemodynamic compromise with poor cerebrovascular reserve, which can be evaluated using a number of imaging modalities. Our institutional protocol relies on a combination of magnetic resonance (MR) imaging consisting of quantitative MR angiography with and without diamox challenge, global blood oxygen level dependent (BOLD) imaging with hypercapnic challenge and regional BOLD imaging using functional MR imaging paradigms. The aggregate information is used to determine if there is reduced or absent cerebrovascular reserve.
3. Adequate donor and recipient vessels to perform the STA–MCA direct anastomosis; this can be an issue in very young pediatric patients, in which case, indirect procedure alone can be pursued.

The combined STA–MCA with EDAS can also be considered the preferred option for pediatric patients if direct bypass is feasible; the greatest barrier to performing direct bypass is posed by the very young pediatric patients (<5 years old), dependent on donor and recipient vessel size, in which case, indirect procedure alone can be pursued. For pediatric patients, even an asymptomatic hemisphere affected by moyamoya warrants consideration for surgery if there is presence of hemodynamic compromise on imaging, as progression to symptoms and stroke is prevalent in this population.

The advantage of the STA–MCA bypass in combination with EDAS, as opposed to in combination with other indirect procedures such as EMS or EDAMS, relate to the relative disadvantages of harvesting and using muscle on the brain surface. Although muscle can be a very effective source of collaterals, its use typically entails a larger craniotomy to expose more brain surface area for muscle contact, entails potential cosmetic issues related to transposition of the muscle underneath the bone flap, and has a higher risk of postoperative hematoma from oozing of muscle fibers over the brain surface, particularly when patients are on aspirin to optimize the patency of direct bypass. The EDAS procedure is more straightforward, combines naturally with the STA–MCA bypass requiring little alteration to the approach that would already be applied for the direct procedure, and provides effective collaterals without the potential disadvantage of muscle use.

## 18.3 Key Principles

The STA–MCA bypass with EDAS provides both immediate revascularization through direct bypass and longer term growth of additional collaterals through indirect EDAS. In fact, there is frequently a reciprocal relationship between direct STA bypass flow and indirect EDAS collaterals that provide durable temporally complementary revascularization.[6] Key concepts that are critical in this procedure are as follows:

- Identification of the vascular territory in most need of flow augmentation, and choosing the skin incision, craniotomy, and donor vessel choice and configuration to optimize direct and indirect bypass.
- Preserving the middle meningeal artery (MMA) when performing the craniotomy and opening the dura, particularly if it is already providing extracranial–intracranial (EC–IC) collaterals (as evident from preoperative angiographic imaging).
- Use of flow-assisted surgical technique[7,8] (as described further) to measure cut flow and cut flow index in order to assess direct STA–MCA bypass.

## 18.4 SWOT Analysis

### 18.4.1 Strengths

- Direct bypass allows for immediate flow augmentation and revascularization.
- Indirect bypass is simple/fast and can be integrated easily with direct bypass.
- Combined procedure provides complementary short- and long-term revascularization.

### 18.4.2 Weaknesses

- Dual STA branch harvest can lead to wound healing problems.
- Longer procedure than indirect EDAS alone.
- Potential risk for hyperperfusion from direct STA–MCA bypass.
- Need for temporary vessel occlusion.

### 18.4.3 Opportunity

- Extension of combined revascularization concept to anterior and posterior cerebral artery territories.

### 18.4.4 Threat

- Lack Class I evidence for comparative efficacy to indirect or direct procedures alone.

## 18.5 Contraindications

The primary contraindication is recent stroke within the last 7 to 14 days, primarily due to higher risk of reperfusion hemorrhage with the direct STA–MCA portion of the procedure, and also in general due to heightened risk of anesthesia and surgery in the setting of a recent ischemic event. Additional contraindications for direct component of the procedure would be poor quality or caliber of the STA donor vessel, or existing spontaneous collaterals from the donor STA which would be disrupted by harvesting and cutting the vessel for direct anastomosis. In such a scenario indirect arterio-synangiosis, using the intact STA which is kept in continuity and apposed to the brain surface, would still be feasible, as long as harvesting the vessel in situ would not directly result in disruption of collaterals.

## 18.6 Special Considerations

For the STA–MCA with EDAS operation the preoperative imaging is critical in planning. Catheter angiography allows the best assessment of the course and caliber of the donor STA vessels, and allows evaluation of spontaneous EC–IC collaterals from the MMA or other sources which must be preserved while performing the operation. The angiogram should provide dedicated internal and external carotid injections to allow the optimal evaluation of these features. The angiogram, in conjunction with blood flow imaging, is also important in determining the vascular territory that is most compromised and most in need of flow augmentation.

In the preoperative arrangements, admission of the patient prior to day of surgery to ensure overnight intravenous hydration while the patient is not allowed oral intake is an important safety measure to reduce the risk of hypovolemia and hypotensive episode during induction of anesthesia. Preoperative administration of aspirin, if the patient is not already routinely taking the medication, is advisable as a maneuver to enhance patency of direct STA–MCA anastomosis, and checking aspirin sensitivity assay to ensure that the medication is effective preoperatively can be performed. For patients with comorbid diseases, it is essential to optimize the management of the condition prior to surgery, for example, in patients with sickle cell disease, use of exchange transfusions and reduction of hemoglobin S levels, or in patients with diabetes, strict glucose regulation, and controlled hemoglobin A1C levels. Otherwise, such conditions can affect either the success of the revascularization or healing and recovery from the surgery.

## 18.7 Pitfalls, Risk Assessment, and Complications

The primary risk associated with STA–MCA bypass with EDAS is similar to any revascularization surgery in patients with MMD, namely the risk of perioperative ischemic stroke. The addition of direct STA–MCA bypass to the EDAS operation ought not to increase this risk, given that temporary occlusion of the cortical MCA branch required for direct anastomosis is extremely well tolerated. However, it does add some additional operative time which could potentially elevate risk, as period of time under anesthesia may be a risk contributor. Direct bypass also can engender a risk for postoperative hyperperfusion or reperfusion hemorrhage which is not encountered with indirect EDAS alone, and requires postoperative vigilance and blood pressure management to avoid. Other general risks include postoperative seizures, and short-term prophylactic anticonvulsants are thus reasonable.

One feature of the STA–MCA with EDAS operation is the dual harvest of both STA branches, using one for direct anastomosis and the other for indirect arterio-synangiosis. The dual harvest however can lead to devascularization of the scalp tissue and incisional healing problems, which in turn can result in wound dehiscence or infection.

## 18.8 Special Instructions, Position, and Anesthesia

As noted above, aspirin is administered preoperatively to patients, typically at full dose of 325 mg for adults and 81 mg for pediatric patients, and aspirin sensitivity is confirmed by platelet function assay prior to the surgery. During the surgery, low-dose heparin (10 units/mL) is used for flushing the donor STA and recipient MCA vessel for direct anastomosis, but no systemic anticoagulation is used.

General endotracheal anesthesia is utilized. The primary considerations are maintenance of blood pressure at or above the patient's baseline blood pressure throughout, especially during the induction of anesthesia when there is most risk of lability and hypotension. Arterial line placement is mandatory for monitoring of the blood pressure during the surgery and for access to draw arterial blood gas samples. End-tidal carbon dioxide levels should be monitored and correlated with arterial levels, to avoid hyperventilation, which reduces cerebral blood flow. The anesthetic regimen is chosen to allow titration to achieve burst suppression during the temporary clipping time for direct anastomosis. Both electroencephalography (EEG) and somatosensory-evoked potential (SSEP) leads are placed prior to positioning for neuromonitoring. EEG allows determination of burst suppression when needed during the operation, and along with SSEP can also alert to hypoperfusion and brain ischemia as both reflect integrity of cortical activity. It is important to assess baselines in these modalities, as prior strokes may affect the symmetry, amplitude, or latency; the relevant concern would be changes noted relative to baseline. Since the EEG and SSEP monitoring utilize scalp electrodes, it is advisable to map the STA prior to placement of these needle or corkscrew electrodes to avoid inadvertent injury to the STA.

During the surgery, the anesthesiologist must also maintain euvolemia for the patient; use of the typical brain relaxation agents such as mannitol and furosemide must be avoided due to risk for hypovolemia, hypotension and subsequent hypoperfusion in the already tenuous and compromised vascular territory undergoing surgery, or even the contralateral side in patients with bilateral disease.

The patient is positioned with the surgeon at the head of the bed, anesthesiologist to the left of the patient and the operating nurse to the right of the patient so that instruments can be easily handed to the right hand of the surgeon during the operation. The patient's head is turned to the right or left dependent on the side that needs to be operated.

## 18.9 Patient Position with Skin Incision and Key Surgical Steps

### 18.9.1 Position

The patient is positioned supine, with pin fixation to place the head into lateral position. Dependent on neck mobility and girth, a roll under the ipsilateral shoulder may be necessary to avoid overrotation of the neck and jugular vein compromise. The Sugita head holder is particularly suitable for the case as it accommodates a ring retractor system with hooks which can be used for both anterior and posterior retraction of the skin edges. Although this head holder allows placement of four pins for stability, in MMD patients where bilateral surgery may ultimately be needed, it is best to utilize only three pins for fixation to avoid the fourth pin which would otherwise be located in the contralateral scalp and risk injuring the contralateral STA (▶ Fig. 18.1**a**).

### 18.9.2 Skin Incision and STA Harvest

The STA anterior (frontal) and posterior (parietal) branch are mapped with Doppler and marked on the skin. After sterile preparation and draping, a straight incision is then created over the parietal branch using needle tip bovie electrocautery on a low setting, and the STA branch is exposed using blunt dissection with a mosquito instrument. The exposed STA is then dissected free with a cuff of attached tissue for a length of approximately 8 to

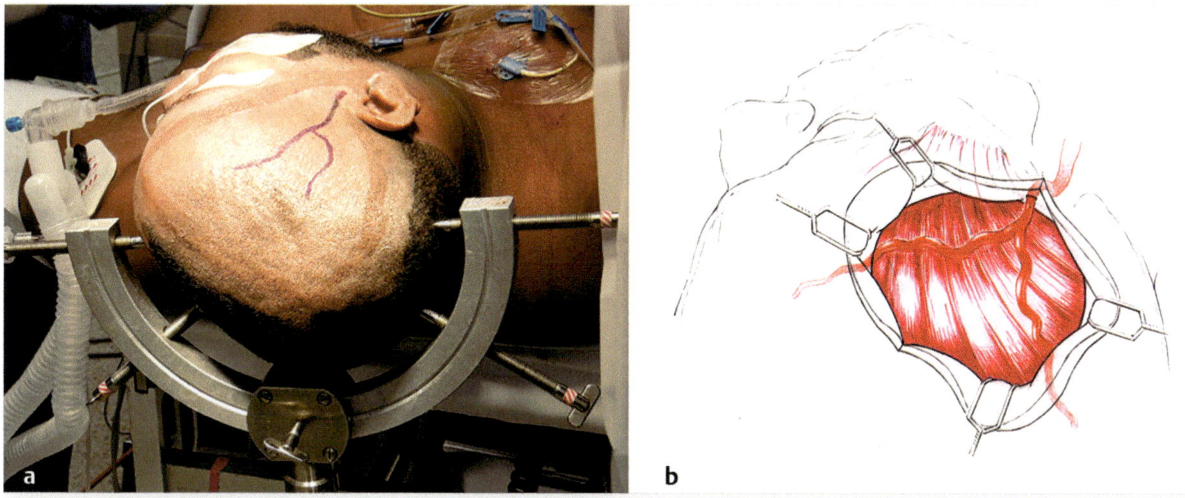

**Fig. 18.1** Positioning and skin incision. **(a)** Patient positioned with head turned lateral, and pinned in a Sugita head frame. The frontal and parietal branches of the STA have been marked. Three rather than four pins can be utilized for fixation to avoid risk of injury to the contralateral superficial temporal artery (STA) in moyamoya disease (MMD) patients. **(b)** Illustration demonstrating the skin flap to expose and harvest the STA branches: as linear skin incision is placed over the parietal branch and then curved anteriorly to allow the frontal STA branch for be dissected from beneath the skin flap. (Panel **(a)** is from Macdonald R.L. Neurosurgical Operative Atlas: Vascular Surgery, 3rd edition. Copyright © 2018. Thieme.)

10 cm. The STA bifurcation and anterior branch are also identified and followed. In pediatric patients, skin elasticity allows the anterior skin edge to be lifted allowing harvest of the frontal branch through the existing linear incision. In adults this is typically not feasible, and the linear incision is curved anteriorly into a skin flap; the frontal branch is then harvested from the undersurface of the flap (▶ Fig. 18.1**b**). The frontal branch will typically be utilized for direct anastomosis and the parietal branch for the in situ indirect arterio-synangiosis. Thus, the former is cut distally, and occluded with a temporary clip proximally, while the latter is left in continuity. The cut frontal branch is flushed with heparin solution (10 units/mL, ensuring to release the clip momentarily to flush proximal to it in order to reduce risk of thrombus formation from stagnant flow). Both frontal and parietal branch ae then wrapped in a papaverine soaked cottonoid to keep them hydrated and relieve any vasospasm created from manipulation during the harvest.

## 18.9.3 Craniotomy

The temporalis muscle and fascia are opened in a T-shaped fashion below the intact STA branch (▶ Fig. 18.2), and the muscle edges retracted both anteriorly and posteriorly to expose the underlying cranium. While protecting the STA branches, burr holes are placed inferiorly and superiorly beneath the proximal and distal aspects of the parietal STA branch, and a craniotomy is elevated with a power drill straight bit attached to a foot plate. The craniotomy placement spans both anterior and posterior to the parietal branch, to allow the vessel to have good exposure to the underlying brain for indirect bypass. Care is taken in the anterior aspect of the planned craniotomy to strip the dura in order to avoid injury to the MMA; if necessary this aspect of the boney opening is performed by sequential biting of the bone under direct vision rather than removing it with the remainder of the bone flap. The dura is tacked to the edges of the bone with sutures for epidural hemostasis, again with care to avoid dural vessel branches. The dura is then opened in a cruciate fashion but avoiding the MMA and any major dural branches, which are instead preserved as bridges of dura across the craniotomy field as needed (▶ Fig. 18.2).

## 18.9.4 Recipient Vessel Preparation

At this point of the surgery, the intraoperative microscope is utilized. In preparing both for STA–MCA bypass and EDAS, the arachnoid over the cortical vessels is opened with an arachnoid knife. Different potential recipients for direct anastomosis are evaluated based on size, vascular territory (e.g., superior vs. inferior division of MCA) and orientation/location in the operative field. The ideal orientation for a right handed surgeon is a vessel laying from 10:30 to 4:30 on a clock face, with ideal location being central within the boney opening rather than close to a bone or dural edge. The chosen vessel is dissected more extensively and very small perforating branches are sacrificed if needed to prevent back-bleeding into the vessel during anastomosis. The recipient is then separated from the surrounding brain, by placing a small rubber dam beneath the vessel, and Gelfoam beneath this to elevate the artery out of its sulcus

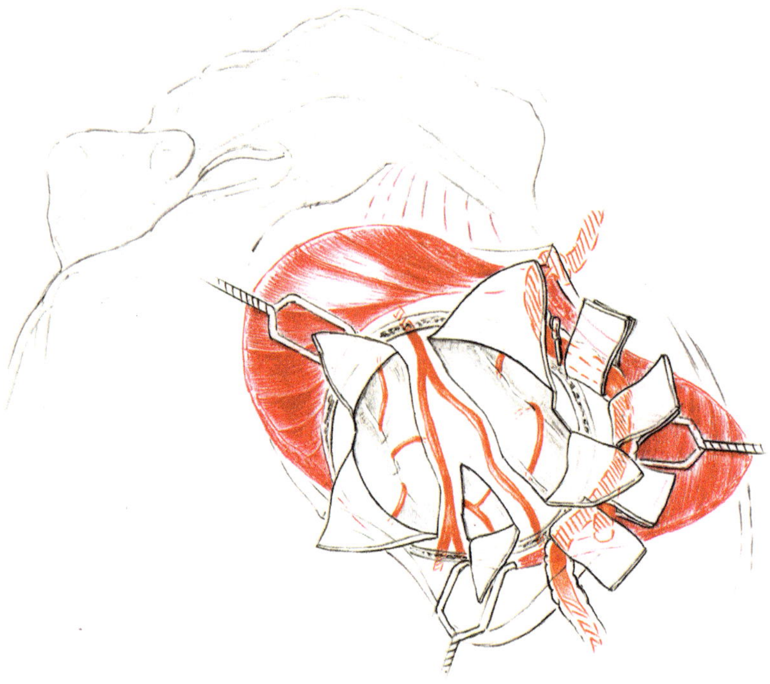

**Fig. 18.2** Craniotomy and dural opening. Illustration demonstrating the muscle opening, the craniotomy, and dural opening.

(▶ Fig. 18.4**a**). Papaverine cottonoids are applied to the recipient briefly as needed to relieve any vasospasm created by the dissection.

## 18.9.5 Donor Vessel Preparation

The frontal branch which is being prepared for direct anastomosis is first prepared distally by dissecting away the surrounding cuff of tissue using microscissors; any small branch vessels encountered are coagulated gently to prevent bleeding after flow is restored. Once the vessel has been adequately prepared, the cut flow is measured.[9,10] This entails releasing the proximal temporary clip and measuring the flow within the free-flowing artery using an ultrasonic transit-time flow probe (the Transonic Charbel micro-flow probe) in cc/min (▶ Fig. 18.3). Following the measurement, the vessel is again flushed with heparinized saline and a clip is reapplied proximally. The donor vessel end is then cut in a beveled fashion and fish mouthed in preparation for anastomosis. A marker is used to mark the vessel circumferentially prior to cutting the vessel for improved visualization of vessel edges during the anastomosis.

## 18.9.6 STA–MCA Bypass

A marking pen is utilized to mark the surface of the recipient cortical vessel where the arteriotomy will be placed in order to improve visualization of the vessel edges during anastomosis (▶ Fig. 18.4**a**). After confirming that the patient is in burst suppression, temporary vessel clips are placed on the recipient vessel and a fine microblade is utilized to create the arteriotomy which is then extended with fine microscissors until it matches the length of the opening of the beveled and fish-mouthed donor vessel. The internal lumen of the recipient is flushed with heparinized saline and a small silastic stent can be placed inside the recipient vessel lumen to hold the vessel walls apart, as needed.

To perform the anastomosis, a 10–0 nylon suture is placed between the heel of the donor vessel and one end of the arteriotomy (▶ Fig. 18.4**b**); the suture is tied to create the first apical stitch. At the other side of the arteriotomy, the suture is placed from the toe of the donor vessel to the other apex of the arteriotomy. Having placed the apical stitches, the remaining suture from the apical stich can be used to close the arteriotomy on each side in a running to or interrupted fashion. If performed in a running fashion, the suture loops are kept loose until all the stitches have been places and then tightened sequentially while keeping the pulled suture taut, in order to create even tension along the entire suture line (▶ Fig. 18.4**c**). If closed in an interrupted fashion, stitches can be placed from each end towards the center and the subsequent stitch placed before tying the prior suture (▶ Fig. 18.4**e**); both maneuvers allow maximal visualization of needle placement in the donor and recipient vessel edges during suturing. After one side of the arteriotomy is complete, the lumen should be checked form the other side to ensure none of the stitches have caught the “back” wall

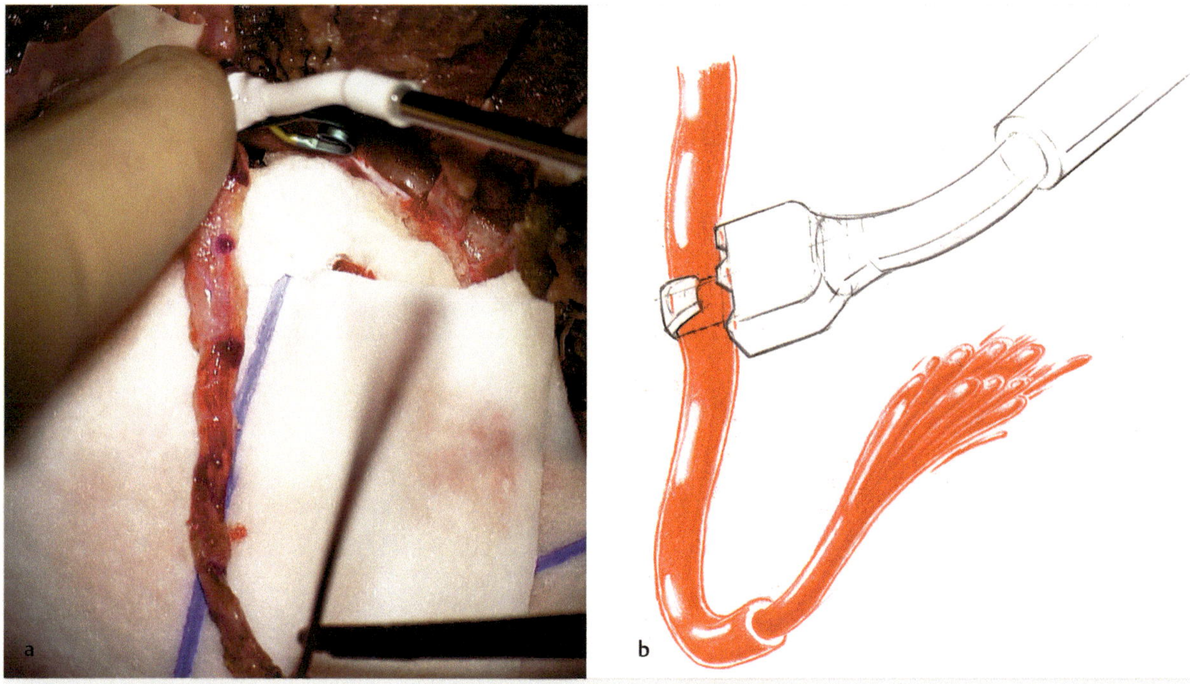

**Fig. 18.3** Measurement of cut flow. Intraoperative photograph **(a)** and illustration **(b)** demonstrating the cut flow being measured in the frontal superficial temporal artery (STA) donor branch.

(▶ Fig. 18.4**d**). Once confirmed, the remaining side of the anastomosis is completed (▶ Fig. 18.4**f**), making sure to remove the stent, if one has been used, prior to placement of the final stitches. Once the anastomosis is complete, the distal and then proximal temporary clips are removed from the recipient vessel and the anastomosis line is observed for hemostasis, prior to then removing the temporary clip from the proximal donor STA.

The final maneuver is then to measure the bypass flow using the ultrasonic microflow probe. The cut flow index (CFI), that is, the bypass flow/cut flow, can then be determined, with a CFI of less than 0.5 indicating a well-functioning bypass. The flow measurements should be made under similar anesthetic conditions related to blood pressure, burst suppression and end-tidal carbon dioxide, as these factors alone can impact blood flow. High bypass flows, such as greater than 80 cc per minute, should prompt judicious blood pressure control to avoid hyperperfusion.

## 18.9.7 Encephalo-arterio-synangiosis

To perform the arterio-synangiosis, the parietal branch of the STA, which is still intact, is laid over the brain surface (▶ Fig. 18.5), ensuring that the arachnoid has been opened particularly in areas where the vessel apposes the brain surface. Then, 10–0 nylon sutures are used to suture the cuff of tissue along the STA to the arachnoid to maintain good apposition between the artery and the brain. Three to four such sutures are placed along the length of the STA as it travels over the brain surface. Care is taken to avoid stitches near the edge of the craniotomy in order to avoid kinking of the vessel as it travels in and out of the surgical field.

## 18.9.8 Encephalo-duro-synangiosis

The final step in the revascularization procedure is the dural synangiosis. This can be performed simply be inverting the cut dural leaflets onto the brain surface, such that the outer more vascular dural surface is in direct contact with the brain surface. Alternatively, the dura can be split into two layers with forceps, exposing the vasculature within the dura, and then inverting the inner layer over the pia while laying the outer layer onto the pia (▶ Fig. 18.5). This has the advantage of providing a greater surface area of contact between the dura and the brain.

## 18.9.9 Closure

The dural opening and remaining exposed brain surface can be covered with dural substitute or hemostatic layer such as Gelfoam. The bone flap is thinned and trimmed to avoid pressure or kinking of the STA branches. The flap is replaced such that the parietal branch serving as indirect bypass enters and exists through the inferior and superior burr hole sites.

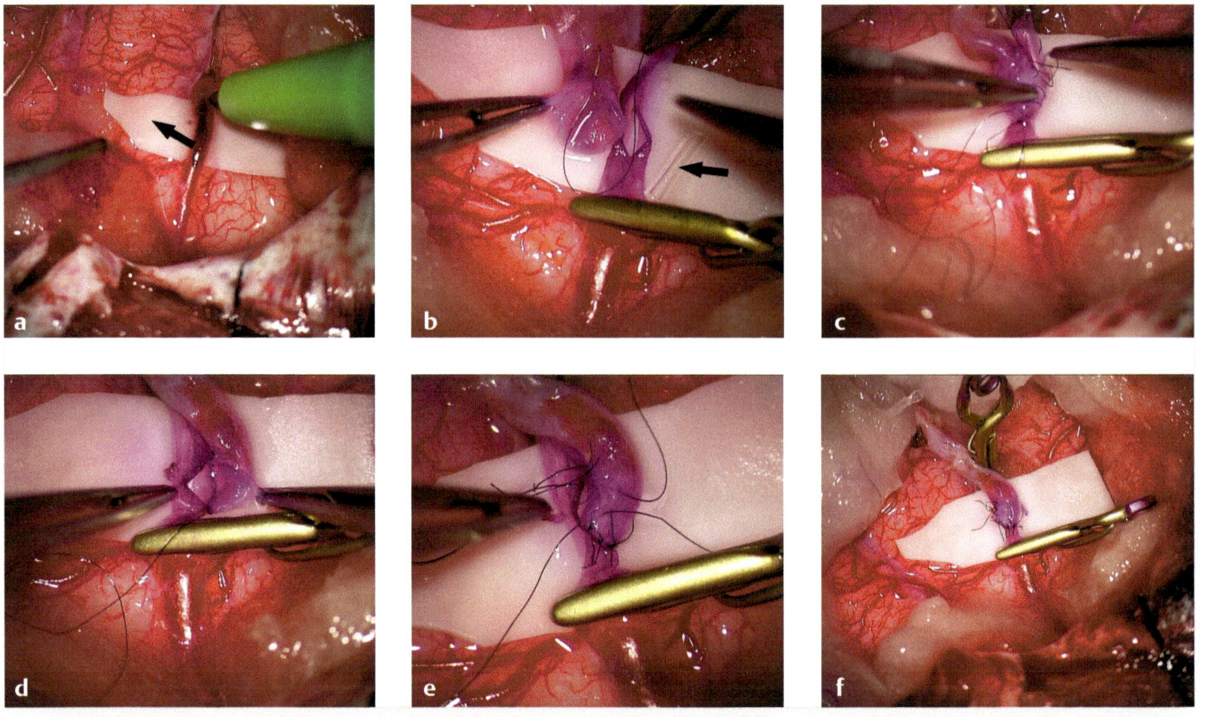

**Fig. 18.4** Anastomosis: intraoperative photographs. **(a)** The recipient vessel dissected free of arachnoid, and elevated from the sulcus using a rubber dam; a marking pen is utilized to mark the planned arteriotomy site. A small perforator (*arrow*) has been coagulated and cut to allow isolation of the vessel segment. **(b)** First suture placed at the apex of the recipient and through heel of the donor superficial temporal artery (STA). Note that the donor STA branch has been cleaned distally, marked, cut at a bevel and fish-mouthed. A stent (*arrow*) is nearby to be inserted into the recipient lumen. **(c)** Suturing is initiated on the first side of the anastomosis after both apical stitches have been placed. The running suture line is shown with the suture loops left loose and now being tightened sequentially to be tied to the contralateral apical stitch in order to complete this side of the anastomosis. **(d)** The lumen of the anastomosis is checked from the other side prior to commencing suturing of this side. **(e)** Interrupted sutures have been placed on this side of the anastomosis, closing towards the center for better visualization and leaving one suture form each knot long in case of need to tie adjacent stitches together if leakage. Note that the subsequent stich is being places prior to tying the prior stitch, also for better visualization of the lumen as the suture is placed. The stent is visible through the thin translucent wall of the recipient vessel. **(f)** Final anastomosis after removal of the stent, and prior to release of the temporary clips.

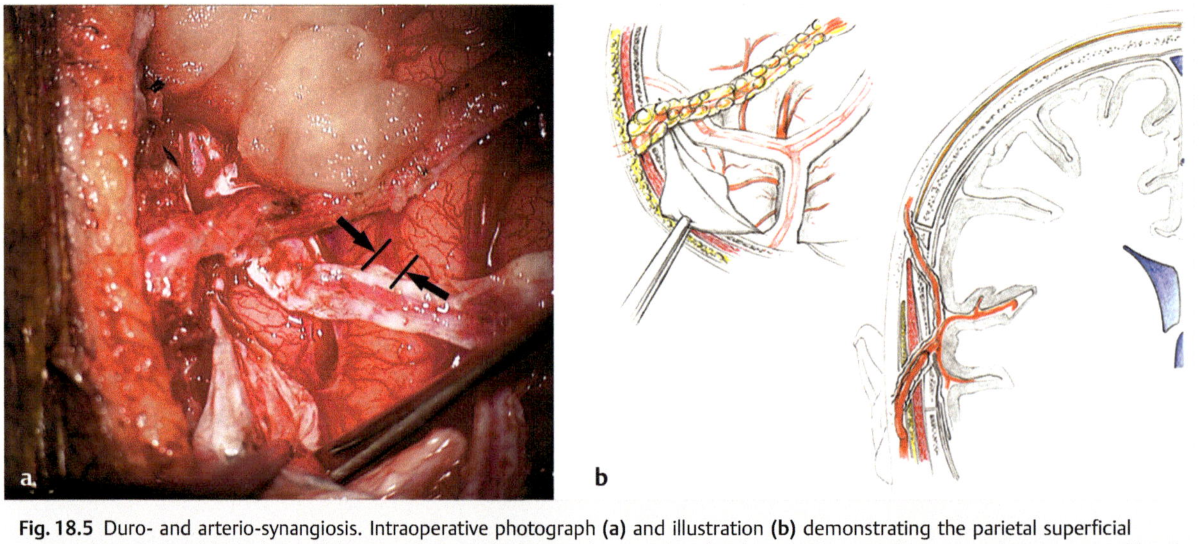

**Fig. 18.5** Duro- and arterio-synangiosis. Intraoperative photograph **(a)** and illustration **(b)** demonstrating the parietal superficial temporal artery (STA) branch on the brain surface to which it has been apposed with several 10–0 nylon sutures between its cuff and the arachnoid. A dural bridge across the opening is evident, created to spare the middle meningeal artery (MMA) branches within the dura (*arrows*). A dural leaflet has been split and the inner leaflet is being inverted with a Penfield instrument over the brain surface just beyond the craniotomy edge. Inset demonstrates cross-sectional view of dural inversion. (Panel **(b)** is modified after Mr. Peter Roth; Department of Neurosurgery; University Hospital Zurich; Zurich, Switzerland.)

The temporal fascia and muscle is stitched but the proximal portion is not closed to avoid kinking or pressure on the STA stump and branches. After bone flap replacement and muscle closure, the bypass flow is remeasured to ensure patency has been maintained. A nonadherent Gelfilm layer is placed over the STA stump to prevent adhesion and scarring in this location in case of any future need to reopen the incision. The skin is then closed with galeal stitches after placement of a short closed-system subgaleal drain. A nylon suture is placed in the skin; in pediatric patients, absorbable suture instead of nylon can be used to avoid the need for subsequent suture removal. In adults, healing of the incision is generally slower, compounded by the devascularization of the scalp by the dual STA harvest and the longer curved incision in adults; these factors favor the use of permanent suture material which can be removed when the surgeon chooses based on inspection and verification of healing, rather than absorbable sutures which lose integrity at a pre-determined interval.

## 18.10 Difficulties Encountered

If the frontal STA branch which is typically used for the STA–MCA bypass is discovered to be inadequate during surgery or has poor cut flow, the parietal branch can be used as an alternative. In such a scenario the parietal branch alone will serve as both direct bypass and the source for arterio-synangiosis along the course of the vessel, where it is apposed to the brain surface, proximal to the anastomosis.

Pitfalls and mistakes to remain vigilant for and avoid include the following:

### 18.10.1 Donor Vessel

- Injuring STA during harvest or craniotomy.
- Failing to coagulate side branches leads to leakage after bypass.
- Failing to flush and irrigate vessel leads to desiccation.
- Creating a dissection in the vessel wall during harvest or flushing.

### 18.10.2 Craniotomy/Durotomy

- Inadequate craniotomy size, location.
- Sacrifice of the MMA during craniotomy or dura opening.
- Poor hemostasis prior to starting bypass—continuous oozing disrupts visualization.

### 18.10.3 Recipient Vessel

- Injuring or coagulating recipient which is friable.
- Failure to coagualate perforating branches which will cause back bleeding during anastomosis.

### 18.10.4 Anastomosis

- Catching back wall during suturing of the anastomosis.
- Inadequate number of sutures leads to leakage of anastomosis.
- Failure to remove stent.
- Revascularizing wrong territory (superior vs. inferior MCA division).

### 18.10.5 Closure

- Strangulating STA during bone flap replacement or muscle reapproximation.
- Catch STA stump in suture line during skin closure.

For the STA–MCA bypass, if a poor bypass flow or cut flow index (e.g., $<0.5$) is encountered, several factor can be contributing:

- Poor patient selection (no hemodynamic compromise): this problem is best averted by careful attention to preoperative hemodynamic imaging and careful patient selection.
- Donor problem: avoid by not injuring or coagulating vessel during harvest, keeping the branch moist and wrapped in a papaverine soaked cottonoid, flushing with heparinized saline, cleaning the adventitial cuff well, and making sure the vessel wall is not dissected prior to anastomosis.
- Anastomosis problem: avoid by checking back wall during suturing (and using a silastic stent), flushing with heparinized saline prior to completion, and making sure no sutures are protruding into the lumen.
- Recipient or distal bed problem: avoid by choosing adequate size recipient, flushing with heparinized saline, and recognizing that the vascular territory may require double STA bypass if recipient beds are isolated by proximal occlusive disease.

## 18.11 Bailout, Rescue, and Salvage Maneuvers

It is best to avoid the potential pitfalls by careful attention to detail, rather than manage them after occurrence, but in some cases, salvage strategies are necessary.

If the donor STA becomes injured, for example, the parietal branch, which is kept intact is caught in the drill during craniotomy, that branch can still potentially be salvaged and used as a direct bypass if it can be cut proximal to the area of injury.

If direct STA–MCA anastomosis thromboses, it is important to check the suture line and massage the vessels and anastomosis site gently as a small clot may dislodge and regain patency. Otherwise, if a problem with the suture line is suspected, the anastomosis can be reopened and revised using heparin and small flushes of tissue plasminogen activator (tPA) to fully dissolve any thrombus prior to resuturing. Unfortunately if thrombus has formed in the anastomosis for any reason, this is frequently white platelet rich clot which is less responsive to heparin and tPA and is prone to reaccumulation. Even if patency cannot be restored, direct bypass should be kept in place as the bypass occasionally recanalizes over time to deliver flow.

If the anastomosis suture line has leakage after release of temporary clips, the first maneuver is to apply gentle pressure with a cotton ball which frequently abates the issue. If unsuccessful, an additional stitch may be required, although there is risk of suboptimal placement as visualization is impaired compared to during the anastomosis. Another strategy if interrupted sutures have been used is to leave one suture end long for each stitch during the anastomosis; if a leak is subsequently evident between sutures after the temporary clips are removed, the long ends of each can then be tied together to cinch the leakage area avoiding the need for placement of a new stich.

# 18.12 Tips, Pearls, and Lessons Learned

Tips and key elements can be categorized as relevant to different phases of the operation as outlined below.

## 18.12.1 Preoperative Management

- Good preoperative patient selection.
- Study angiographic imaging and plan case (assess the best donor/recipient territory, assess for spontaneous MMA collaterals).

## 18.12.2 Intraoperative Anesthetic Management

- No mannitol, lasix, hyperventilation during surgery.
- Burst suppression during temporary clipping.
- Anticonvulsant prophylaxis.
- SSEP/EEG monitoring to detect, and thus avoid, intraoperative ischemia.
- Strict blood pressure maintenance during induction and anesthesia.

## 18.12.3 Intraoperative Technique

- Attention to details throughout—from skin incision to closure.
- Avoid all thrombogenic material—flush vessels, create perfect field hemostasis, avoid Floseal.
- Keep STA moist and wrapped in papaverine soaked cottonoid until used.
- If there's leakage at anastomosis site, irrigate copiously and apply gentle pressure (rare to require additional stich); for interrupted sutures, tie long end of adjacent stitches together.

Additionally, close postoperative monitoring and management is critical. Blood pressure should be controlled to patient's baseline range and the patient should be observed in the intensive care unit for the first 24 to 48 hours postoperatively. Postoperative head CT to rule out any hemorrhage, and assessment of bypass function and patency with quantitative magnetic resonance angiography (▶ Fig. 18.6), and angiogram during the hospital stay as a baseline is useful. Reassessment of hemodynamics

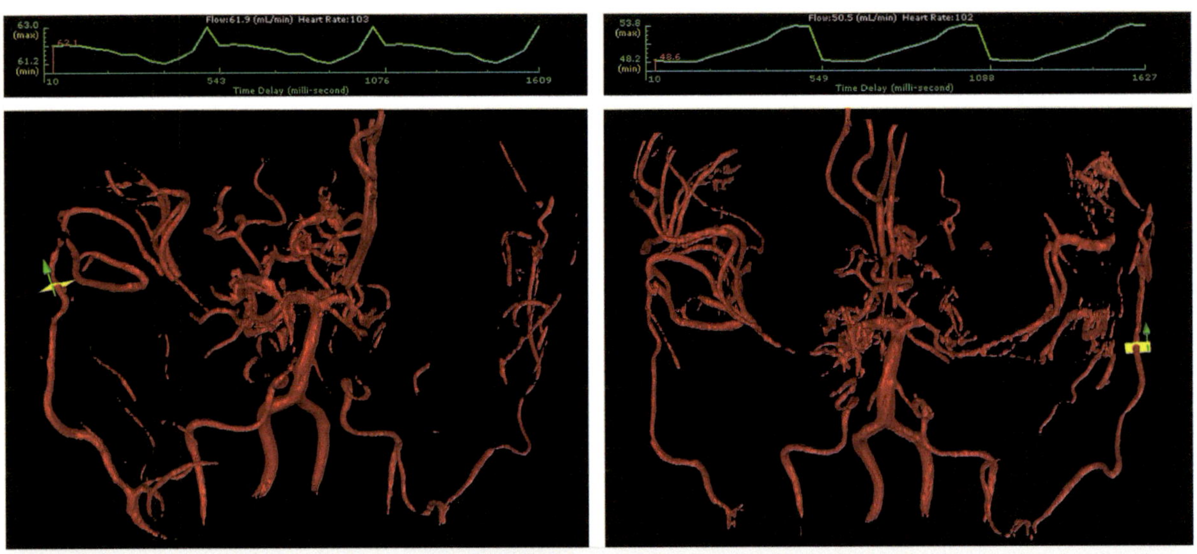


**Fig. 18.6** Quantitative magnetic resonance angiography (QMRA) imaging demonstrating blood flow of 62 cc and 50 cc per minute in the right and left superficial temporal artery (STA), respectively, of a patient with moyamoya disease (MMD) following bilateral STA–MCA bypass with encephalo-duro-arterio-synangiosis (EDAS).

with imaging at 6 weeks, 6 months, and 12 months is our standard protocol and annually thereafter, along with neuropsychological testing. If bilateral surgery is needed these are generally separated by 4 to 6 weeks to allow interim recovery.

## Acknowledgment

The author would like to acknowledge Christa Wellman and Ziad Hage, MD, for assistance in preparation of the figures, and Fady T Charbel, MD, for the development of the flow-based approach to STA–MCA bypass.

## References

[1] Cahan LD. Failure of encephalo-duro-arterio-synangiosis procedure in moyamoya disease. Pediatr Neurosci. 1985–1986; 12(1):58–62

[2] Miyamoto S, Kikuchi H, Karasawa J, Nagata I, Yamazoe N, Akiyama Y. Pitfalls in the surgical treatment of moyamoya disease. Operative techniques for refractory cases. J Neurosurg. 1988; 68(4):537–543

[3] Matsushima T, Fujiwara S, Nagata S, Fujii K, Fukui M, Hasuo K. Reoperation for moyamoya disease refractory to encephalo-duro-arterio-synangiosis. Acta Neurochir (Wien). 1990; 107(3–4):129–132

[4] Houkin K, Kamiyama H, Takahashi A, Kuroda S, Abe H. Combined revascularization surgery for childhood moyamoya disease: STA–MCA and encephalo-duro-arterio-myo-synangiosis. Childs Nerv Syst. 1997; 13(1):24–29

[5] Matsushima T, Inoue T, Suzuki SO, Fujii K, Fukui M, Hasuo K. Surgical treatment of moyamoya disease in pediatric patients—comparison between the results of indirect and direct revascularization procedures. Neurosurgery. 1992; 31(3):401–405

[6] Amin-Hanjani S, Singh A, Rifai H, et al. Combined direct and indirect bypass for moyamoya: quantitative assessment of direct bypass flow over time. Neurosurgery. 2013; 73(6):962–967, discussion 967–968

[7] Amin-Hanjani S. Cerebral revascularization: extracranial-intracranial bypass. J Neurosurg Sci. 2011; 55(2):107–116

[8] Amin-Hanjani S, Charbel FT. Flow-assisted surgical technique in cerebrovascular surgery. Surg Neurol. 2007; 68 Suppl 1:S4–S11

[9] Amin-Hanjani S, Du X, Mlinarevich N, Meglio G, Zhao M, Charbel FT. The cut flow index: an intraoperative predictor of the success of extracranial-intracranial bypass for occlusive cerebrovascular disease. Neurosurgery. 2005; 56(1) Suppl:75–85, discussion 75–85

[10] Charbel FT, Meglio G, Amin-Hanjani S. Superficial temporal artery-to-middle cerebral artery bypass. Neurosurgery. 2005; 56(1) Suppl: 186–190, discussion 186–190

# 19 Individualized Extracranial–Intracranial Revascularization in the Treatment of Late-Stage Moyamoya Disease

*Bin Xu*

**Abstract**

Late stage moyamoya disease is defined as the one at stage 5 to 6 of Suzuki's grading system, despite of spontaneous collaterals from branches of external carotid artery, cerebral revascularization is still necessary in most patients. But the diversity and complexity of collateral paths make it difficult to preserve the already-formed collaterals, which is the principle of this kind of surgical procedure. Individualized revascularization seems to be an effective solution. Here we will introduce a set of strategies, including individualized designation of skin flap, temporal muscle flap, bone flap, dura matter flap, and target revascularization. The set of strategies is proved to be safe and effective in our single institution case series.

*Keywords:* moyamoya disease, Suzuki stage, extracranial-intracranial revascularization, spontaneous collaterals, individualized revascularization

## 19.1 History and Initial Description

Late-stage moyamoya disease (MMD) is defined as the one at stage 5 to 6 of Suzuki's grading system and is characterized by spontaneous collaterals from branches of external carotid artery. In a series of 336 patients affected by late-stage MMD treated in the Department of Neurosurgery of Huashan hospital from 2005 to 2015, spontaneous collaterals are fully developed in only 3 cases (1% of the entire series) without any symptoms or cerebral hemodynamic impairment who need no surgical treatment (▶ Fig. 19.1). About 333 patients of late-stage MMD were operated for cerebral ischemia or intracranial hemorrhage, or both, with impaired hemodynamics which could be detected by CT perfusion (CTP) or single-photon emission computed tomography (SPECT) routinely.

## 19.2 Indications

The indication of individualized extracranial–intracranial (EC–IC) revascularization in late-stage MMD is carefully analyzed. Microsurgical treatment of the patients is planned with attention to any preexisted spontaneous collaterals, ischemic symptoms, and hemorrhagic history.

## 19.3 Key Principles

The key principle of the surgery is to use all the three layered external carotid artery (ECA) branches including superficial temporal artery (STA), posterior auricular artery (PAA) or occipital artery (OA) that are feeding the scalp, deep temporal artery (DTA) feeding the temporal muscle, and middle meningeal artery (MMA) feeding the dura, meanwhile preserving the already-formed collaterals.

## 19.4 SWOT Analysis

### 19.4.1 Strength

- Combined direct and indirect approach allows the full use of all the branches coming from the ECA, while preserving preexisted spontaneous collaterals.

### 19.4.2 Weaknesses

- Due to poorer MCA vessel networks of late-stage MMD, the recipient artery may not distribute blood flow as efficiently as in early stage MMD with heathier MCA vessel network.
- The mean blood flow in bypass is reduced compared with those bypass flow performed in patients with early stage of MMD.
- There can be a competition between the bypass flow and the original flow in MCA network that may cause blood flow congestion and edema of the cortex, which have consequently higher occurrence of postoperative transient neurological deficit.

### 19.4.3 Opportunities

- Carefully designed revascularization, based on a comprehensive understanding of clinical symptoms, spontaneous collaterals, hemodynamic characters, and recipient artery networks, could replace the blood flow to most suffering ischemic area of the brain cortex.
- Late stage of MMD already has some spontaneous stomas from ECA branches with a better potential to form new stomas by encephalo-duro-myo-synangiosis (EDMS), the indirect part of the surgery.

### 19.4.4 Threats

- Due to the barrier of ventricles, although the ischemic condition of deep structure such as thalamus and basal

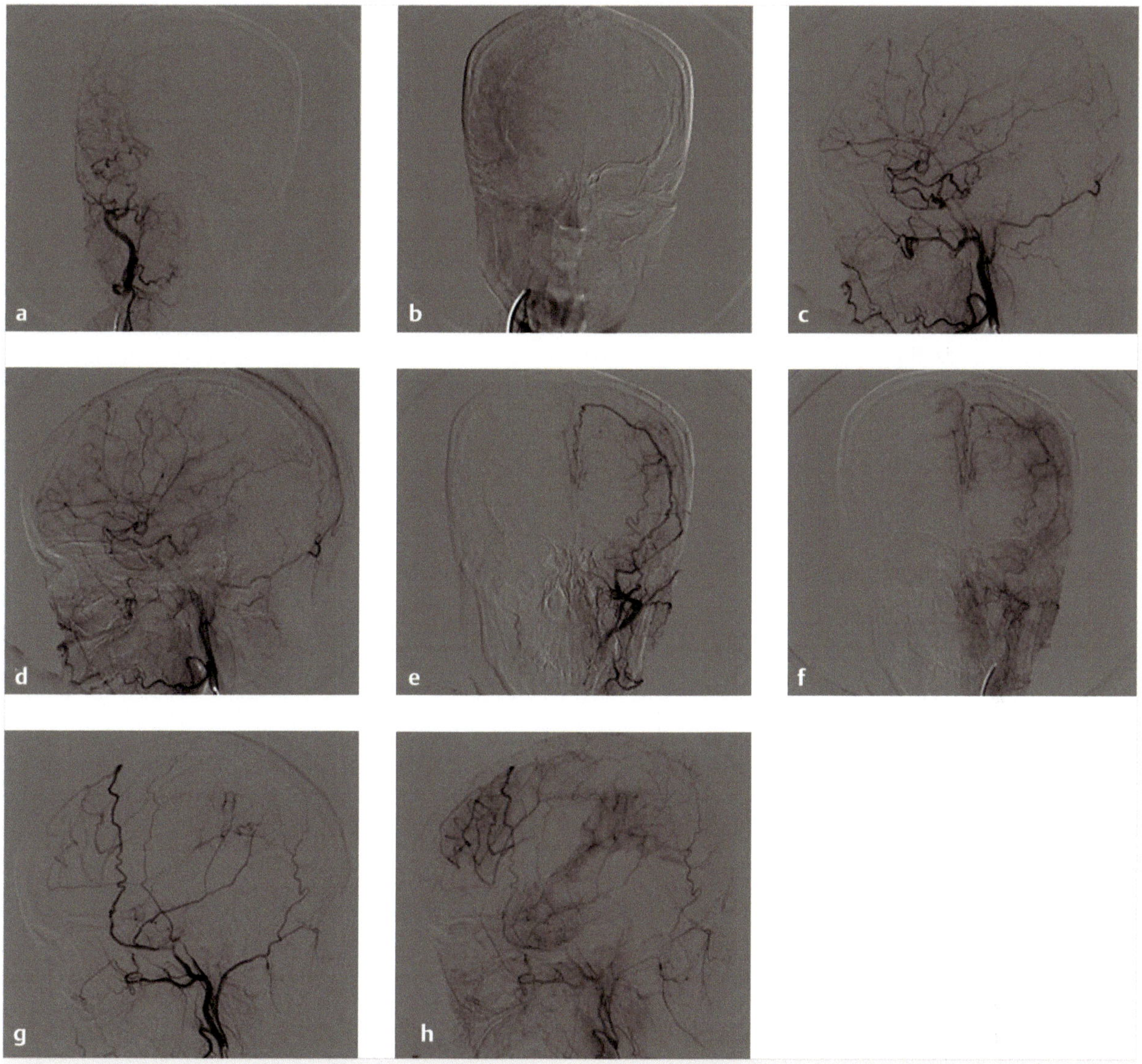


**Fig. 19.1** Angiography of patients with well-developed spontaneous collaterals where revascularization considered unnecessary. **(a–h)** Case 1, anteroposterior projection and lateral projection of bilateral external carotid arteries (**[a–d]** right ECA; **[e–h]** left ECA) indicated well-developed transdural spontaneous collaterals. (*Continued*)

ganglion could be improved, the blood flow via the moyamoya vessels is still needed in most cases.

- The occurrence of rehemorrhage cannot be totally obliterated.

## 19.5 Contraindications

The contraindications to perform this technique are when the ECA already developed full collateral blood flow.

## 19.6 Special Considerations

Neurosurgeons should analyze the spontaneous collaterals in the preoperative digital subtraction angiography (DSA) very carefully (▶ Fig. 19.2). Main collateral paths in the abovementioned group of 336 cases are listed in ▶ Table 19.1.

MMA is the most common source of spontaneous collaterals. It enters the floor of the middle cranial fossa through the foramen spinosum, passes laterally on to the temporal bone, and curves anteriorly over the great wing of sphenoid. Thereafter, it divides into anterior and posterior branch. MMA can provide important collateral flow through dura mater. Normally, it is the anterior (frontal) branch that provides collateral blood flow to anterior cerebral artery (ACA) territory through falx. MMA could be originated from ophthalmic artery in anatomic variated cases. MMA is vulnerable to the routine pterional

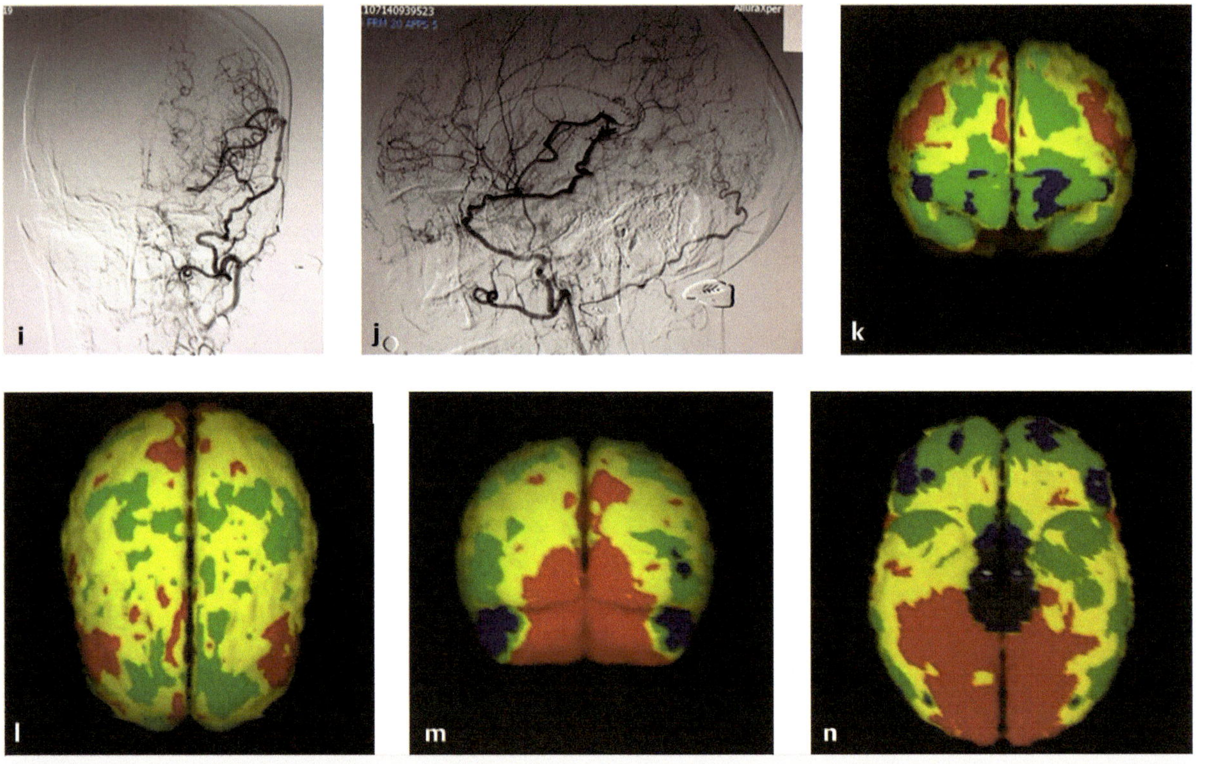

**Fig. 19.1** (*Continued*) **(i–n)** Case 2, angiography of left ECA revealed spontaneous collaterals from ECA perfused middle cerebral artery territory, where SPECT showed mild hemodynamic impairment (**[k]** anterior view; **[l]** superior view; **[m]** posterior view; **[n]** inferior view).

**Table 19.1** Main collateral paths in our case series

| Collateral paths | MMA | STA | OA | EVD[a] | Others[b] |
|---|---|---|---|---|---|
| n | 297 | 17 | 10 | 14 | 7 |

Abbreviations: EVD, external ventricular drainage; MMA, middle meningeal artery; OA, occipital artery; STA, superior temporal artery.
[a]Spontaneous collaterals developed in the burr holes of external ventricular drainage.
[b]Spontaneous collaterals of other paths, such as ophthalmic artery to anterior meningeal artery path.

craniotomy because hyperplasia MMA may be located deep in the cranial sulcus, increasing the risk of damage, causing post-procedural ischemic stroke.

Scalp arteries, such as STA, OA, and sometimes PAA, are rare sources of spontaneous collaterals, but in patients with any kind of craniotomy history like cerebral hematoma evacuation or external ventricular drainage, the proportion is greatly increased. In this situation, individualized designation of scalp flap is of great importance.

Heparin saline irrigation is recommended only during anastomosis; we do not recommend a general heparinization.

## 19.7 Pitfalls, Risk Assessment, and Complications

- In some cases, direct bypass may not be feasible due to the small size of recipient artery.
- Sometimes the dimeter ratio of donor–recipient artery is larger than 2.5 times, the operator may quit direct bypass because of the high possibility of postoperative hemorrhage.
- The recipient MCA network is very poor on DSA and MR angiography (MRA). There is poor blood flow in some branches of MCA that looks pale and poorly filled under microscope. It is also a contradiction for direct bypass.
- The EC–IC revascularization holds the potential risk of postoperative transient neurological deficits, seizure, and postoperative hemorrhage.

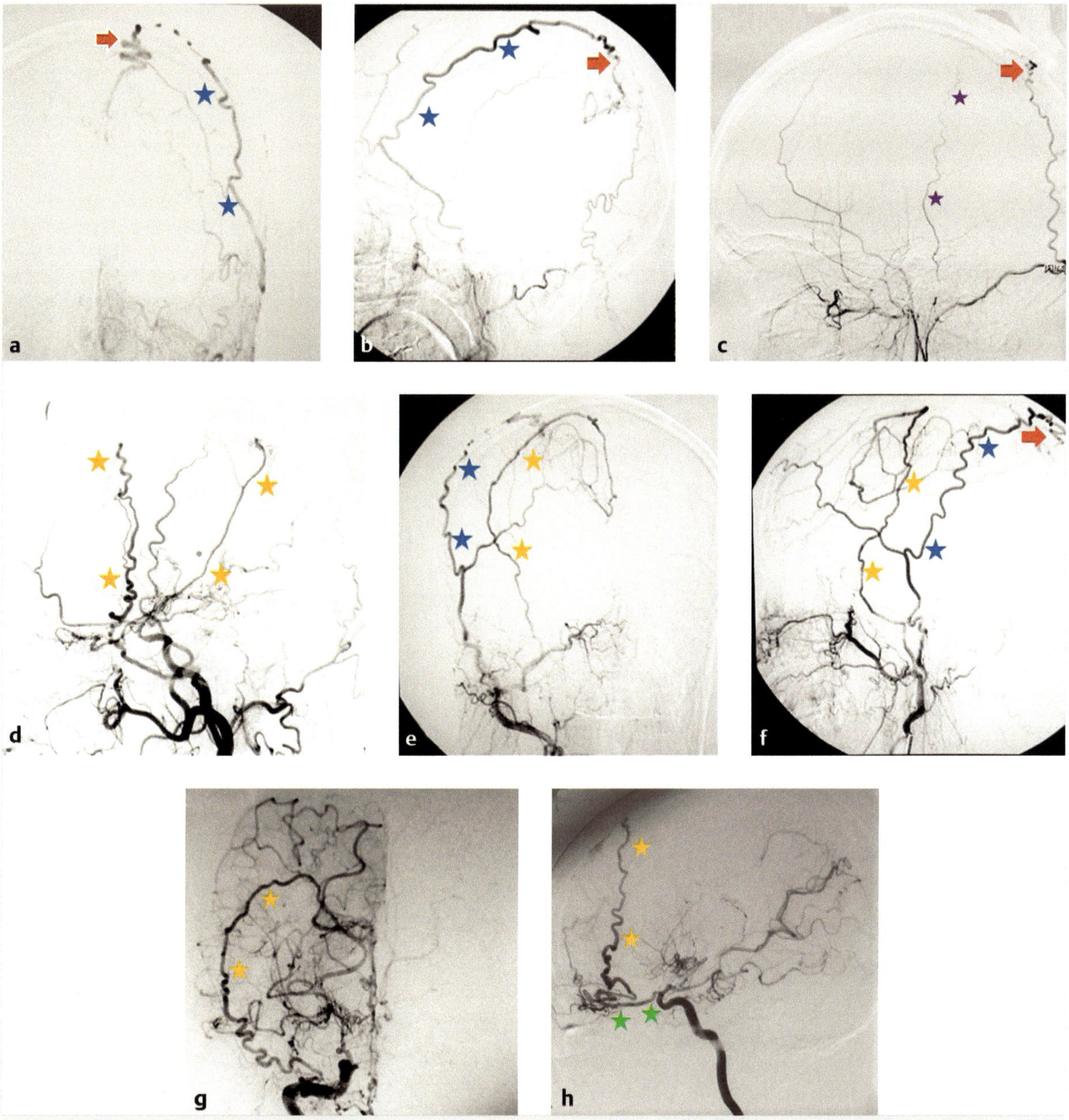


**Fig. 19.2** Different collateral paths. **(a, b)** Collaterals from STA. **(c)** Collateral from occipital artery. **(d)** Collaterals from MMA trunk and branches. **(e, f)** Collaterals from MMA and STA. **(g, h)** Special MMA originated from ophthalmic artery. *Red arrow,* transcranial segment of collaterals from skin arteries STA or occipital artery; *blue star,* STA; *purple star,* posterior auricular artery; *yellow star,* MMA trunk and branches; *green star,* ophthalmic artery.

## 19.8 Special Instructions, Position, and Anesthesia

Supine position was used as a routine for STA-MCA or PAA-MCA bypass. Park-bench position was used for OA-PCA bypass. The use of head clamp should be avoided to protect contralateral STA. Blood pressure was maintained within the patient's baseline range throughout the surgical procedural. Hyperventilation was avoided in order to prevent vasoconstriction. During the perioperative period, blood volume was expanded using crystalloid, normally 1.25 to 1.4 times maintenance through postoperative day 2.

## 19.9 Patient Position with Skin Incision and Key Surgical Steps

### 19.9.1 Skin Incision

The main concern of individualized designation of skin incision is to recognize the preexisted spontaneous anastomosis; meanwhile, the bone flap should cover the ischemic area. Selected ECA angiogram is routinely performed before surgery; MRA or CT angiography (CTA) could not provide all the necessary details of spontaneous collaterals.

In our routine procedure, an extended pterional skin incision is adopted to make full use of DTA of temporal muscle and of STA branches located in the scalp flap. The incision is extended by 1.0 to 1.5 cm above the superior temporal line. Individualized adjustments would be made in the following situations (▶ Fig. 19.3):

1. Spontaneous collaterals from STA branch are carefully identified in the angiography. The area of ischemic cortex is defined by CT perfusion or SPECT. Scalp incision should be adjusted forward or backward so as to avoid injury of scalp artery with preexisted spontaneous collaterals and to cover the ischemic cortex.
2. When routine pterional craniotomy cannot cover ischemic region, the procedure can be planned differently. For example, in patients with ischemic bilateral ACA territory, bilateral frontal lobe should be covered in the way that a coronal incision is adopted (▶ Fig. 19.1; ▶ Fig. 19.8). When the ischemic area is located in the occipital lobe, horseshoe-shape scalp incision covering the temporal-parietal-occipital lobe is adopted.

### 19.9.2 Temporal Muscle

Spontaneous anastomosis from temporal muscle could be formed only in patients with a history of craniotomy, and rest part of temporal muscle outside bone window could still be used as donor tissue. The temporal muscle is dissected from the temporal bone without using monopolar so that the entire DTA network is kept intact (▶ Fig. 19.4). DTA normally is small and the distal part could not be recognized clearly in preoperative DSA. Any incision of the temporal muscle could hurt the DTA network and result in poor collateral flow. We therefore avoid temporal muscle incision except in very thick ones.

### 19.9.3 Bone Flap

MMA is the most common source of spontaneous collaterals in late-stage MMD, and it is vulnerable in craniotomy. Kuroda analyzed the relationship between MMA and pterion and divided it into the following: (1) bridge, (2) monorail, and (3) tunnel types. The extent of difficulty to preserve MMA integrity increases from type a to c. In routine single-window pterional craniotomy, it is very difficult and time-consuming to preserve MMA; we thus developed another double-window craniotomy.

Preoperative localization of MMA is of paramount importance. The groove of MMA in cranium could be seen in DSA mask images clearly (▶ Fig. 19.7**a**), and the relationship between MMA groove and coronal suture is of great help in localizing MMA in craniotomy. The relation between MMA and STA is also helpful. The course of MMA is approximately parallel to that of STA parietal branch, by 2 to 3 cm anteriorly (▶ Fig. 19.5**a**).

1. Single-window bone flap.
   When MMA groove is shallow and vague in DSA mask images, a single-window heart-shape craniotomy is performed. The bone window is expanded carefully towards sphenoidal crest to the site where MMA perforated from the bone, preserving the lesser wing of sphenoid bone (▶ Fig. 19.5).
   When transdural collaterals could be identified on the convexity of frontal lobe, there's no ischemic area in frontal lobe, a single-window bone flap posterior to MMA would be adopted (▶ Fig. 19.6).
2. Double-window bone flaps.
   When MMA groove is deep and clear in DSA mask images, we prefer double-window bone flaps-anterior and posterior to MMA respectively, a bone bridge is left to cover the course of MMA. We created a complex of dura, MMA, middle meningeal vein (MMV), and covered-bone bridge (▶ Fig. 19.7). We believe that this is the best way to protect MMA and the distal spontaneous stomas.
   In patients with ischemia of bilateral ACA territory, bilateral frontal lobe should be covered, a coronal incision and bifrontal bone flaps should be adopted (▶ Fig. 19.8).

### 19.9.4 Dura Mater

The integrity of MMA network is the most important aspect in order to preserve the vascular support. Since the potential of MMA as donor is great, every single branch of MMA should be preserved. Dura mater would be incised along each main branch of MMA separately. Radial incisions were made on the remaining part of the dura mater. After hemostasis, dura mater is flipped over with its outer surface being in close contact with the cortex (▶ Fig. 19.9).

Sometimes, the bleeding of accompanying MMV is difficult to control. The coagulation using bipolar could damage MMA. In this condition, keeping the patency of MMA and hemostasis of accompanying MMV could be attained simultaneously by means of barrel-suturing (▶ Fig. 19.9**f, g**), which is what we call “Chinese spring roll.” The margin of the dura mater was sutured into a shape of barrel with the inner surface facing outside. The

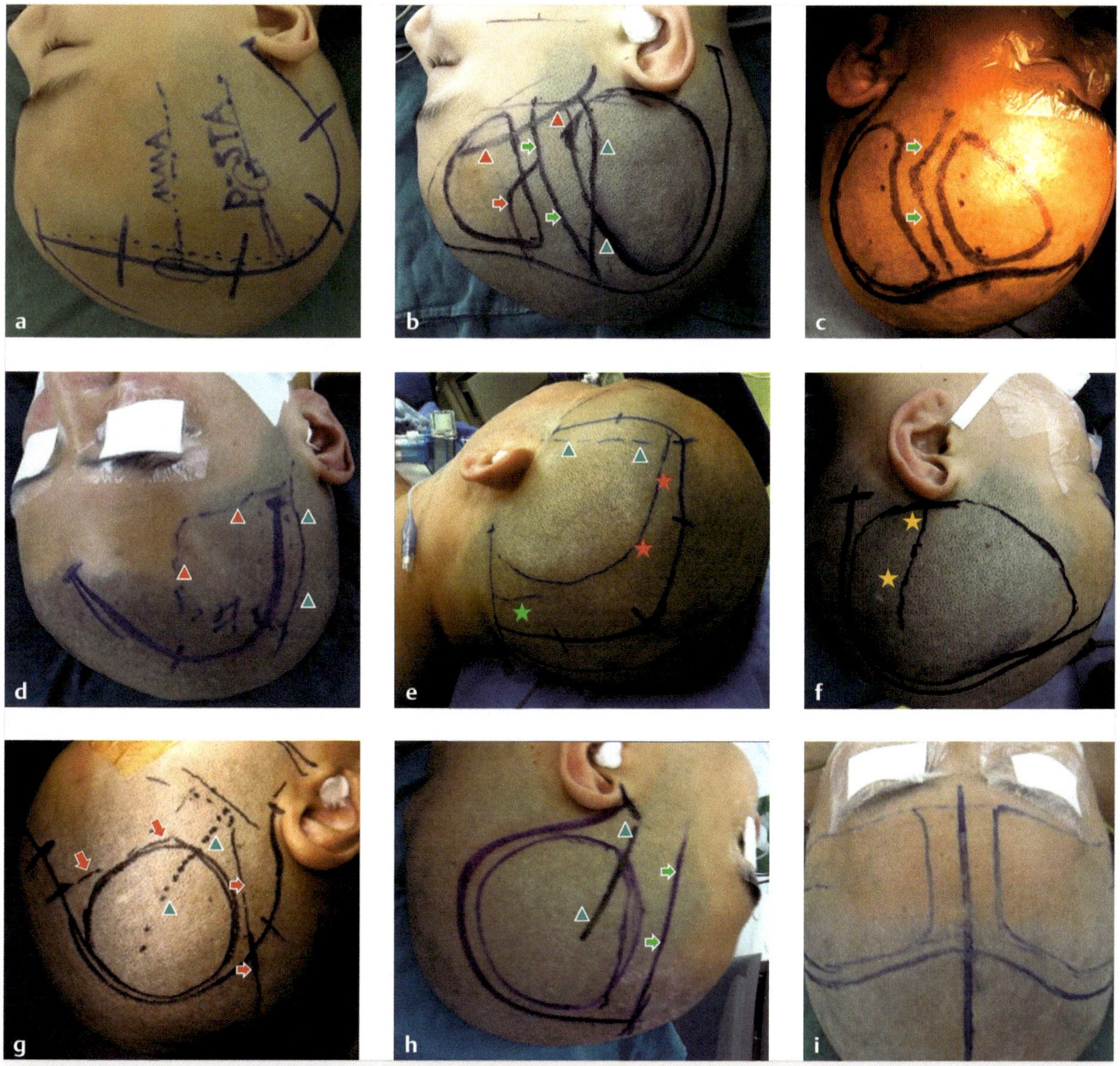


**Fig. 19.3** Individualized skin incision and surgical plan. **(a)** Routine skin incision in our case series, middle meningeal artery (MMA, body surface projection) and superficial temporal artery (STA) parietal branch (p-STA) is localized. **(b)** Double-window craniotomy is planned to protect MMA with spontaneous collaterals. **(c)** Individualized bone flaps in accordance with MMA course. **(d)** Forwarded skin incision to protect p-STA with spontaneous collaterals. **(e)** Back-warded incision to cover ischemic occipital lobe. **(f)** Posterior auricular artery (PAA) was used because there is no parietal branch of STA in this case. **(g)** Bone flap was made between MMA branches (*red arrows*) with collaterals, p-STA was used as donor artery. **(h)** Partly bone flap posterior to MMA to protect collaterals, using p-STA as donor artery. **(i)** Coronal incision in a patient with bilateral anterior cerebral artery (ACA) region ischemia. *Blue triangle*, posterior STA branch; *red triangle*, anterior STA branch; *green arrow*, MMA trunk; *red arrow*, MMA branches; *red star*, superior temporal line; *green star*, occipital artery; *yellow star*, posterior auricular artery.

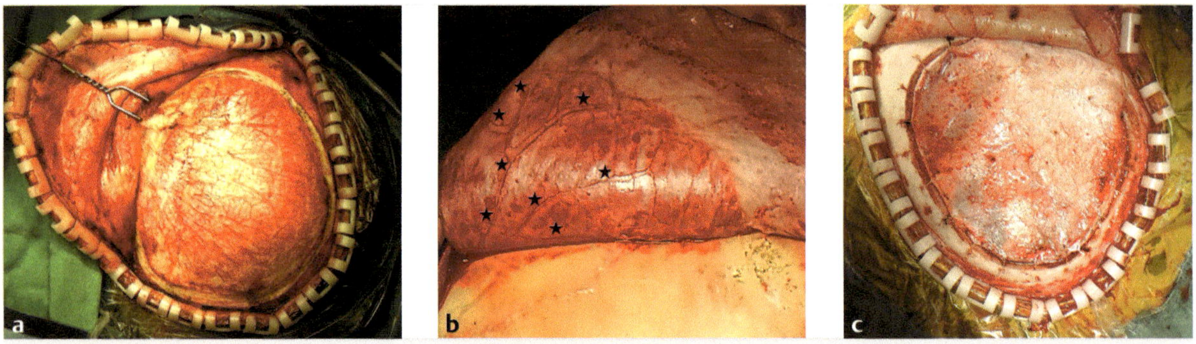

**Fig. 19.4** Handling of temporal muscle. **(a)** Temporal muscle was dissected. **(b)** The entire DTA network was kept intact (*black stars*). **(c)** Encephalo-duro-myo-synangiosis (EDMS), temporal muscle was sutured with the dura mater and fixed to the bone window, covering the cortex without any tension.

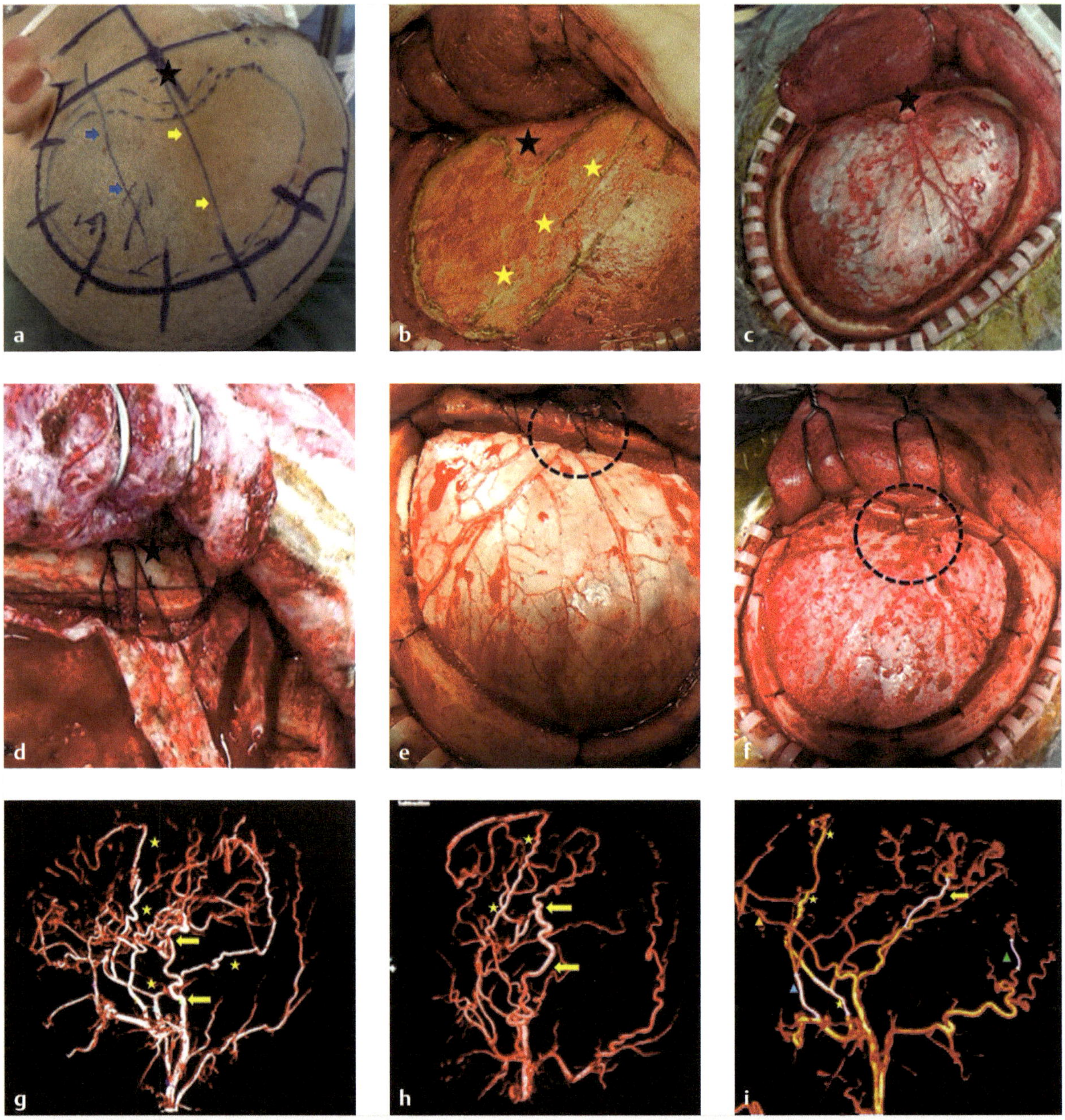

**Fig. 19.5** Single-window bone flap and follow-up angiography. **(a)** Single-window bone flap was planned, the courses of MMA (body surface projection, *yellow arrows*) and STA (*blue arrows*) were identified. **(b, c)** Heart-shape bone window, superior temporal line (*yellow stars*), sphenoidal crest residue (*blue stars*). **(d)** Dura mater on both sides of the sphenoidal crest residue was fixed to avoid potential avulsion or rupture of the MMA trunk. **(e, f)** When MMA groove is shallow and vague in DSA mask images, sphenoidal crest could be removed as well (*black circles*). **(g–i)** Follow-up three-dimensional angiography in different patients showed intact MMA (*yellow stars*), patent thickened direct bypass (*yellow arrows*), and indirect anastomosis from STA frontal branch (*yellow triangle*), DTA (*blue triangle*), and occipital artery (*green triangle*).

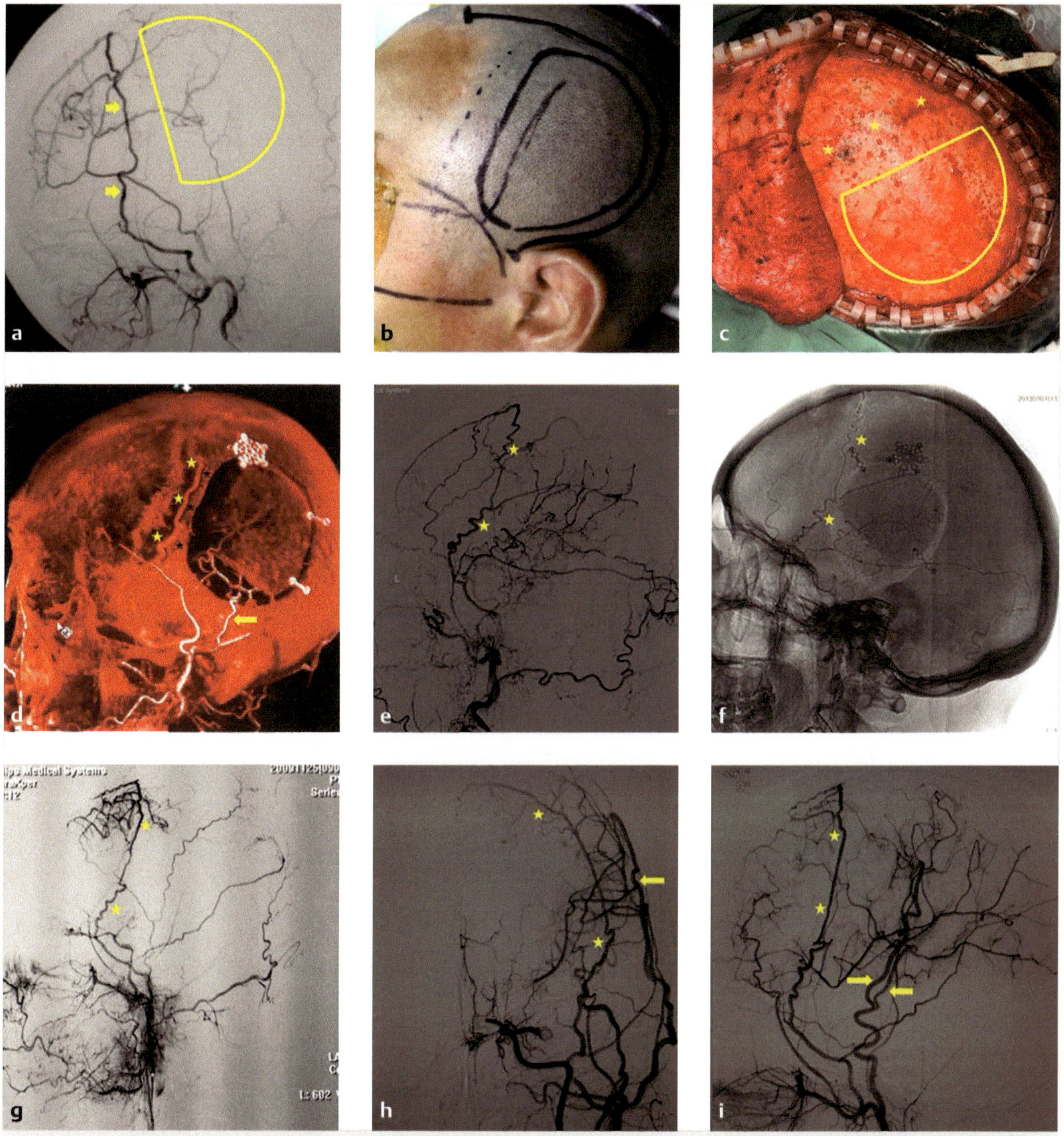


**Fig. 19.6** Individualized single-window bone flap and follow-up angiography. **(a)** Lateral projection of ECA revealed pre-existed collaterals from MMA (*yellow arrows*) and trans-dual anastomosis on the convexity of pre-frontal lobe. **(b, c)** Bone flap posterior to MMA was adopted, a deep MMA groove could be recognized from outside ([c] *yellow stars*). **(d)** Follow-up 3D angiography confirmed the patency of MMA and direct bypass, a deep MMA groove could be recognized easily (*yellow stars*). **(e, f)** Indirect anastomosis developed in the bone window, while MMA was preserved well in another patient with similar pre-existed collaterals. **(g–i)** Case 3, pre-surgical ECA lateral projection Image in **(g)** revealed well-developed spontaneous collaterals from MMA, follow-up angiogram **(h, i)** showed three STA (*yellow arrows*) branches were patent after triple direct bypasses, as well as intact MMA (*yellow stars*).

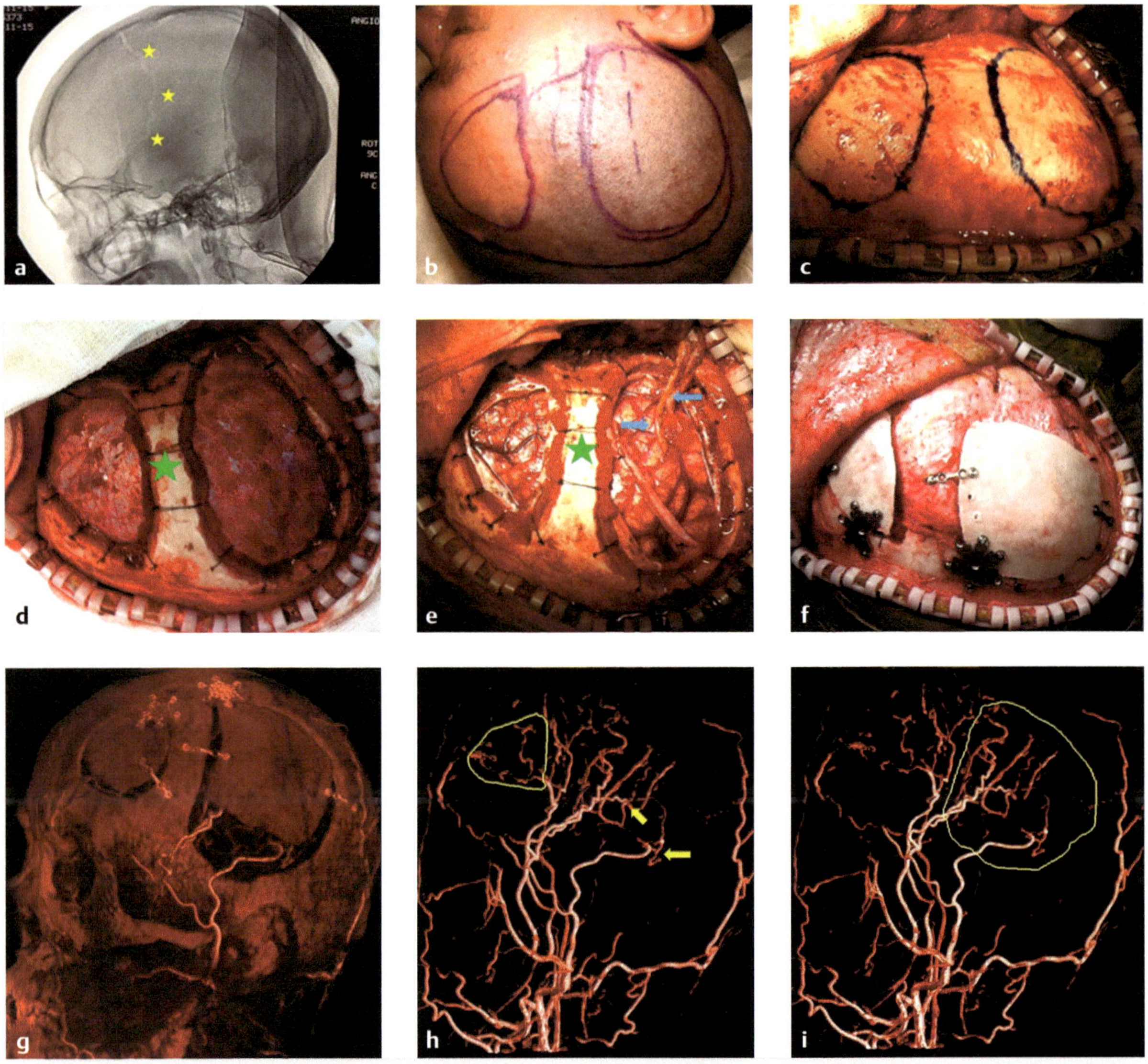

**Fig. 19.7** Double-window bone flaps and follow-up angiography. **(a)** DSA mask images showed deep MMA groove (*yellow stars*). **(b, c)** Double-window bone flaps were designed. **(d)** Dura mater was sutured at the margin of bone flap and along the "bone bridge (*green stars*)", a complex was created consisted of dura, MMA, middle meningeal vein (MMV), and covered bone bridge. **(e)** Double direct bypass (blue arrows), **(f)** Temporal muscle was sutured with the dura mater and fixed to the bone window, the inferior edge of bone flaps were trimmed into compatible shape and elevated a little to reduce compression of STA and temporal muscle. **(g–i)** Follow-up 3D angiography with/without cranium revealed patent double bypass (*yellow arrows* indicated the stomas), as well as indirect anastomosis both anterior and posterior to MMA (*circles*).

barrel is exactly like a "Chinese spring roll," containing MMA, accompanying veins, and some gelfoam strip.

## 19.9.5 Target Revascularization

Ischemic area could be defined by hemodynamic evaluation as CTP or SPECT. Spontaneous collaterals in late-stage MMD created some normal-perfused island in the ischemic hemisphere. If the recipient artery located in this kind of normal perfused area, the pressure difference between donor and recipient ($\Delta P$ of Poiseuille's Law, $Q = \pi \times r^4 \times \Delta p / 8\eta l$, $\Delta P$ is the only explanation for driving the blood flow) could be too small to form a sustainable bypass. $\Delta P$ is a dynamically changing parameter after surgery until achieving a balanced condition after all the spontaneous stoma formed. This progress may take 6 months or even longer. The competitive blood flow for bypass comes not only from the internal carotid artery system, but also progressively from the collateral blood flow via the spontaneous stoma originated from MMA

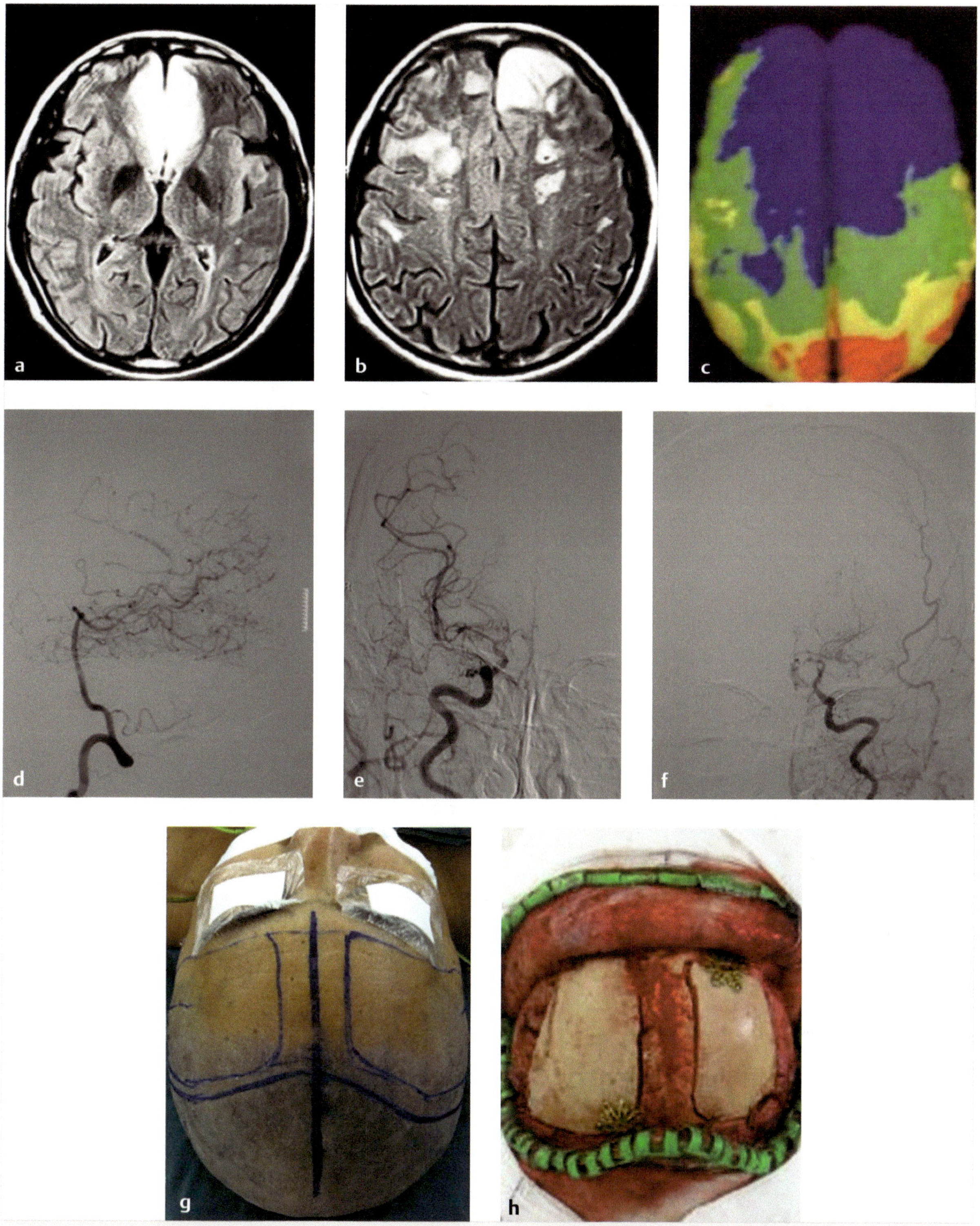


**Fig. 19.8** Individualized Double-window bone flaps in cases with bilateral pre-frontal lobe infarction **(a, b)** and impaired hemodynamic (**[c]** brain SPECT) in ACA territory, angiography (**[d–f]** lateral projection of vertebral artery and AP projection bilateral ICA) revealed poor perfusion and no collaterals from posterior circulation in this area, a coronal incision **(g)** with bilateral prefrontal bone flaps **(h)** was designed.

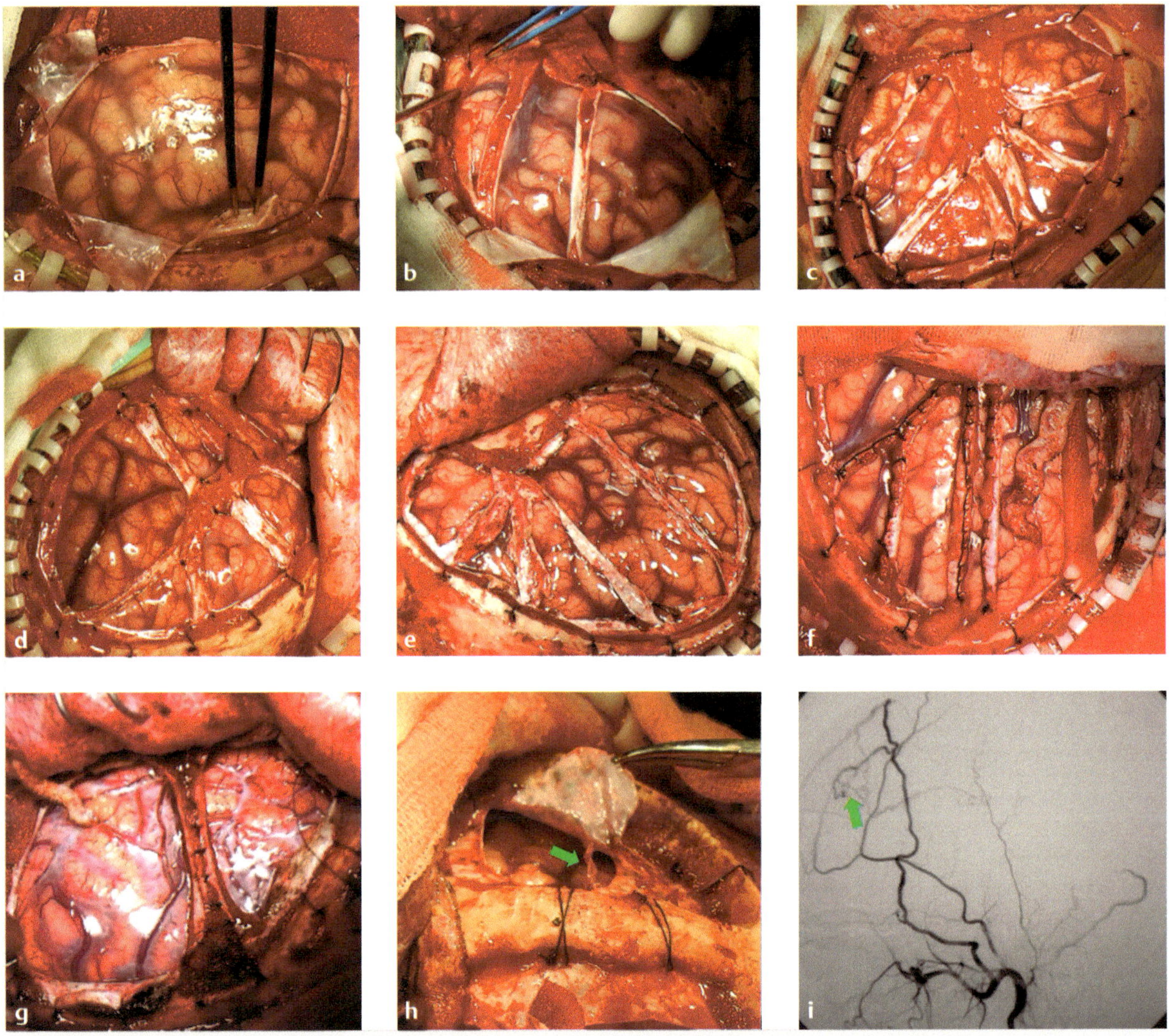


**Fig. 19.9** Individualized processing of dura mater. **(a–e)** Dura mater was incised along each main branch of MMA, radial incisions were made on the remaining part of dura mater **(b)**, after hemostasis, dura valves were flipped over with its outer surface being in close contact with cortex **(a)**. **(f, g)** Barrel-suturing, also called as "Chinese spring roll," the margin of dura mater was sutured into a shape of barrel with the inner surface facing outside. **(h, i)** Trans-dural anastomosis on brain surface (*green arrows*).

and DTA. On the basis of these two facts, target revascularization is reasonable, which may facilitate blood flow to where it is mostly demanded with greatest ΔP. There are two different blood flow pressure gradients in MCA networks. One is still keeping the physiological direction from proximal to distal. The pressure gradient is $P_{proximal} > P_{distal}$. The other is reversed, $P_{proximal} < P_{distal}$ (▶ Fig. 19.10). Operators could recognize the different pressure gradient after careful scrutinize of DSA and SPECT (▶ Fig. 19.11**a–d**). Intraoperative indocyanine green (ICG) angiogram is also helpful in localizing the recipient area. In cases of good MCA network, which can bear more blood flow from donor arteries, double barrel bypass would be considered, sometimes only using single branch of STA (▶ Fig. 19.11 **f**). The totally infarcted area should be avoided as revascularization is in vain.

## 19.9.6 The Simplest Anastomosis Techniques

The recipient artery of late-stage MMD is usually fragile and with a lot of small branches. The vessel wall is very thin. We use two or three curved mini temporal clips to occlude the recipient artery. In this way, we can preserve all the small branches without using bipolar. No rubber mat or silicon rubber tube is needed. Interrupted suturing is adopted to guarantee the possibility of the stoma's

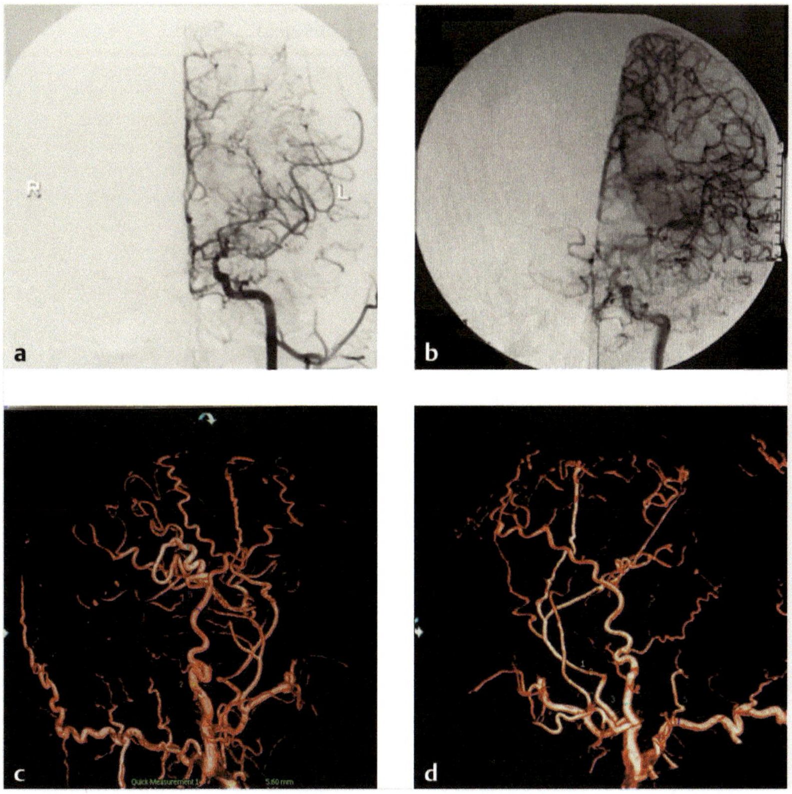

**Fig. 19.10** MCA networks and blood flow pressure gradients. **(a)** Frontal angiogram of a left ICA showed blood flow from proximal to distal, the pressure gradient is $P_{proximal} > P_{distal}$; **(b)** frontal angiogram of another left ICA showed blood flow from distal to proximal, the pressure gradient is $P_{proximal} < P_{distal}$. **(c)** Follow-up angiogram showed enlarged bypass in a hemisphere with good MCA network; **(d)** follow-up angiogram showed shrink bypass in another hemisphere with poor MCA network.

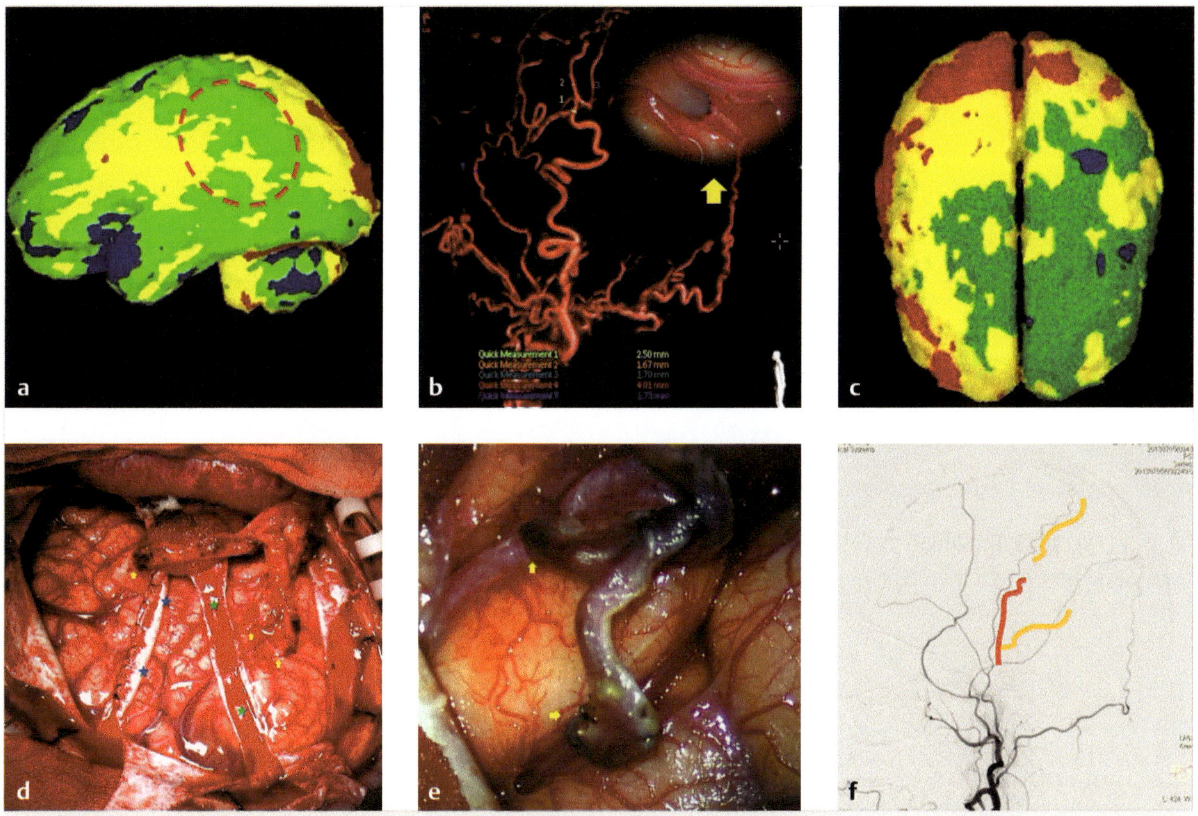

**Fig. 19.11** Individualized target revascularization. **(a)** Brain SPECT showed normal-perfused islands in a hypo-perfused hemisphere, a misery-perfused region (*red circle*) was considered responsible for clinical symptoms. **(b)** Targeted direct bypass was introduced to this misery-perfused region, stoma (*yellow arrow*), follow-up 3D angiography revealed thickened STA (2.5 mm in diameter) and recipient artery (1.67 mm and 1.70 mm in diameter, respectively). **(c)** Brain SPECT showed a case with global hypo-perfusion in left hemisphere. **(d)** Triple bypass (*yellow arrows*) to different regions could increase blood flow globally, Chinese spring roll (*blue stars*), MMA branch (*green stars*). **(e, f)** In a similar case, only one single STA parietal branch (p-STA) was suitable for direct bypass, distal p-STA (*yellow line*) was cut and anastomosis to proximal part (*red line*) in an end-to-side way, thus two donor arteries could be created (*red and proximal yellow lines*).

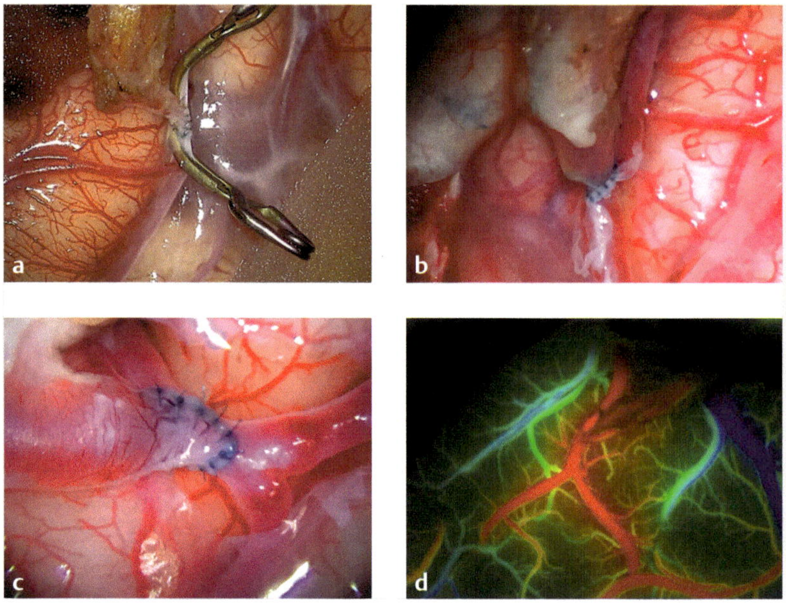


**Fig. 19.12** The simplest anastomosis technique. **(a)** Two curved mini temporal clips were used to occlude the recipient artery; **(b)** a small piece of arachnoid membrane was sutured to the anastomosis site, as a scarf for supporting the stoma, which is helpful to stop the hemorrhage from the needle hole; **(c, d)** the stoma location near a bifurcation is preferred because it can distribute the blood flow more efficiently.

expanding. Square knot is carefully made without any kinking of the suture. The vascular intima is never touched in anastomosing. The stoma location near a bifurcation is preferred because it can distribute the blood flow more efficiently (▶ Fig. 19.12).

In some cases, the wall of recipient artery is almost transparent under microscope. A tiny perforator could be left open on purpose to let small amount of blood flow reflux into the cavity of the recipient artery. This maneuver can give the recipient artery a small pressure. The stoma is kept opening for facilitating the anastomosing. With the different color of blood, the vessel wall could be seen more clearly under microscope. The irrigating of heparin saline by assistant could prevent the thrombosis.

## 19.10 Difficulties Encountered

A challenge encountered is extremely thin vessel wall of the recipient artery, which not only raise the difficulty of anastomosis, but also increase the risk of hemorrhage from the needle hole. We use a small piece of arachnoid membrane as a scarf for supporting the stomas (▶ Fig. 19.12**b**).

## 19.11 Bailout, Rescue, and Salvage Maneuvers

The hemorrhage from the needle holes or some small teared holes of the extremely thin recipient artery wall is really difficult to treat. It needs some extra autologous tissue for fixing as a patch outside of the vessel wall. We normally use arachnoid membrane or fat tissue as a patch.

Postoperative complications, such as hemorrhage in distant location, status epilepticus, and severe edema, are often considered to be results of hyperperfusion, in a few cases, sacrifice of the direct bypass is maybe the only choice. In case of postoperative cerebral infarction in contralateral hemisphere, emergent combined revascularization surgery could be considered.

## 19.12 Tips, Pearls, and Lessons Learned

To dissect STA from the inner side of scalp is a safe and fast way. Closing the incision of superficial temporal fascia from inner side of the scalp could prevent delayed scalp healing or infection effectively.

We could create double barrel bypass with one single parietal STA in cases with good MCA network, which may introduce STA blood flow to a wider area but keeping the frontal branch for feeding scalp flap.

Double-window craniotomy, with a complex consisted of dura, MMA, MMV, and bone bridge, is the best way to keep the integrity of MMA and distal spontaneous stomas.

“Chinese spring roll” containing MMA, accompanying veins, and some gelfoam strip are the solution for keeping the patency of MMA and hemostasis of accompanying MMV simultaneously.

The simplest anastomosis technique is effective in shortening average temporary occulting time, while preserving all branches of the recipient artery.

The autologous tissue such as arachnoid membrane and fat tissue could be used as a “patch” outside of the extremely thin recipient vessel wall for hemostasis and strengthening the stoma.

A tiny perforator could be left open on purpose to let small amount of blood flow reflux into the cavity to keep the recipient artery open for facilitating the anastomosing.

Determinants of blood flow after bypass are including: carrying capacity of STA, $\Delta P = P(\text{donor}) - P(\text{recipient})$, carrying capacity of recipient artery and integrity of MCA network.

# Suggested Readings


Suzuki J, Takaku A. Cerebrovascular "moyamoya" disease. Disease showing abnormal net-like vessels in base of brain. Arch Neurol. 1969; 20(3):288–299

Kuroda S, Houkin K. Moyamoya disease: current concepts and future perspectives. Lancet Neurol. 2008; 7(11):1056–1066

Matsushima T, Inoue K, Kawashima M, Inoue T. History of the development of surgical treatments for moyamoya disease. Neurol Med Chir (Tokyo). 2012; 52(5):278–286

Kuroda S, Houkin K. Bypass surgery for moyamoya disease: concept and essence of surgical techniques. Neurol Med Chir (Tokyo). 2012; 52(5):287–294

Xu B, Song DL, Mao Y, et al. Superficial temporal artery-middle cerebral artery bypass combined with encephalo-duro-myo-synangiosis in treating moyamoya disease: surgical techniques, indications and midterm follow-up results. Chin Med J (Engl). 2012; 125(24):4398–4405

Xu B, Song DL, Mao Y, Xu H, Gu YX, Chen G. Use superficial temporal artery-middle cerebral artery bypass combined with encephalo-duro-myo-synangiosis to treat moyamoya disease. Chin J Cerebrovasc Dis (Chin). 2007; 4:445–448

Shimizu S, Hagiwara H, Utsuki S, Oka H, Nakayama K, Fujii K. Bony tunnel formation in the middle meningeal groove: an anatomic study for safer pterional craniotomy. Minim Invasive Neurosurg. 2008; 51(6):329–332

Ma S, Baillie LJ, Stringer MD. Reappraising the surface anatomy of the pterion and its relationship to the middle meningeal artery. Clin Anat. 2012; 25(3):330–339

Hori S, Kashiwazaki D, Akioka N, et al. Surgical anatomy and preservation of the middle meningeal artery during bypass surgery for moyamoya disease. Acta Neurochir (Wien). 2015; 157(1):29–36

Chen L, Xu B, Wang Y, Liao Y, Pan H, Wang Y. Preoperative evaluation of moyamoya spontaneous anastomosis of combined revascularization donor vessels in adults by duplexultrasonography. Br J Neurosurg. 2017 (Nov):1360–1366

Wang Y, Chen L, Wang Y, et al. Hemodynamic study with duplex ultrasonography on combined (direct/indirect) revascularization in adult moyamoya disease. J Stroke Cerebrovasc Dis. 2014; 23(10):2573–2579

# Part 5

## Rescue Strategies for Repeat Surgery



5

# 20 Omental–Cranial Transposition

*Mario Teo, Jeremiah N. Johnson, and Gary K. Steinberg*

**Abstract**
Selective moyamoya disease (MMD) patients have progressive neurological deterioration despite previous revascularization, and many have exhausted typical sources for bypass or have wide ischemic areas needing further revascularization. Omental–cranial transposition, a technique used sparingly, can be performed efficiently and safely. In this chapter, we highlight the steps and nuances in performing the laparoscopic omental harvest (which is better tolerated than laparotomy), the techniques used to ensure a thin, homogeneous, pedicled omental flap to provide wide cerebral hemispheric coverage, and illustrate with the appropriate case examples. We also include the preoperative workup, intraoperative strategies with step-by-step descriptions of key procedures, and postoperative management with long-term clinical and radiological outcome. With this method, we can achieve excellent angiographic revascularization and symptoms resolution for selective patients with resistant MMD.

*Keywords:* omental–cranial transposition, laparoscopic omental harvest, pedicled omental flap, resistant MMD, wide revascularization

## 20.1 Background

Revascularizations for moyamoya disease (MMD), either by direct or indirect procedures, are an accepted and effective treatment for the prevention of future ischemic events. However, small subsets of patients have persistent or new symptoms due to inadequate collateralization, hence, repeat revascularizations are performed. These repeat surgeries are technically more challenging due to scar tissue from the previous surgery, the meticulous attention required to avoid violating the previous bypass donor and its collateralization, and the lack of suitable local donor grafts. We describe the omental–cranial transposition as one of the rescue strategies that could be employed in these circumstances.

### 20.1.1 History

- 1936—O'Shaughnessy sutured a pedicle of omentum to the heart.
- 1962 to 1975—Vineberg explored clinical omental transposition to the heart.
- 1973—Goldsmith et al described the first experimental omental–cranial flap in dogs to promote brain revascularization.
- 1974 and 1977—Yasargil, Yonekawa, and their colleagues explored the use of omentum transplantation in animal models for the treatment of hydrocephalus and cerebral ischemia.
- 1980—Karasawa et al described the first use of an omental flap in a patient with MMD who presented with ischemic symptoms. Anastomoses were made between the corresponding artery and vein of the superficial temporal and gastroepiploic vessels. The patient was free of ischemic attacks at 2 years follow-up.

## 20.2 Indications

- Revascularization of MMD in the absence of superficial temporal artery (STA), occipital artery or muscle donor.
- Large cortical surface areas to be revascularized, including bilateral hemispheres.
- Commonly employed strategy for repeat revascularization of MMD.

## 20.3 Key Principles

- Laparoscopic omental graft harvest in conjunction with the general surgeon.
- Preservation of gastroduodenal artery/vein and right gastroepiploic artery/vein blood supply.
- Careful delivery of the omentum to the cranial compartment.

## 20.4 SWOT Analysis

### 20.4.1 Strength

- Stretches and conforms easily to cover a large cortical area.

### 20.4.2 Weakness

- Technically challenging, potential associated morbidity with abdominal surgery.

### 20.4.3 Opportunity

- Stem cells in omentum produce angiogenesis-promoting cytokines, for example, vascular endothelial growth factor (VEGF) and basic fibroblast growth factor (bFGF).

### 20.4.4 Threat

- The viability of the omental graft could be compromised if the gastroepiploic artery is not preserved during harvest, or significant graft torsion occurs in the process of extraperitoneal omental delivery or tunneling to the cranial compartment.

## 20.5 Contraindications

- Previous complex abdominal surgery.
- Abdominal adhesion (peritonitis, peritoneal dialysis).
- Scarred down chest wall, difficulty with tunneling (relative contraindication).

## 20.6 Special Considerations

- History of previous major abdominal surgery should be carefully considered when contemplating omental–cranial harvest.
- Cortical areas to be revascularized: if located superior in the cerebral hemispheres (difficulty revascularizing using donor vessels due to inadequate length and small size of distal vessel), or a wide cortical surface area is to be reperfused (including bilateral hemispheres), the omental graft is a very good option.

## 20.7 Risk Assessment: Our Experience

At Stanford, we have performed 25 omental–cerebral transpositions for MMD (with 10 additional for non-MMD stroke patients).

- 1991 to 2000: 9 cases with laparotomy for omental graft harvest (3 pedicled and 6 free grafts).
- 2011 to 2016: 16 cases with laparoscopic harvesting of pedicled omental grafts.
- In our laparoscopic omental–cranial transposition experience, 17 hemispheres in 16 patients were revascularized.
- Ages ranged from 5 to 45 years old, mean follow-up of 10.8 years (range: 1–27 years).
- Three patients had small postoperative diffusion weighted imaging (DWI) plus infarcts on MRI of the brain associated with contralateral arm and/or hand weakness, which recovered to preoperative baseline over 2 to 3 months. Two additional patients developed transient neurological deficits (TNDs) in the 30-day postoperative period that resolved.
- At the last follow-up, angiographic and MR findings of all cases showed patent grafts as well as viable omentum, and all patients experienced preoperative symptom resolution or improvement.

## 20.8 Preoperative Workup

Preoperatively, patients undergo a thorough medical, cardiac, and anesthetic assessment with routine preoperative labs and the relevant diagnostic imaging, including five-vessel cerebral angiogram, MRI of the brain, and cerebral perfusion imaging with and without Diamox (positron emission tomography, MR perfusion, CT perfusion, single-photon emission computed tomography [SPECT], transcranial Doppler). At our institution, we perform MR perfusion with and without Diamox, and patients who demonstrate poor cerebrovascular reserve (CVR) with steal phenomenon (indicating that the affected vascular territory is already maximally vasodilated to promote flow) are considered, especially patients of high risk for ongoing ischemia without treatment. These patients are also at higher risk for perioperative ischemic complications; thus, particular care is taken to avoid hypotension perioperatively and during the recovery period. Intraoperatively, each patient's blood pressure is maintained at or above the preoperative baseline at all times.

### 20.8.1 Specific Consideration with Anticoagulation

- For patients with mechanical heart valves or recent venous thromboembolism, we would restart anticoagulation at 2 to 4 weeks postoperatively after a head CT confirmed no significant hemorrhage.
- Aspirin is continued through the preoperative day and restarted on postoperative day 1.

## 20.9 Patient Preparation

### 20.9.1 Patient Position with Skin Incision (▶ Fig. 20.1)

- The laparoscopic surgical and neurosurgical teams work simultaneously.
- The patient is positioned supine.

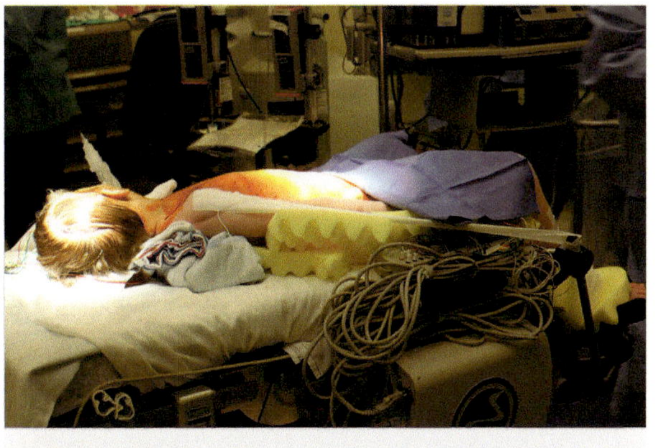

**Fig. 20.1** Patient positioned with the neurosurgical and pediatric laparoscopic surgical team working simultaneously. (Used with permission from Navarro R, Chao K, Gooderham PA, Bruzoni M, Dutta S, Steinberg GK. Less invasive pedicled omental-cranial transposition in pediatric patients with moyamoya disease and failed prior revascularization. Neurosurgery. 2014;10:1–14.)

- The head is positioned on a doughnut headrest to bring the cortical area to be revascularized uppermost.
- A transverse lower neck incision is made for tunneling of the omental graft from the peritoneal cavity to the cervical region over the chest wall. A retroauricular pocket is also created to connect the craniotomy site to the cervical incision.
- A lithotomy position is used.
- Laparoscopic port site insertion (three times), a subxiphoid incision is made to deliver the omentum after harvest.

## 20.10 Surgical Steps

### 20.10.1 Key Procedural Step 1: Omental Harvest (▶ Fig. 20.2)

- ▶ Fig. 20.2**a–c** illustrates the key anatomical landmarks of the omental harvest stage. ▶ Fig. 20.2**d–f** shows the senior author's early technique with open omental harvest.
- Laparoscopic omental harvest through working ports.
- Omentum dissected off the transverse colon, then splenic flexure (avoiding splenic vessel injury), and hepatic flexure.
- Dissection is along the greater curve of the stomach, preserving the right gastroepiploic artery and vein; the left gastroepiploic is cut.
- The pedicle is preserved at the pylorus.

### 20.10.2 Key Procedural Step 2: Delivery and Tunneling (▶ Fig. 20.3)

- Subxiphoid incision (3–4 cm) for omental delivery under direct vision, once the omentum is maximally mobilized.
- Omentum is inspected to identify its vascular supply and confirm patency of the arterial anastomotic arch of Barkow.
- To create a thin, homogeneous omental flap, the omentum is carefully divided between the epiploic arcades with step cuts.
- Subcutaneous tunnel from subxiphoid incision to a lower cervical incision is created using long lighted retractors and dissectors.
- Copious lubrication is used to facilitate the delivery of the omental graft to the low cervical area, then to the craniotomy site in step wise fashion.
- The subxiphoid incision is closed in multiple layers: abdominal fascia, subcutaneous tissue, and skin. The remaining abdominal port site incisions are closed in a subcuticular fashion.

### 20.10.3 Key Procedural Step 3: Craniotomy (▶ Fig. 20.4)

- The incision and craniotomy should be designed to avoid damage to previous revascularization.
- A horseshoe cranial flap is performed for a large craniotomy.
- Dura is opened widely followed by wide opening of the arachnoid, and thin omental flap is placed over the entire exposed cortical surface area and secured to the dural edges using 4–0 sutures.
- If the contralateral hemisphere also undergoes revascularization, the remaining omental flap can be mobilized subcutaneously, and the same procedure repeated.
- Omental flow is demonstrated using a Doppler probe and indocyanine green (ICG) angiogram.
- The craniotomy bone flap is trimmed on the inferior aspects, and thinned on the inner table to avoid strangulation of the vasculature and mass effect over the cortex.
- The bone flap is secured using titanium miniplates, and the scalp closure is performed in multiple layers.

## 20.11 Tips, Pearls, and Lessons Learned

- Omentum is excellent for secondary revascularization in difficult MMD cases.
- Work with an experienced laparoscopic surgeon to ensure a safe omental harvest.
- A thin omental covering of cortex is best in order to avoid mass effect on the brain parenchyma; drill off the inner table of the skull plate to be replaced during closure.
- A postoperative angiogram should include gastroduodenal or celiac artery injection to assess graft patency. However, sometimes the omental graft parasitizes blood supply from chest or cervical arteries, decreasing the filling from the gastroepiploic artery.

## 20.12 Pitfalls

- An inadequate omental harvest due to injury to gastroepiploic or gastroduodenal arteries.
- Possible pedicle twisting during extraperitoneal delivery or the tunneling stage to the cranial compartment.
- Omentum that is too thick to place on the cerebral cortex, which could result in mass effect on the brain parenchyma when replacing the bone flap. We routinely thin the inner table of the skull flap, leaving only the outer table.

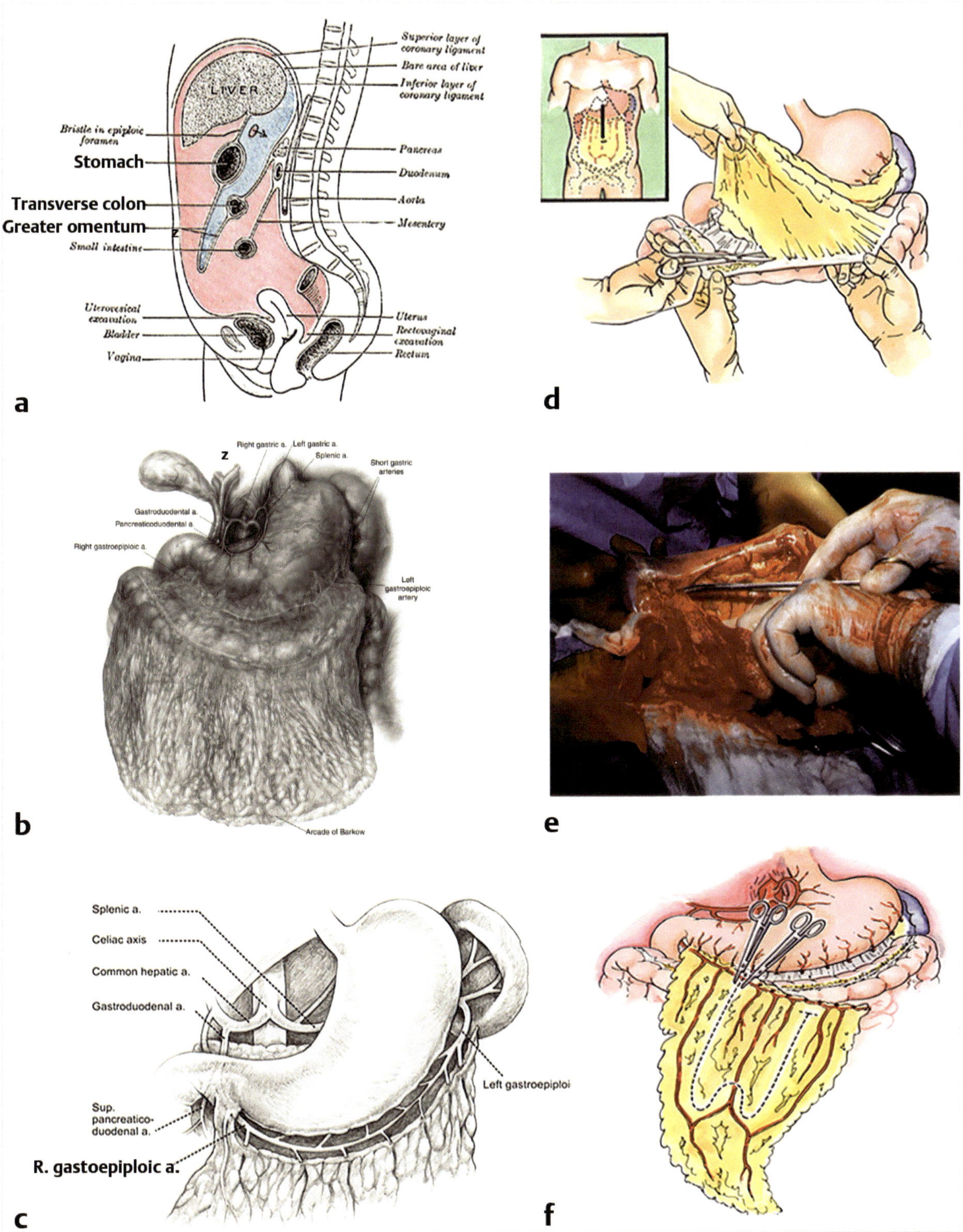


**Fig. 20.2** **(a)** Anatomy of the greater omentum relative to the greater curve of the stomach and transverse colon. **(b)** Blood supply to the greater omentum including the gastroepiploic artery and the arch of Barkow. **(c)** The course of the right gastroepiploic artery along the greater curve of the stomach, and subsequent division at the left gastroepiploic artery during the omental harvest. **(d)** The open omental harvest technique as performed in the senior author's early experience, dividing the greater omentum from the transverse colon. **(e)** Division of the greater omentum from the greater curve of stomach, preserving the right gastroepiploic artery, and dividing the left gastroepiploic artery. **(f)** An illustration of how to lengthen the omental graft and preserving the blood supply by dividing along the arches of the anterior epiploic branches. Panel **(a)** is from Henry Gray (1918) Anatomy of the Human Body. Available at: Bartleby.com: Gray's Anatomy, Plate 1035. Panel **(b)** is reprinted from The Technique of Omentum Harvest for Intrathoracic Use. Boulton BJ and Force S. 2010, with permission from Elsevier. Panel **(c)** is with permission from Jensen, Surgical Anatomy and Mastery of Open Operations: A Multimedia Curriculum for Training Residents, Wolters Kluwer. Panels **(d–f)** are used with permission from Cockroft KM, Mahoney ME, Cobb LF, Steinberg GK: Omental Cerebral Transposition. In: Steinberg GK, (Ed.). Techniques in Neurosurgery: Cerebral Revascularization Techniques. Philadelphia, PA: Lippincott Williams and Wilkins, 2000 (vol. 6, issue 2), pp. 172–181.

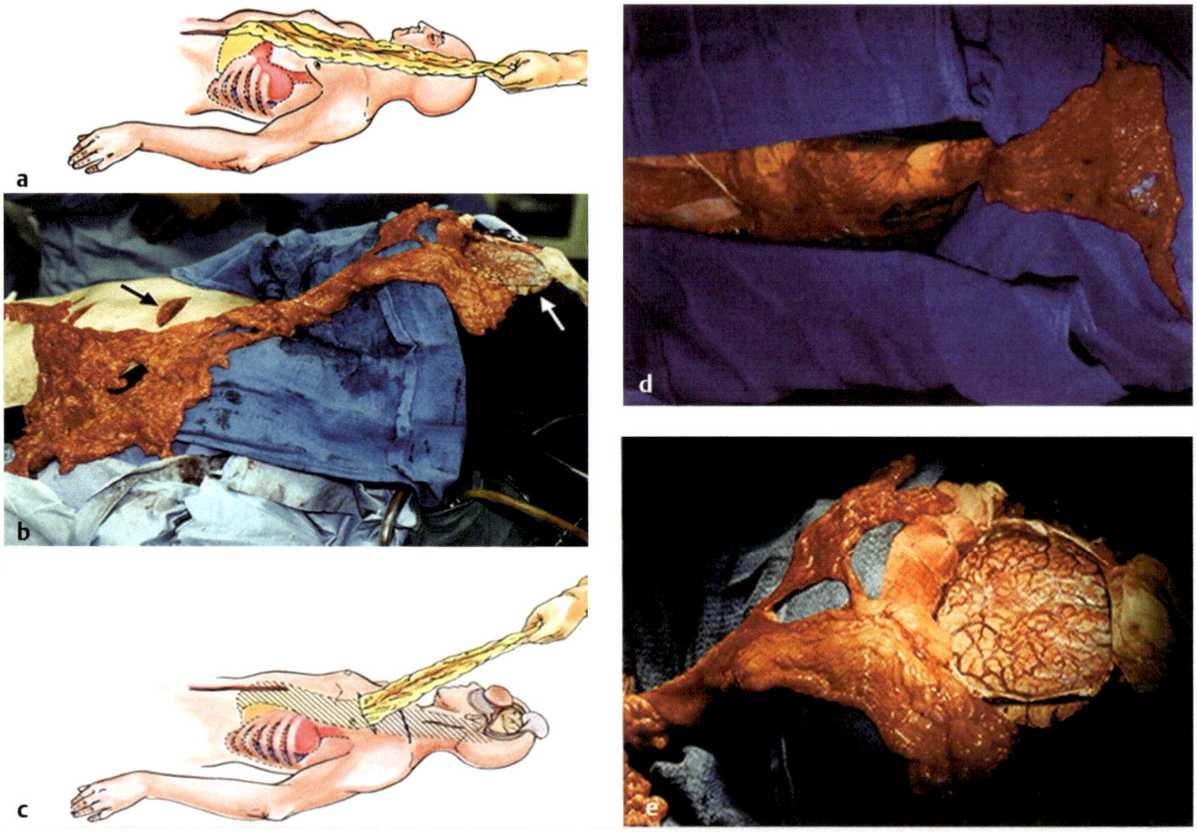

Fig. 20.3 **(a)** Illustration of omental delivery to the cranial compartment. **(b)** Intraoperative view of omental delivery to the cranial compartment (*white arrow*) shows adequate length for the revascularization. Incision (*black arrow*) to ease the tunneling process and avoid strangulation or excessive traction on the omental graft. **(c)** Use of the release incision to aid the tunneling process. **(d)** Intraoperative view of the omental graft delivered to the cervical region. **(e)** Craniotomy exposed with the omental graft ready for the transposition stage. (Used with permission from Cockroft KM, Mahoney ME, Cobb LF, Steinberg GK. Omental cerebral transposition. In: Steinberg GK, ed. Techniques in Neurosurgery: Cerebral Revascularization Techniques, Philadelphia, PA: Lippincott Williams and Wilkins, 2000 (vol. 6, issue 2): pp. 172–181.)

- Challenge of preserving the omental blood supply when trimming the omental flap for smaller cortical placement.

## 20.13 Bailout, Rescue, and Salvage Maneuvers

- Work with an experienced laparoscopic surgeon.
- Deliver and tunnel omental pedicle under direct vision to avoid twisting.
- Irrigate frequently to avoid dehydration and shrinkage of the omental flap.

## 20.14 Postoperative Care

### 20.14.1 Patient Surveillance

- First 24 hours after surgery:
  - Patient is in the intensive care unit with regular neuro checks.
  - Closely monitor hemodynamic status (fluid intake, output, electrolyte, and gastrointestinal function).
  - Maintain thresholds for blood pressure (mean arterial pressure goals 90–110 to prevent hypoperfusion, TND, and hyperperfusion with potential postoperative hematoma).

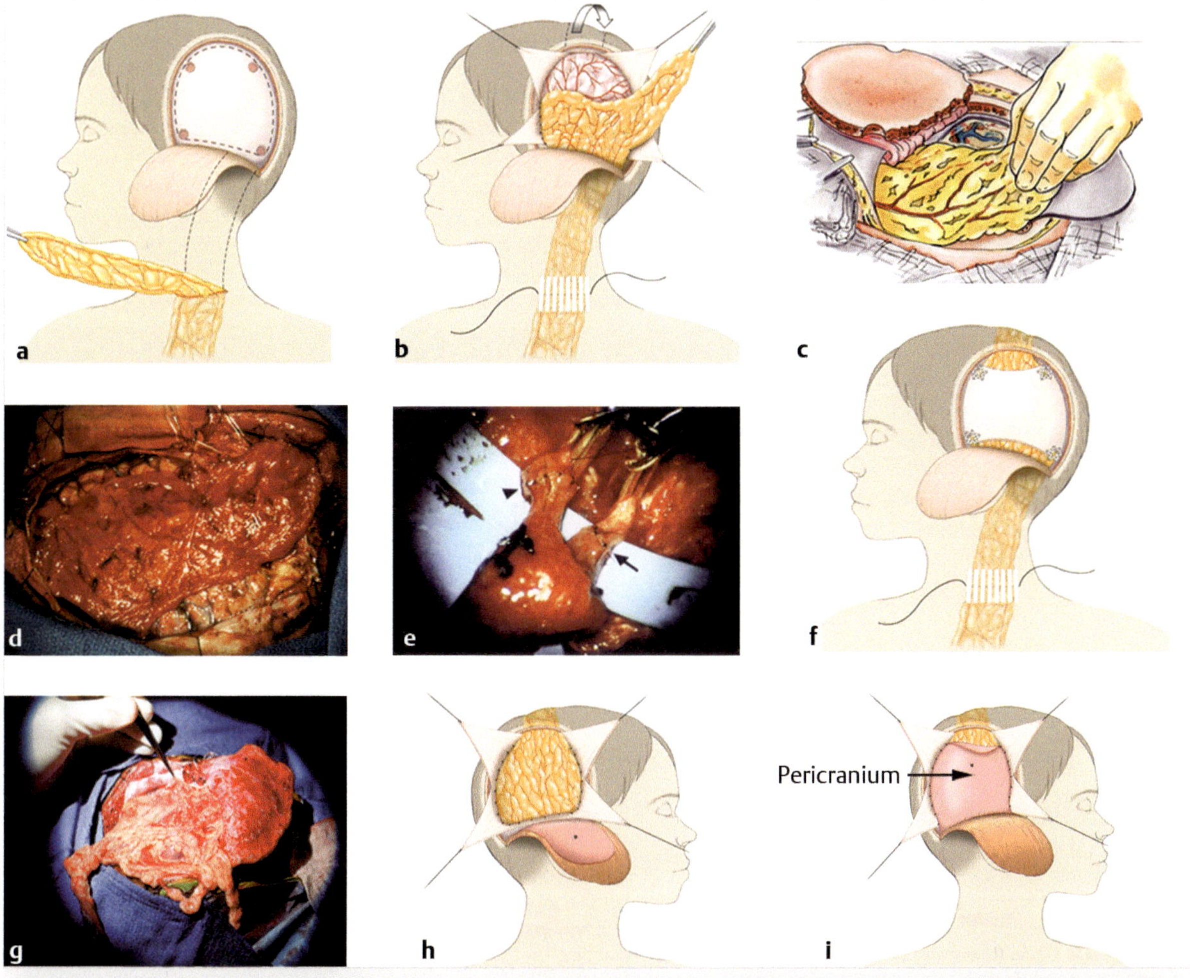


**Fig. 20.4** **(a)** Maximal craniotomy performed over the brain territory to be revascularized, preserving the underlying collateralization from previous bypass surgery. **(b)** The exposed dura is excised and the microscope is brought in to widely dissect open the arachnoid. A subgaleal tunnel connecting the bilateral craniotomies is made. The omentum is then pulled up as far as possible, and the proximal portion laying over the left-sided craniotomy is trimmed. **(c)** For unilateral revascularization, the omentum is laid gently on the exposed brain, and excessive tissue tucked under the bone edges under visualization. **(d)** Omental graft lying neatly on the brain surface, not exerting mass effect. **(e)** In the event that a free omental graft is to be used (as in the senior author's earlier experience), anastomosis of the gastroepiploic artery (*arrow*) and vein (*arrowhead*) is performed to the superficial temporal artery and vein on the corresponding site. **(f)** Prior to replacing the bone flap, the inner table is shaved to reduce the mass effect caused by the omentum on the brain. The bone at the inlet and outlet for the omentum is also widely removed with a craniotome drill to accommodate the flap. Then, the bone is fixed to the rest of the skull with titanium plates. **(g)** Intraoperative image shows excessive omental graft that could be used to revascularize the contralateral hemisphere. **(h)** The dura is then opened widely on the contralateral side. Through similar steps, the omental flap is secured to the dura and laid over the exposed brain. **(i)** To provide an additional source for indirect revascularization, the previously harvested pericranium (*asterisk*) is laid on top of the omental flap and secured to the dura. The bone is contoured as described and secured to the skull with plates, followed by multilayer scalp closure. Panels **(a, b, f–i)** are used with permission from Navarro R, Chao K, Gooderham PA, Bruzoni M, Dutta S, Steinberg GK. Less invasive pedicled omental-cranial transposition in pediatric patients with moyamoya disease and failed prior revascularization. Neurosurgery. 2014;10:1–14. Panels **(c, d)** are from Cockroft KM, Mahoney ME, Cobb LF, Steinberg GK: Omental Cerebral Transposition. In: Steinberg GK (ed), Techniques in Neurosurgery: Cerebral Revascularization Techniques, Lippincott Williams and Wilkins, Philadelphia, 2000, vol. 6(2):172–181.

- Analgesia and antiemetic.
- Day 2: Mobilize, observe oral intake, and transfer to regular ward care.
- Discharge from hospital when deemed to be safe by the neurosurgical and general surgical team (4-day average hospital stay).
- Post discharge: Educate and inform about TND, wound care, and subsequent follow-up plans.

### 20.14.2 Bypass Function Assessment

- Intraoperative omental bypass graft assessment using ICG angiogram and Doppler probe.
- Six-month postoperative digital subtraction angiogram including injection of celiac trunk, gastroduodenal artery and five-vessel cerebral angiograms, MRI brain including fluid-attenuated inversion recovery/DWI sequence, MRI perfusion without/with Diamox (to assess CVR), and neuropsychological testing.
- Long-term follow-up at 3, 10, 20, and 30 years with clinical and radiological surveillance (investigations performed as listed at 6 month check).

## 20.15 Case Illustrations

### 20.15.1 Case 1

A 7-year-old girl had bilateral direct STA–middle cerebral artery (MCA) bypasses, after initially presenting with a left hemispheric stroke manifested by aphasia and right hemiparesis, and became asymptomatic for 5 years. She subsequently developed new-onset, left-body transient weakness with intermittent choreiform movements affecting her left arm and foot. MRI of the brain showed no new strokes but significantly reduced perfusion in the right MCA territory, posterior and superior to the region of her previous STA–MCA bypass. Her SPECT cerebral blood flow studies showed impaired perfusion and poor augmentation of the right hemisphere, including basal ganglia, consistent with impaired hemodynamic reserve after Diamox study. Cerebral angiography showed excellent revascularization of her left hemisphere with a patent bypass graft, and a right hemisphere mainly supplied by meningeal collateral vessels, with poor revascularization in the areas posterior and superior to the prior bypass graft (▶ Fig. 20.5**a, b**). She underwent an uneventful right craniotomy and laparoscopic omental–cranial transposition to revascularize her right parietal region.

At 3 months after surgery she was free of transient ischemic attacks (TIAs) with resolution of the choreiform movements. A 6-month angiogram showed a gastroepiploic arterial supply along the course of the subcutaneous tunnel and excellent collateralization of the high right parietal area (▶ Fig. 20.5**c, d**). An MRI of the brain at 6 months also showed reduced thickness of the omental flap compared to the immediate postoperative scan (▶ Fig. 20.5**e, f**). A postoperative SPECT study at 6 months showed more symmetrical augmentation bilaterally after Diamox administration (▶ Fig. 20.5**g**). She remained symptom free at the latest follow-up, and a delayed angiogram at 4 years showed that the underlying right STA–MCA bypass graft (▶ Fig. 20.5**h**) and the omental–cranial transposition graft remained patent (▶ Fig. 20.5**i–k**).

### 20.15.2 Case 2

A 5-year-old girl presented with progressive neurological deterioration 6 months after bilateral direct STA–MCA/encephalo-duro-arterio-myo-synangioses (EDAMS) that were performed at an outside institution. Despite her previous treatment, she had persistent headaches with worsening motor and sensory (TIAs involving bilateral hemispheres). MRI and SPECT studies showed new bilateral ischemic lesions and reduced perfusion in the watershed areas, worse on the left. A cerebral angiogram showed progression of bilateral MMD, limited MCA collateralizations from previous bypasses, and lack of revascularization in bilateral high frontoparietal regions (▶ Fig. 20.6**a–d**). She continued to deteriorate despite efforts to optimize her fluid status and blood pressure, and underwent bilateral omental–cranial transposition using a single pedicled, laparoscopic-harvested, vascularized omental flap.

She made an uneventful recovery, and was discharged on day 4 postoperatively. Her TIAs markedly reduced in frequency and severity 2 months after the omental–cranial transposition, and her 6-month angiogram showed excellent revascularization from the omental flap supplying bilateral superior MCA territories, and the gastroepiploic artery along the subcutaneous tunnel (▶ Fig. 20.6**e, f**). Robust collateralization between the external carotid systems and the omental graft's arterial supply was also seen.

She was symptom free at her 3.5 year follow-up with hypertrophy of the gastroepiploic artery supplying the brain parenchyma (▶ Fig. 20.6**g–j**), and a thin layer of omental graft visible on an MRI of the brain (▶ Fig. 20.6**k**).

## 20.16 Conclusion

Omental–cranial transposition as a rescue strategy for MMD patients with persistent or new symptoms after previous revascularizations is a versatile option with very good clinical outcome. Laparoscopic harvest of the omentum reduces the abdominal morbidity associated with the procedure, and the omental graft provides coverage for a large surface area of the brain hemisphere to be revascularized.

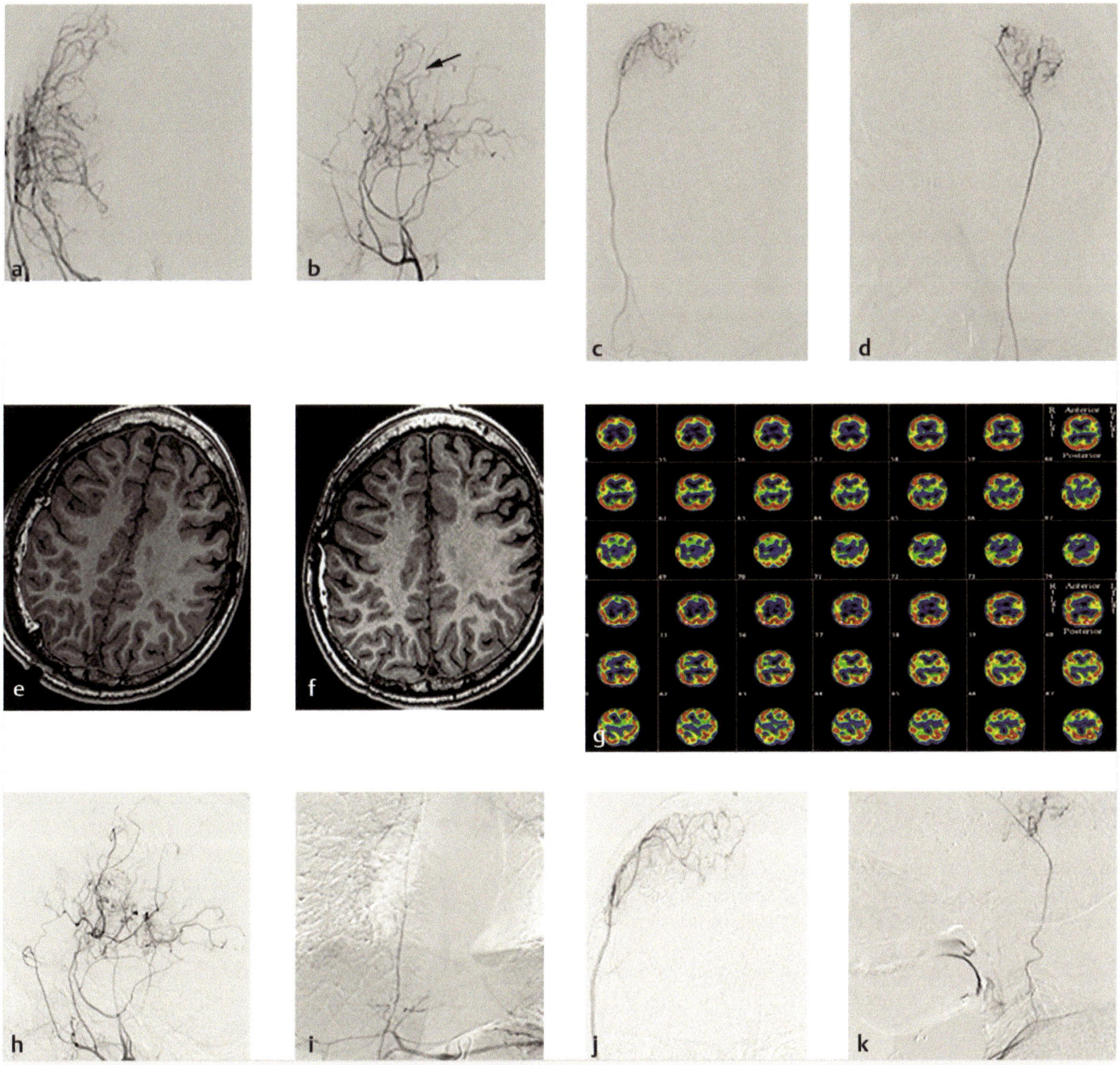

**Fig. 20.5** A 7-year-old girl with bilateral STA–MCA direct bypass was symptom free for 5 years, then presented with right hemispheric symptoms consisting of left-sided choreiform movements and left-sided TIAs. **(a)** Cerebral angiogram (anteroposterior [AP] view) of the right ECA shows a patent bypass graft with extensive collateralization with right MCA, supplying the majority of the right hemisphere. **(b)** Cerebral angiogram (lateral view) of the right ECA shows a patent bypass graft supplying much of right hemisphere mainly but with poor revascularization in the areas posterior and superior to the prior bypass graft (*arrow*). **(c)** Right gastroduodenal artery injection angiogram (AP view) at 6 months after right-sided laparoscopic omental cranial transposition shows a gastroepiploic arterial supply along the course of the subcutaneous tunnel and excellent collateralization of the high right parietal area. **(d)** Right gastroduodenal artery injection angiogram (lateral view) at 6 months shows excellent revascularization to the area marked with deficient collateralization in 5a. **(e)** Immediate postoperative MRI brain shows the omental graft overlying the right parietal region. **(f)** MRI brain at 6 months shows reduced thickness of the omental flap compared to the immediate postoperative scan. **(g)** Postoperative SPECT study at 6 months shows improved cerebral blood flow to the right hemisphere and more symmetrical augmentation bilaterally after Diamox administration (top three rows are pre-Diamox, bottom three rows are post-Diamox), signifying improved cerebrovascular reserve. **(h)** The patient remained symptom free at the latest follow-up with the delayed angiogram (right ECA injection, lateral view) at 4 years showing a patent underlying right STA–MCA bypass graft with extensive MCA collateralization. **(i)** A 4-year delayed angiogram with right gastroduodenal injection shows the gastroepiploic artery coursing along the right anterior chest wall. **(j)** The delayed angiogram of the right gastroduodenal injection (AP view) also shows the robust and patent right omental-cranial transposition graft supplying the high parietal region remained patent. **(k)** Lateral view of right omental–cranial graft with the same findings as above. (Used with permission from Navarro R, Chao K, Gooderham PA, Bruzoni M, Dutta S, Steinberg GK. Less invasive pedicled omental-cranial transposition in pediatric patients with moyamoya disease and failed prior revascularization. Neurosurgery. 2014;10:1–14.)

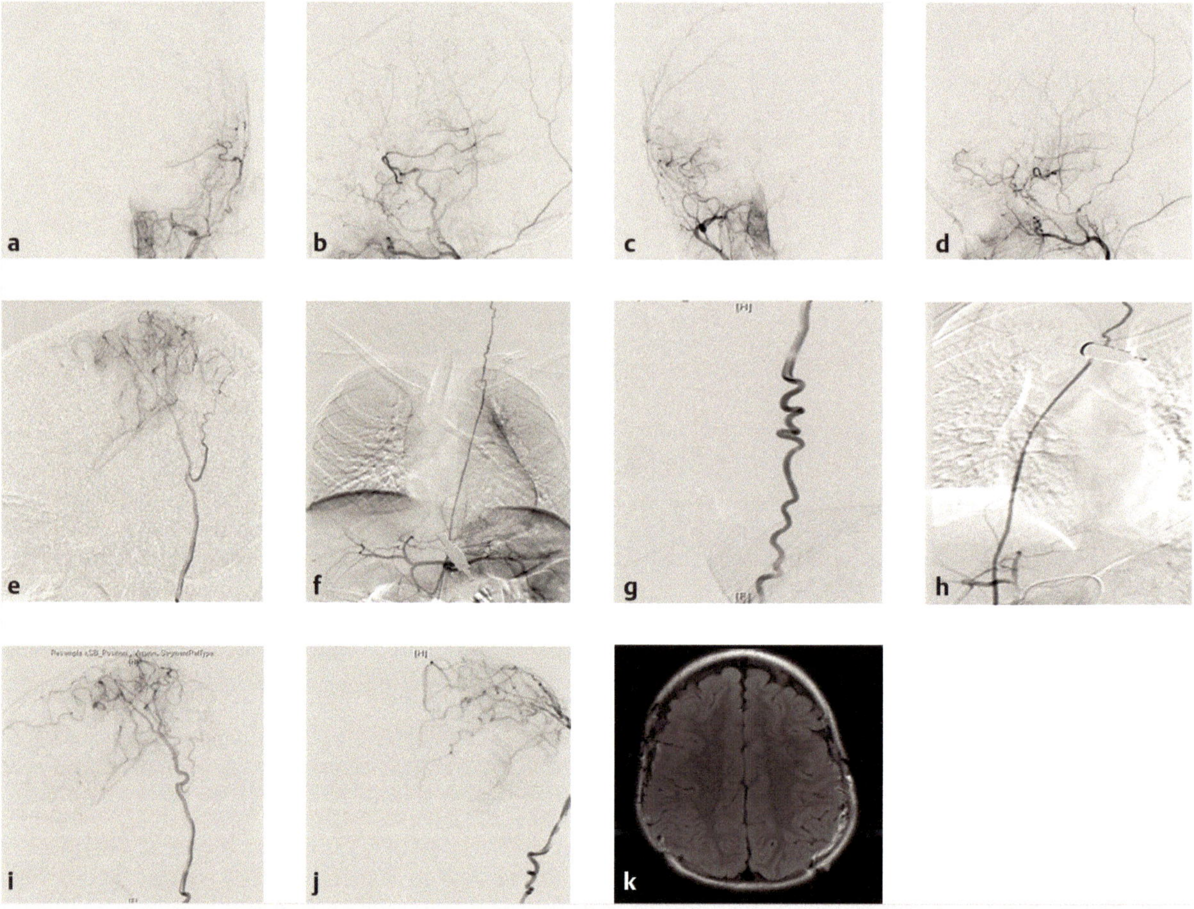

**Fig. 20.6** A 5-year-old girl with progressive neurological deterioration 6 months after bilateral direct STA–MCA and EDAMS that was performed at an outside institution. MRI brain and SPECT studies show new bilateral ischemic lesions and reduced perfusion in the watershed areas, worse on the left. Cerebral angiogram—**(a)** left CCA injection (AP view); **(b)** left CCA injection (lateral view); **(c)** right CCA injection (anteroposterior [AP] view); **(d)** right CCA injection (lateral view)—shows progression of bilateral MMD, limited MCA collateralizations from previous bypasses, and lack of revascularization in bilateral high frontoparietal regions. The patient underwent bilateral omental-cranial transposition using a single pedicled, laparoscopic-harvested, vascularized omental flap. **(e)** Her 6-month angiogram of the gastroduodenal artery (lateral view of the skull) shows excellent revascularization from the omental flap supplying bilateral superior MCA territories. **(f)** The gastroepiploic artery is seen in the chest wall along the subcutaneous tunnel. She was symptom free at her 3.5 year follow-up. **(g–j)** Delayed angiogram of the gastroduodenal artery—**(g)** AP view over the abdomen, **(h)** AP view over the chest wall, **(i)** lateral view of the skull, and **(j)** AP view of the skull—shows hypertrophy of the gastroepiploic artery coursing along the epigastrium, chest wall, neck and supplying the major portion of the brain parenchyma. **(k)** MRI brain shows a thin layer of omental graft visible over the cerebral cortex. (Used with permission from Navarro R, Chao K, Gooderham PA, Bruzoni M, Dutta S, Steinberg GK. Less invasive pedicled omental-cranial transposition in pediatric patients with moyamoya disease and failed prior revascularization. Neurosurgery. 2014;10:1–14.)

## Suggested Readings


Goldsmith HS, Chen WF, Duckett SW. Brain vascularization by intact omentum. Arch Surg. 1973; 106(5):695–698

Karasawa J, Kikuchi H, Kawamura J, Sakai T. Intracranial transplantation of the omentum for cerebrovascular moyamoya disease: a two-year follow-up study. Surg Neurol. 1980; 14(6):444–449

Karasawa J, Touho H, Ohnishi H, Miyamoto S, Kikuchi H. Cerebral revascularization using omental transplantation for childhood moyamoya disease. J Neurosurg. 1993; 79(2):192–196

Lee J, Steinberg GK. Omental to cerebral transposition for the treatment of cerebral ischemia. In: Goldsmith HS, ed. The Omentum. Woodbury, CT: Ciné-Med, Inc.; 2010:137–149

Navarro R, Chao K, Gooderham PA, Bruzoni M, Dutta S, Steinberg GK. Less invasive pedicled omental-cranial transposition in pediatric patients with moyamoya disease and failed prior revascularization. Neurosurgery. 2014; 10(1) Suppl 1:1–14

Yaşargil MG, Yonekawa Y, Denton I, Piroth D, Benes I. Experimental intracranial transplantation of autogenic omentum majus. J Neurosurg. 1974; 40 (2):213–217

Yonekawa Y, Yaşargil MG. Brain vascularization by transplanted omentum: a possible treatment of cerebral ischemia. Neurosurgery. 1977; 1(3):256–259

# 21 ECA–MCA Bypass with Radial Artery Graft

*Satoshi Hori and Peter Vajkoczy*

**Abstract**

This chapter presents the concept and technique of external carotid artery to middle cerebral artery (ECA–MCA) bypass with radial artery grafts as a rescue strategy for the patients with moyamoya disease (MMD) who failed conventional revascularization.

Failure of direct revascularization with superficial temporal artery (STA) to MCA bypass for MMD is comparatively rare. However, for those cases where a bypass fails to prevent further ischemic attack, safe and efficient rescue strategies are needed.

The indications for rescue revascularization are symptomatic, and the proof of bypass graft failure and impaired cerebrovascular reserve capacity (CVRC) by digital subtraction angiography (DSA) and cerebral blood flow (CBF) study, respectively. As an escape strategy, the radial artery graft bypass from the ECA to M3 or M2 portion is performed.

This strategy may be technically infeasible due to recipient vessel mismatch and high fragility of MMD vessels. Furthermore, there is potential risk for graft occlusion due to thrombosis and hyperperfusion syndrome. To prevent these problems, meticulous surgical manipulation, dilatation of the graft vessel with hydrostatic pressure as a preparation, use of heparin when opening the anastomosis and strict blood pressure control have to be remembered to perform.

The revascularization with radial artery graft provides immediate and reliable augmentation of blood supply. It could be a reasonable option for rescue revascularization, providing satisfying clinical and functional results. However, the number of patients who undergo this technique are so limited because MMD is an uncommon disease and STA–MCA bypass graft failure is rare.

*Keywords:* moyamoya disease, STA–MCA bypass, hyperperfusion syndrome, radial artery graft, rescue revascularization

## 21.1 History and Initial Description

Surgical revascularization for moyamoya disease (MMD) has shown to improve cerebral hemodynamics and prevent further cerebrovascular events. Especially, direct bypass surgery, that is, superficial temporal artery to middle cerebral artery (STA–MCA) bypass, is a potent method to resolve ischemic attacks immediately after surgery.[1]

Late failure of STA–MCA bypass is rare,[2] and most of these cases remain asymptomatic and will not result in reoccurrence of ischemic or hemorrhagic symptoms because either accompanying indirect bypass or endogenous collaterals have taken over.[3] However, rarely, late STA–MCA graft failure may cause persistent or new transient ischemic attacks (TIAs) and new ischemic stroke.[4] For these patients, rescue revascularization strategies are needed and most surgeons would elect indirect revascularizations strategies currently.[5–7]

Large caliber graft bypass using radial artery or saphenous vein grafts for MMD patients has been controversial due to the fear of procedure-related complications, the high fragility of MMD vessels and the potential high risk of hyperperfusion syndrome.[8,9] However, the revascularization with large caliber graft provides immediate and reliable augmentation of blood supply. It could be a reasonable option for rescue revascularization, providing satisfying clinical and functional results at a low complication rate.[10]

This chapter shows the concept and technique of external carotid artery (ECA) to MCA bypass with radial artery graft as a rescue revascularization for the MMD patients who failed conventional revascularization including STA–MCA bypass.

## 21.2 Indications

The patient is symptomatic and has new ischemic lesions. The imaging studies demonstrate STA–MCA bypass graft failure on digital subtraction angiography (DSA) and persisting impaired cerebrovascular capacity (CVRC) on cerebral blood flow (CBF) study. Furthermore, no other extradural pedicled graft vessels are available.

## 21.3 Key Principles

For preparation and harvesting of the radial artery graft, preoperative evaluation of Allen's test, vessel patency, and length (22–23 cm are needed) are essential. The radial artery graft is passed subcutaneously from the craniotomy incision to the cervical incision. The anastomosis is started with proximal side. When doing the anastomosis of distal side, M3 or distal M2 portion of the MCA is selected as a recipient artery after careful observation to avoid hyperperfusion. The quality of these vessels is usually sufficient for anastomosis. When opening the anastomosis, heparin is used to prevent bypass occlusion. The patency of the graft vessel is confirmed by intraoperative indocyanine green (ICG) angiography and quantitative Doppler flow measurements.

## 21.4 SWOT Analysis

### 21.4.1 Strength

- Immediate and reliable augmentation of blood supply is gained.

### 21.4.2 Weaknesses

- The procedure may be technically infeasible due to the recipient vessel mismatch and high fragility of MMD vessels.
- There is a potential high risk for hyperperfusion syndrome.

### 21.4.3 Opportunity

- The procedure improves current ischemic symptoms and prevents further cerebrovascular events.

### 21.4.4 Threat

- There is the risk for graft occlusion due to vasospasm and thrombosis.

## 21.5 Contraindications

The contraindications are the primary surgery when STA is available, the proof of fresh ischemic stroke with diffusion weighted imaging, and occlusion of radial artery due to thrombosis.

## 21.6 Special Considerations

The selected patients have redeveloped ischemic symptoms, although they have benefitted from initial STA–MCA bypass (symptom-free). Imaging studies demonstrate the delayed STA–MCA graft occlusion with lack of collaterals formation.

The individual testing of platelet antiaggregation is needed preoperatively.

To prevent the bypass occlusion, dilatation of the graft vessel with hydrostatic pressure as a preparation and use of 3,000 units heparin when opening the anastomosis have to be remembered to perform.

The distal end of the radial artery graft should be shaped only slight fish mouthing for recipient vessel mismatch.

## 21.7 Pitfalls, Risk Assessment, and Complications

Bypass may be technically infeasible due to recipient vessel mismatch and high fragility of MMD vessels. Bypass graft may be occluded due to vasospasm and thrombosis (5–10%). There is a high risk for perioperative stroke because the patients are hemodynamically unstable (9.3%). Furthermore, there is a high risk for hyperperfusion syndrome, which is increased for MMD patients (16.7–28.1%) compared to patients with another occlusive disease (atherosclerotic disease) (3.7%).

## 21.8 Special Instructions, Position, and Anesthesia

The patients should be maintained under normotensive conditions (systolic blood pressure, 120–140 mm Hg) immediately after anastomosis and postoperatively. Postoperative careful observations at intensive care unit are needed, whether the patients show the symptoms such as headache, seizure, and focal neurological deficit which are suspected of hyperperfusion.

## 21.9 Patient Position with Skin Incision and Key Surgical Steps

The patient is positioned supine and the head is rotated 30 degrees off the vertical axis. The head skin incision is made behind the hairline from the midline to the zygomatic process. Frontotemporal craniotomy is performed, which expanded the initial craniotomy, if necessary. The cervical skin incision where the carotid bifurcation is also outlined (▶ Fig. 21.1).

The position of the radial artery of the forearm is marked (▶ Fig. 21.2). Radial artery is harvested in a typical manner. The graft vessel is dilated with controlled hydrostatic pressure and checked for leakage (▶ Fig. 21.3).

M3 portion of the MCA is observed carefully whether it is suitable for use as a recipient artery. The arachnoid around the recipient artery (M3) is opened (▶ Fig. 21.4).

If M3 portion is not suitable for recipient artery, M2 portion is selected. The sylvian fissure is gently opened to approach the M2 portion of the MCA (▶ Fig. 21.5).

The radial artery graft is passed subcutaneously from the craniotomy incision to the cervical incision, and the proximal end of graft is prepared. The arteriotomy of the ECA is created with the aortic punch (▶ Fig. 21.6). The first anastomosis is performed between the proximal end of the graft vessel and the ECA, just distal to the bifurcation of the common carotid artery (CCA) in end-to-side technique with 7–0 nylon threads. One side of the anastomosis is performed and the lumen is inspected (▶ Fig. 21.7). The first anastomosis is completed (▶ Fig. 21.8).

After distal end of the radial artery is prepared, the arteriotomy of M3 portion is created (▶ Fig. 21.9). The second anastomosis is performed between the distal end of the graft vessel and the M3 portion in end-to-side technique with 10–0 nylon threads (▶ Fig. 21.10). The second anastomosis is completed (▶ Fig. 21.11).

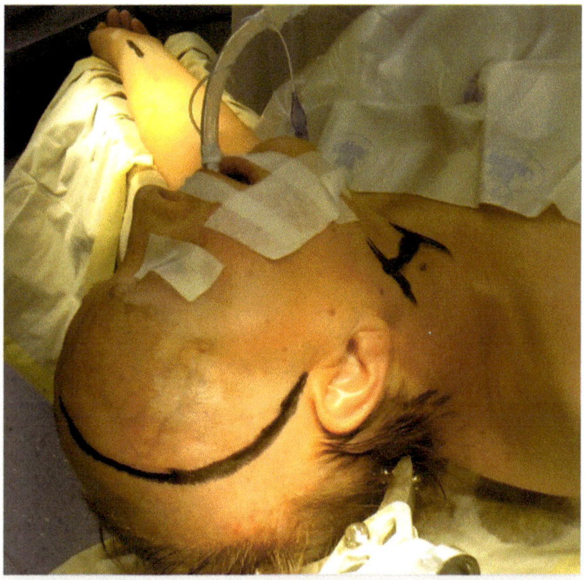

**Fig. 21.1** The patient is positioned supine and the head is rotated 30 degrees off the vertical axis. The head skin incision is made behind the hairline from the midline to the zygomatic process. The cervical skin incision where the carotid bifurcation is also outlined.

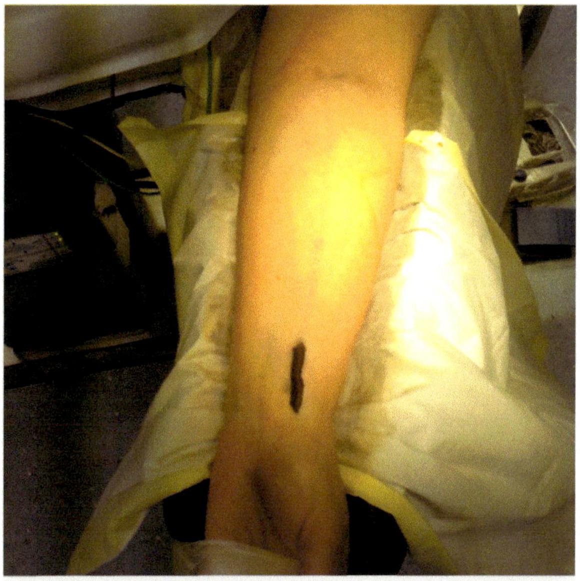

**Fig. 21.2** The radial artery of the forearm is marked.

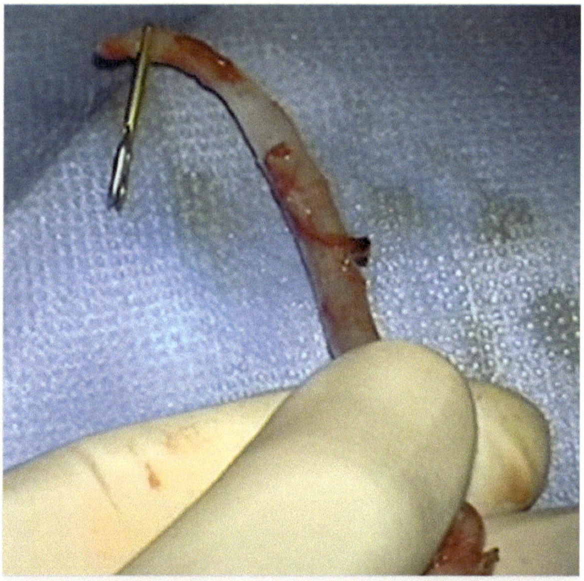

**Fig. 21.3** Radial artery is harvested in a typical manner. The graft vessel is dilated with controlled hydrostatic pressure and checked for leakage.

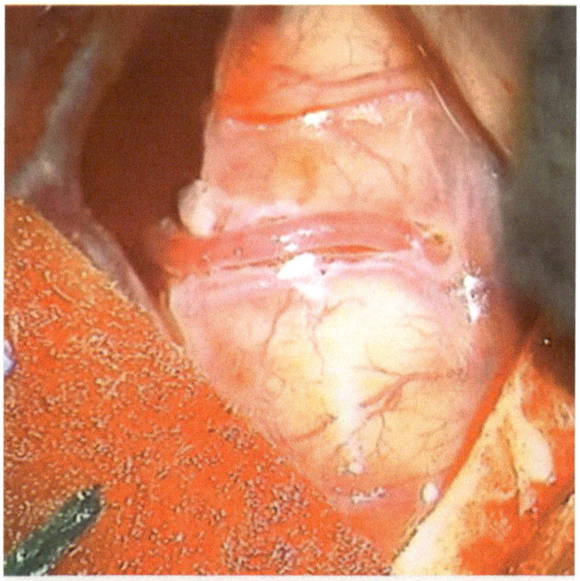

**Fig. 21.4** M3 portion of the middle cerebral artery (MCA) is observed carefully whether it is suitable for use as a recipient artery. The arachnoid around the recipient artery (M3) is opened.

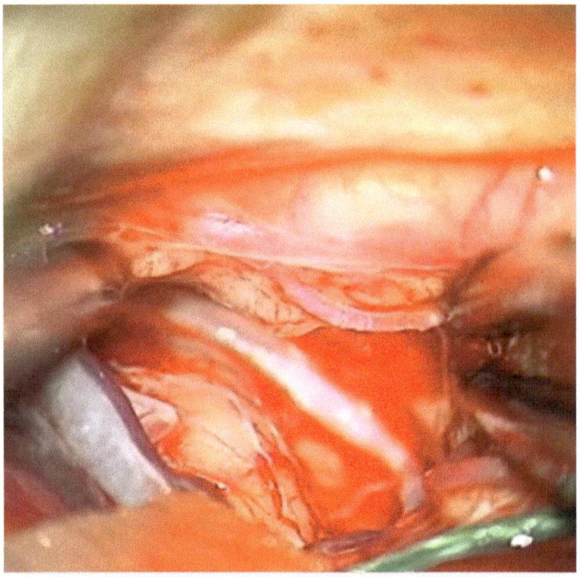

**Fig. 21.5** If M3 portion is not suitable for recipient artery, M2 portion is selected. The sylvian fissure is gently opened to approach the M2 portion of the middle cerebral artery (MCA).

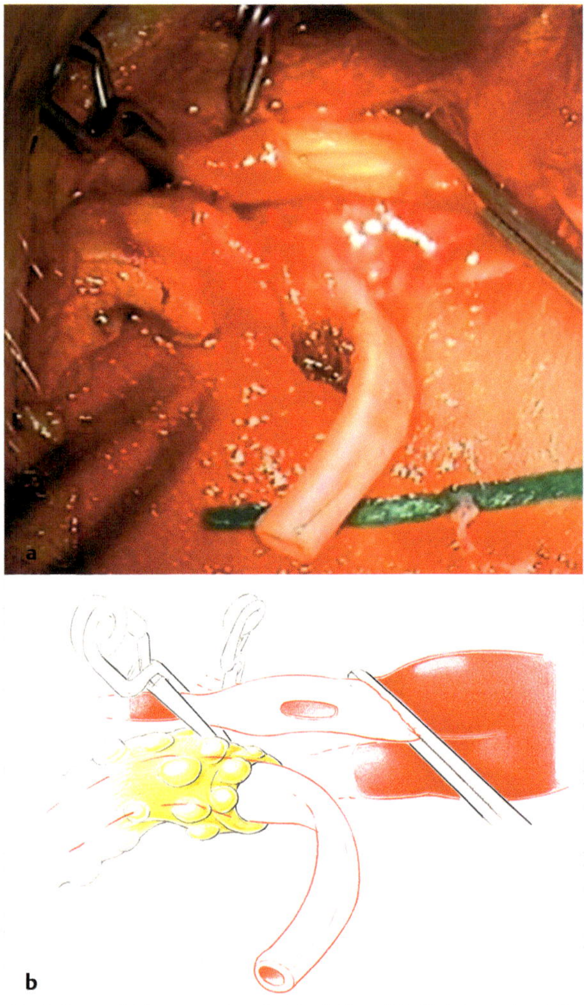

**Fig. 21.6 (a, b)** The radial artery graft is passed subcutaneously from the craniotomy incision to the cervical incision, and the proximal end of graft is prepared. The arteriotomy of the external carotid artery (ECA) is created with the aortic punch

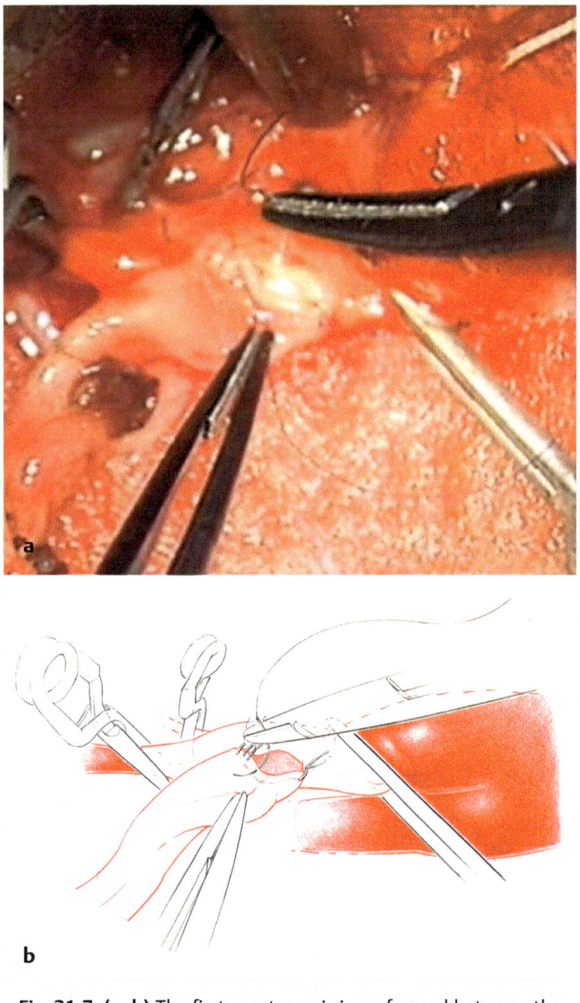

**Fig. 21.7 (a, b)** The first anastomosis is performed between the proximal end of the graft vessel and the external carotid artery (ECA) in end-to-side technique with 7–0 nylon threads. One side of the anastomosis is performed and the lumen is inspected.

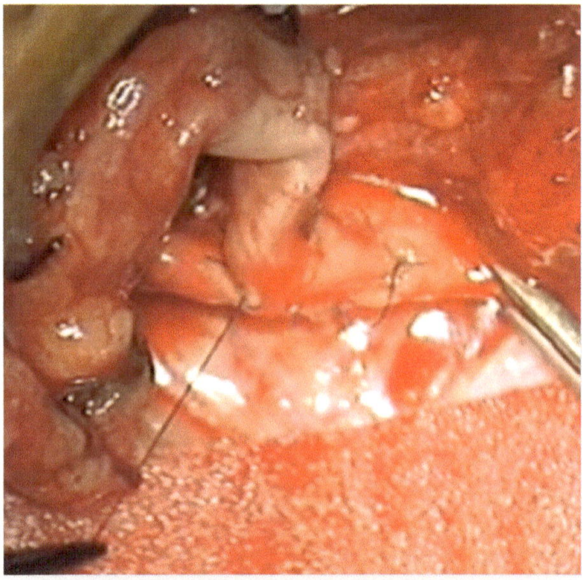

**Fig. 21.8** The first anastomosis is completed.

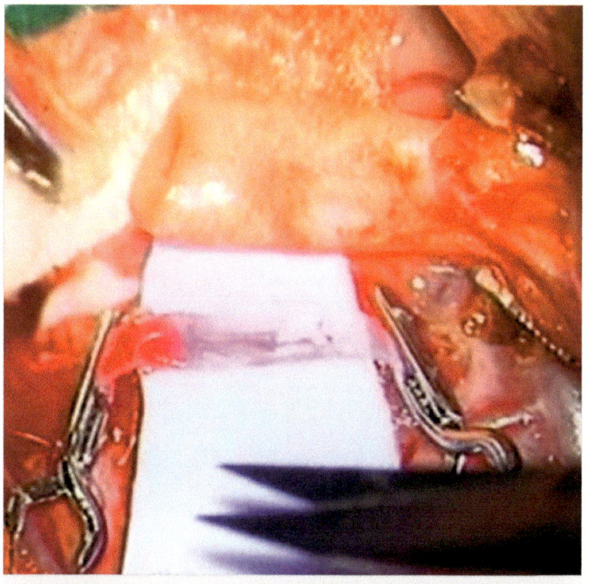

**Fig. 21.9** After distal end of the radial artery is prepared, the arteriotomy of M3 portion is created.

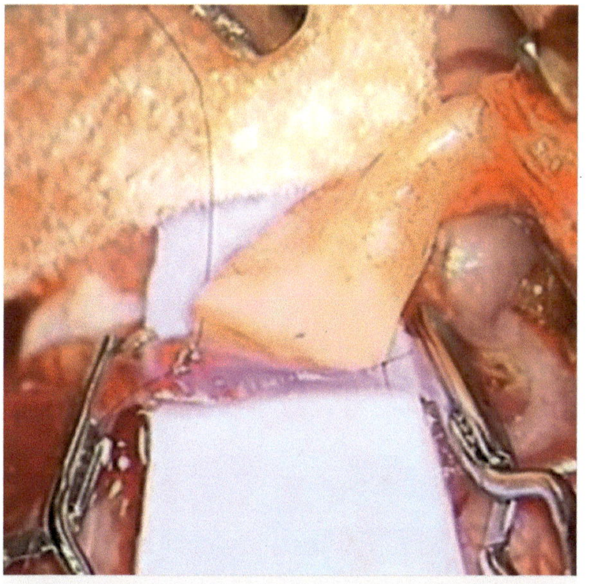

**Fig. 21.10** The second anastomosis is performed between the distal end of the graft vessel and the M3 portion in end-to-side technique with 10–0 nylon threads.

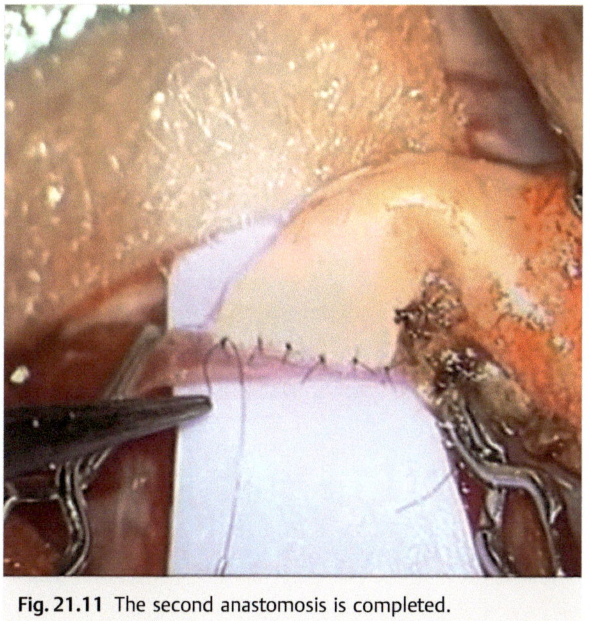

**Fig. 21.11** The second anastomosis is completed.

The radial artery graft is anastomosed to the M3 portion of the MCA with careful attention to avoid graft kinking and distortion in overview of the craniotomy site (▶ Fig. 21.12). The patency of the graft vessel is confirmed by intraoperative ICG angiography (▶ Fig. 21.13) and quantitative Doppler flow measurements (▶ Fig. 21.14).

## 21.10 Difficulties Encountered

- Meticulous surgical manipulation should be performed because the recipient vessel has high fragility.
- Enough orifice of recipient artery which fits the caliber of radial artery graft should be made.
- To avoid the thrombosis of anastomotic site, the proximal anastomosis should be performed first, and the use of heparin while opening the anastomosis has to be remembered.

## 21.11 Bailout, Rescue, and Salvage Maneuvers

Intraoperative bypass occlusion is a serious complication. The graft vessel should be dilated with controlled hydrostatic pressure for preparation to prevent the vasospasm and thrombosis. If the occlusion of anastomostic site is occurred, local injection of heparinized saline should be tried to perform first. If this method is not effective, reopening which followed by resuture of anastomotic site with careful inspection or remove and replace of graft vessel have to be done.

## 21.12 Tips, Pearls, and Lessons Learned

- There is the tendency for vasospasm and easy thrombosis of radial artery graft; therefore, the graft should be handled carefully.

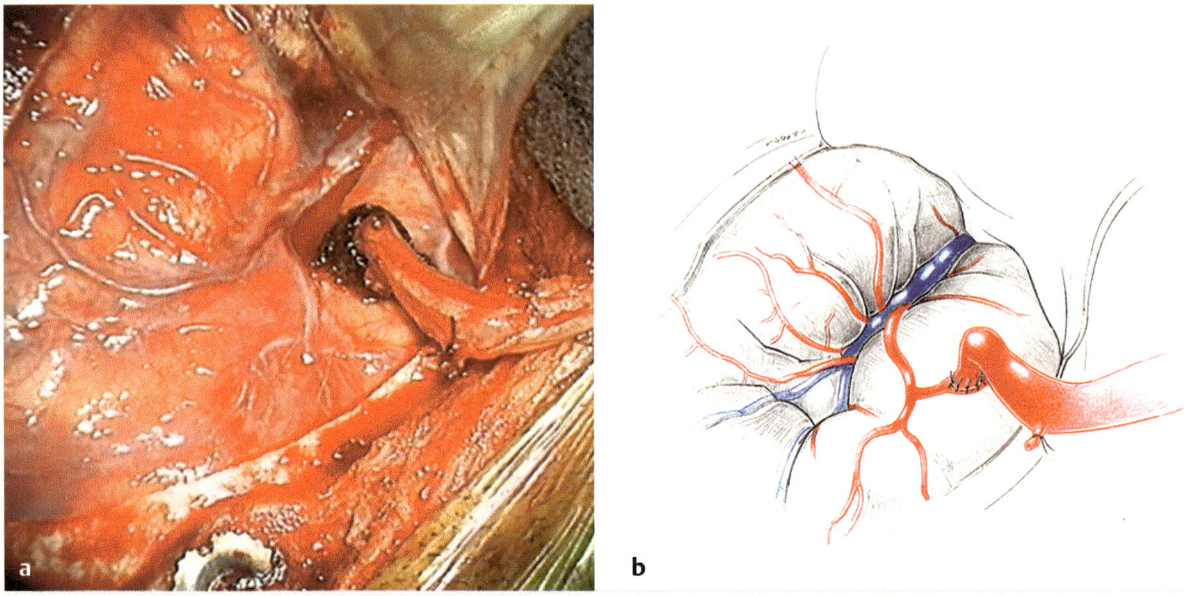

**Fig. 21.12 (a, b)** The radial artery graft is anastomosed to the M3 portion of the middle cerebral artery (MCA) with careful attention to avoid graft kinking and distortion in overview of the craniotomy site.

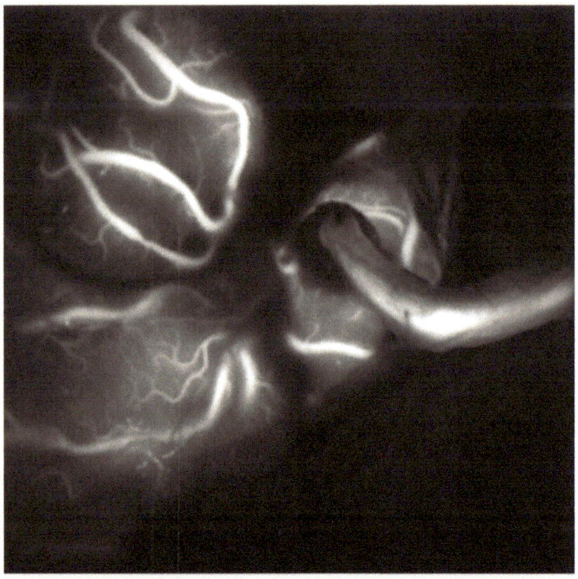

**Fig. 21.13** The patency of the anastomosis is confirmed by intraoperative indocyanine green (ICG) angiography.

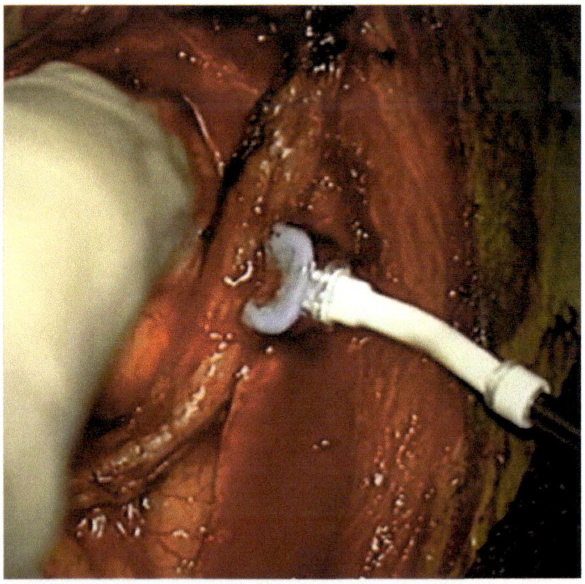

**Fig. 21.14** Quantitative Doppler flow measurement is performed to check the patency of the graft vessel.

- Quality of radial artery graft is usually sufficient even if MMD.
- Starting with proximal anastomosis is recommended for preventing of thrombosis at anastomotic site.
- There is the potential high risk of hyperperfusion; therefore, more distal recipient artery should be selected.
- Doppler flow measurements are needed for checking of graft patency.
- When the flow rates by the Doppler measurements are very high (up to 100 mL/min), it should be paid attention to the high possibility of hyperperfusion.

## References


[1] Kuroda S, Houkin K. Moyamoya disease: current concepts and future perspectives. Lancet Neurol. 2008; 7(11):1056–1066

[2] Schick U, Zimmermann M, Stolke D. Long-term evaluation of EC-IC bypass patency. Acta Neurochir (Wien). 1996; 138(8):938–942, discussion 942–943

[3] Amin-Hanjani S, Singh A, Rifai H, et al. Combined direct and indirect bypass for moyamoya: quantitative assessment of direct bypass flow over time. Neurosurgery. 2013; 73(6):962–967, discussion 967–968

[4] Sandow N, von Weitzel-Mudersbach P, Rosenbaum S, et al. Extra-intracranial standard bypass in the elderly: perioperative risk, bypass patency and outcome. Cerebrovasc Dis. 2013; 36(3):228–235

[5] Karasawa J, Touho H, Ohnishi H, Miyamoto S, Kikuchi H. Cerebral revascularization using omental transplantation for childhood moyamoya disease. J Neurosurg. 1993; 79(2):192–196

[6] Navarro R, Chao K, Gooderham PA, Bruzoni M, Dutta S, Steinberg GK. Less invasive pedicled omental-cranial transposition in pediatric patients with moyamoya disease and failed prior revascularization. Neurosurgery. 2014; 10 Suppl 1:1–14

[7] Touho H, Karasawa J, Tenjin H, Ueda S. Omental transplantation using a superficial temporal artery previously used for encephaloduroarteriosynangiosis. Surg Neurol. 1996; 45(6):550–558, discussion 558–559

[8] Pandey P, Steinberg GK. Outcome of repeat revascularization surgery for moyamoya disease after an unsuccessful indirect revascularization. Clinical article. J Neurosurg. 2011; 115(2):328–336

[9] Sia SF, Davidson AS, Assaad NN, Stoodley M, Morgan MK. Comparative patency between intracranial arterial pedicle and vein bypass surgery. Neurosurgery. 2011; 69(2):308–314

[10] Hori S, Acker G, Vajkoczy P. Radial artery grafts as rescue strategy for patients with moyamoya disease for whom conventional revascularization failed. World Neurosurg. 2016; 85:77–84

# 22 OA–MCA or OA–PCA Bypass

*Mario Teo, Jeremiah N. Johnson, and Gary K. Steinberg*

**Abstract**

When the parietal and frontal superficial temporal arteries are not available as a direct donor to the middle cerebral artery (MCA) territory, the occipital artery (OA) can often be utilized. Additionally, due to significant leptomeningeal collateralization from the posterior circulation to the anterior circulation, progressive steno-occlusion of the posterior cerebral artery (PCA) in advanced moyamoya disease (MMD) can result in inadequate collateralization of the MCA or PCA territory. The OA is also an appealing donor choice for revascularization of these territories due to its close proximity to the target recipient vessels; however, there are challenges associated with this strategy, such as tortuosity, multiple branches, and thick adherent investing tissue, which can result in inadvertent OA injury during vessel harvest. In this chapter, we highlight the steps and nuances in performing the challenging OA–MCA or OA–PCA bypass, the techniques used to troubleshoot inadvertent OA occlusion or injury, and illustrate with appropriate case examples. We also include the preoperative workup, intraoperative patient positioning, a step-by-step description of key procedures, and the long-term clinical and radiological postoperative care and surveillance, all of which contribute to achieving maximal benefits of direct bypass to the posterior MCA or PCA in select patients with MMD vasculopathy.

*Keywords:* OA–PCA or MCA bypass, occipital artery, posterior circulation MMD, inadvertent vessel injury, troubleshooting principles

## 22.1 Background

Moyamoya disease (MMD) is a progressive angiopathy that, over time, can involve the posterior circulation. Because the posterior circulation provides significant collateralization, especially to the anterior circulation, stenosis or occlusion of the posterior cerebral artery (PCA) can also affect the anterior parts of the brain. When the target recipient vessel for bypass is the posterior middle cerebral artery (MCA), or posterior circulation, the occipital artery (OA) is a particularly appealing donor choice.

### 22.1.1 History

- 1970—Yasargil and colleagues reported the first successful extracranial to intracranial (ECIC) bypass.
- 1976—Khodadad reported the first successful OA–posterior interior cerebellar artery (PICA) bypass for a 58-year-old man with posterior circulation ischemic symptoms and a postoperative angiogram confirming bypass graft patency.
- Apart from ischemic neurological disease involving the posterior circulation, OA grafts are frequently used for PICA bypasses in the cases of PICA aneurysms that required parent vessel sacrifice.
- Recently, OA grafts have increasingly been used for posterior MCA or PCA revascularization in MMD.

## 22.2 Indication

- Repeat or initial revascularization for MMD patients with inadequate collateralization of the MCA or PCA territory, when no suitable superficial temporal artery (STA) donor is available.

## 22.3 Key Principles

- The harvest of OA is challenging due to its tortuosity, multiple branches, and thick investing fascia.
- Harvest an adequate length of OA to reach the territory to be revascularized.
- Harvest the main OA trunk, as smaller secondary tributaries are not usually of adequate size for direct bypass.

## 22.4 SWOT Analysis

### 22.4.1 Strength

- Good donor option in the absence of suitable STA, when posterior MCA or PCA territories are to be revascularized.

### 22.4.2 Weakness

- OA is tortuous, has multiple branches, and thick adherent investing tissue.

### 22.4.3 Opportunity

- Stereotactic CT angiography of OA to accurately locate and harvest the OA branch to be utilized.

### 22.4.4 Threat

- Inadvertent injury resulting in occlusion of OA donor during dissection.

## 22.5 Contraindications

- Poor patient medical or neurologic condition excluding patients as candidates for cranial bypass.

- OA with extensive preexisting ECIC collateralization.

### 22.5.1 Relative Contraindications

- Patients with recent cerebral infarct should undergo diffusion-weighted imaging (DWI) on magnetic resonance imaging (MRI) of brain (within 1–2 weeks), as the risk of perioperative strokes is significantly increased.

## 22.6 Special Considerations

- On angiogram, carefully study the OA tributaries and sizes as well as determine the branch to be harvested.
- Assess existing ECIC collateralization provided by OA on cerebral angiograms so as to determine if harvesting OA as a donor graft might lead to more ischemic brain injury.
- Optimize patient positioning for the brain territories to be revascularized, and the OA vessel to be harvested.

## 22.7 Risk Assessment—Stanford Experience

From 1991 to 2016 we have performed 1,440 ECIC bypasses for MMD, of which 1,252 (87%) were direct bypasses. OA-MCA or OA–PCA bypasses were used for repeat revascularization in eight cases.

Age of patients ranged from 8 to 60 years, with a mean follow-up of 6 years (range: 1 to 15 years).

None of the eight patients experienced perioperative infarction. One patient developed a postoperative transient neurologic deficit (TND) that resolved within 10 days.

At last follow-up, all patients had preoperative symptom resolution, with follow-up cerebral angiogram confirming patent bypass grafts of all OA–MCA or OA–PCA revascularizations.

## 22.8 Preoperative Workup

Preoperatively, patients underwent a thorough medical, cardiac, and anesthetic assessment with routine preoperative labs and the relevant diagnostic imaging, which includes 6-vessel cerebral angiogram, MRI brain, and cerebral perfusion imaging with and without Diamox (positron emission tomography, MR perfusion, TCDs). At our institution, we perform MR perfusion with and without Diamox and patients demonstrating poor cerebrovascular reserve or steal (indicating that the affected vascular territory is already maximally vasodilated to promote flow) are considered especially at high risk for ongoing ischemia without treatment. These patients are also at higher risk for perioperative ischemic complications, thus particular care is taken to avoid hypotension perioperatively and during the recovery period. Intraoperatively, the patient's blood pressure is maintained at or above the preoperative baseline at all times.

### 22.8.1 Specific Consideration with Anticoagulation

- For patients with mechanical heart valves or recent venous thromboembolism, we restart anticoagulation at 2 to 4 weeks postoperatively after CT head confirms no significant hemorrhage.
- Aspirin is continued through the day before surgery, withheld on the day of surgery, and restarted on the first postoperative day.

## 22.9 Patient Preparation

### 22.9.1 Patient Position with Skin Incision

- Depending on the vascular territory to be revascularized, positioning options are: (1) prone (for occipital region, PCA territory; ► Fig. 22.1**a**) or (2) supine, head turned with the parietotemporal uppermost (posterior MCA territory).
- A Mayfield head holder secures the head position.
- A Doppler probe is used to map out the course of the OA (► Fig. 22.1**b**)
- Skin incision options include: (1) horseshoe flap (► Fig. 22.1**b**) or (2) linear incision over the vessel to be harvested.

## 22.10 Surgical Steps

### 22.10.1 Key Procedural Step 1: OA Harvest

- Use microscopic guidance.
- For a linear incision, make the superficial skin incision through the epidermis and partial thickness of the dermis starting above the suboccipital muscle over the vessel.
- To avoid damage to the OA, dissect through the remaining dermis and subcutaneous tissue using blunt-tip, fine curve scissors.
- Once the OA is visualized, carefully dissect along the main tributary with meticulous hemostasis to harvest enough length of the vessel to reach the recipient territory.
- For dissection of the OA using a horseshoe flap, the vessel is dissected from the underside of the scalp flap (► Fig. 22.2**a**).

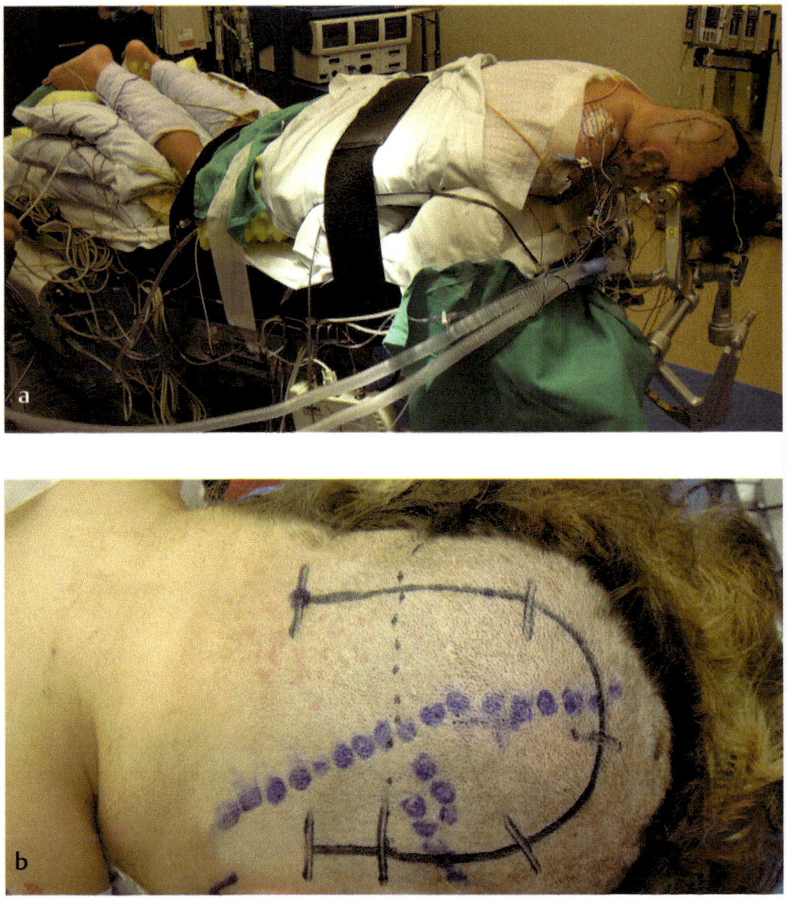

**Fig. 22.1 (a)** Prone position for occipital artery–posterior cerebral artery (OA–PCA) bypass, or alternatively supine, head turned so that the parietotemporal is uppermost to vascularize posterior middle cerebral artery territory. **(b)** Doppler is used to map out the course of OA, and horseshoe flap for the OA harvest. Alternatively, linear incision over the main trunk of OA to be harvested can also be used.

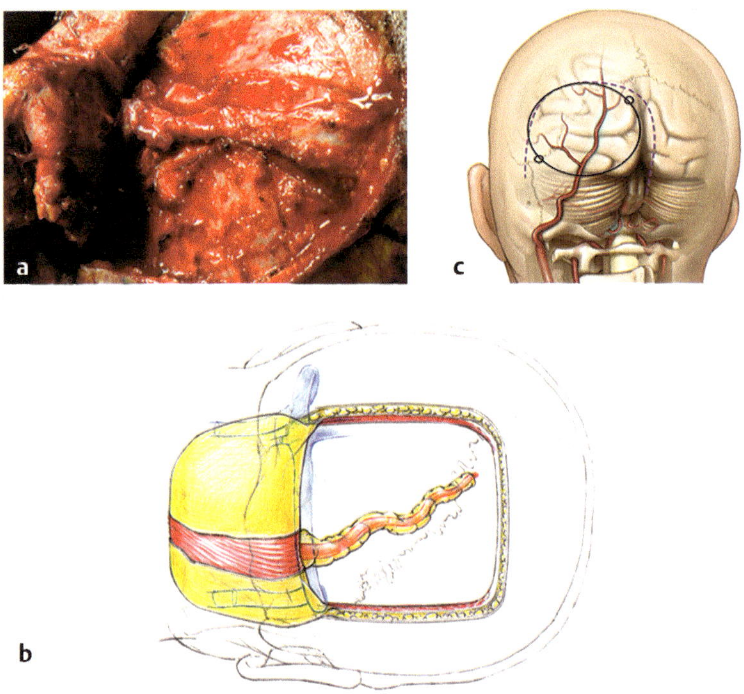

**Fig. 22.2 (a, b)** Using a horseshoe flap, the occipital artery (OA) vessel is dissected from the underside of the scalp flap. Note the thick scalp tissue overlying OA vessel, and the underlying pericranium to be dissected for the craniotomy. **(c)** Craniotomy performed over the parietotemporal or occipital region depending on whether the posterior middle cerebral artery or posterior cerebral artery is being revascularized. It is important to be mindful of the superior sagittal sinus and transverse sinus when raising the bone flap.

### 22.10.2 Key Procedural Step 2: Craniotomy and Dural Opening

- The OA is retracted laterally and protected with a vein retractor.
- The underlying occipitalis, fascia, and pericranium are incised in line with the long axis of the harvested OA.
- Perform subperiosteal dissection of the muscle and pericranial attachment to expose the underlying bone for craniotomy opening.
- Fashion burr holes in the supratentorial compartment, avoiding injury to the torcula, superior sagittal sinus, and transverse sinus.
- Perform the craniotomy over the parietotemporal or occipital region depending on whether the posterior MCA or PCA is being revascularized (▶ Fig. 22.2**b**).
- Open the dura in a cruciate manner or with a flap that is based on the venous sinuses, and use dural tack-ups to obliterate the epidural space.

### 22.10.3 Key Procedural Step 3: Prepare Recipient Vessel

- Open the arachnoid for the recipient vessel with enough length (usually 7–10 mm) exposed to prepare for temporary clipping and anastomoses.
- Size measurement: the minimum diameter for the recipient vessel should be 0.8 mm, but ideally at least 1 mm.
- Measure flow using the Charbel Transonics ultrasonic flow probe.
- Select the position for temporary clip application.
- Choose the site for arteriotomy (parietotemporal or lateral occipital lobe for MCA territory, medial occipital or inferior temporal lobe for PCA territory).

### 22.10.4 Key Procedural Step 4: Prepare Donor Vessel

- Measure the size of the donor OA to ensure its diameter matches the recipient vessel, and is adequate for direct bypass (ideally 1 mm or larger, but at least 0.8 mm; ▶ Fig. 22.3**a**).
- Ensure patency of the donor graft with frequent handheld Doppler checks.
- Apply a temporary clip to the proximal OA, and divide the distal OA at a 45-degree angle (▶ Fig. 22.3**b**). Flush the vessel lumen with heparinized saline to prevent thrombus formation (▶ Fig. 22.3**c**).
- Perform "cut flow" measurement of the donor artery using Charbel Transonics ultrasonic flow probe.
- Fish mouth the donor vessel.
- Ensure well-visualized OA vessel walls.

Techniques used to troubleshoot inadvertent OA occlusion or injury:

- Flush with heparinized saline; regular papaverine or nicardipine drip on the vessel to prevent vasospasm.
- In the event of no blood flow after dividing the OA vessel, pass a 3F pediatric sheath or wire to dislodge any formed thrombus or to locate the area of occlusion (▶ Fig. 22.3**d**).
- If an area of occlusion is identified that cannot be opened easily with the wire or pediatric sheath, excise the occluded segment, flush both proximal and distal cut end with heparinized saline (▶ Fig. 22.3**e**), followed by primary anastomosis of the donor vessel (▶ Fig. 22.3**f**) to restore donor graft patency (▶ Fig. 22.3**g**).

### 22.10.5 Key Procedural Step 5: Microanastomosis

- Anesthetic optimization (hypothermia: 33 °C, $CO_2$: 35 mm Hg, mean arterial pressure [MAP]: 80–90 mm Hg during exposure, MAP: 90–100 mm Hg) and burst suppression using propofol prior to recipient vessel occlusion.
- Apply temporary clips to M4/P4, followed by arteriotomy and flush the lumen with heparinized saline (▶ Fig. 22.4**a**).
- The donor and recipient vessels are tinted with indigo carmine, methylene blue, or a sterile marking pen to better visualize the arteries during the microanastomosis (▶ Fig. 22.4**b**).
- Use 10/0 Prolene for the anastomosis, toe stitch first, then heel stitch, three (sometimes four) interrupted stitches on each side, making sure to avoid incorporating the opposite vessel wall or stenosing the recipient vessel (▶ Fig. 22.4**b–f**).

### 22.10.6 Key Procedural Step 6: Ensure Bypass Graft Patency

- Should observe some blood leakage at the anastomotic site on release of the temporary clips, which will mostly seal with time and irrigation.
- Occasionally, additional sutures are needed to control blood leakage at the anastomosis, but usually not necessary to reocclude the recipient artery.
- To confirm patency and function of the bypass graft we perform: (1) flow measurement (Transonics Charbel Flowmeter) of the OA, proximal, and distal recipient vessels, (2) Doppler probe for flow signal transduction, and (3) intraoperative indocyanine green (ICG) angiogram (▶ Fig. 22.4**g**).

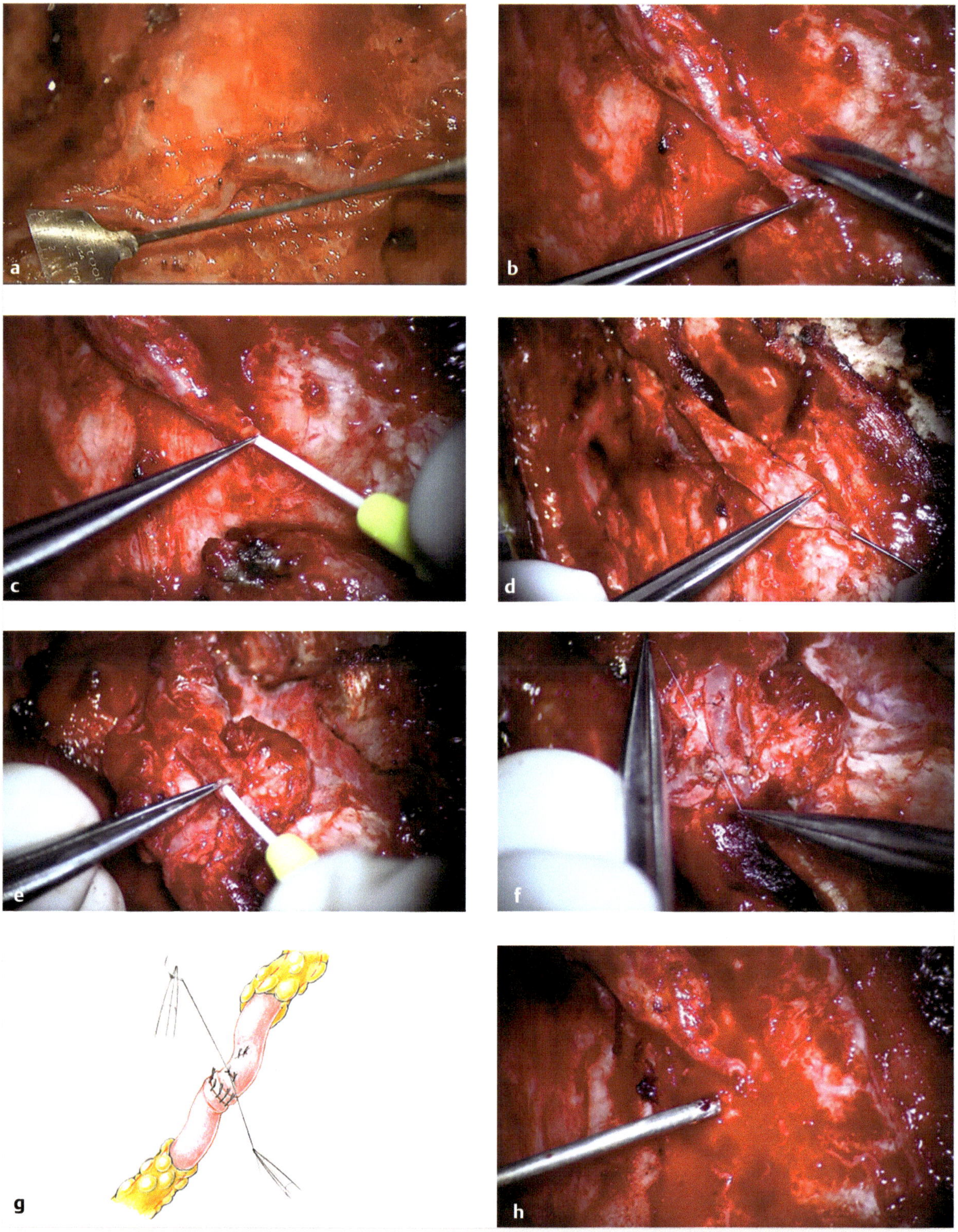

**Fig. 22.3 (a)** Measure the size of the donor occipital artery (OA) to ensure the diameter matches the donor vessel, and is adequate for direct bypass (ideally 1 mm or larger, but bypass can be performed for a vessel 0.8 mm). **(b)** A temporary clip is applied to the proximal OA, and the distal OA is divided at a 45-degree angle. **(c)** After dividing the OA distally, flush the vessel lumen with heparinized saline to prevent thrombus formation. **(d)** In the event of no blood flow after dividing the OA vessel, pass a 3F pediatric sheath or wire to dislodge formed thrombus or locate the area of occlusion. **(e)** Once the area of occlusion is identified, excise the occluded segment, and flush both the proximal and distal cut end with heparinized saline. **(f)** Use 10–0 Prolene for the primary anastomosis of the OA donor vessel to restore continuity of the vessel. **(g, h)** OA donor graft patency is confirmed upon removing the clip on the proximal OA by observing good blood flow distally.

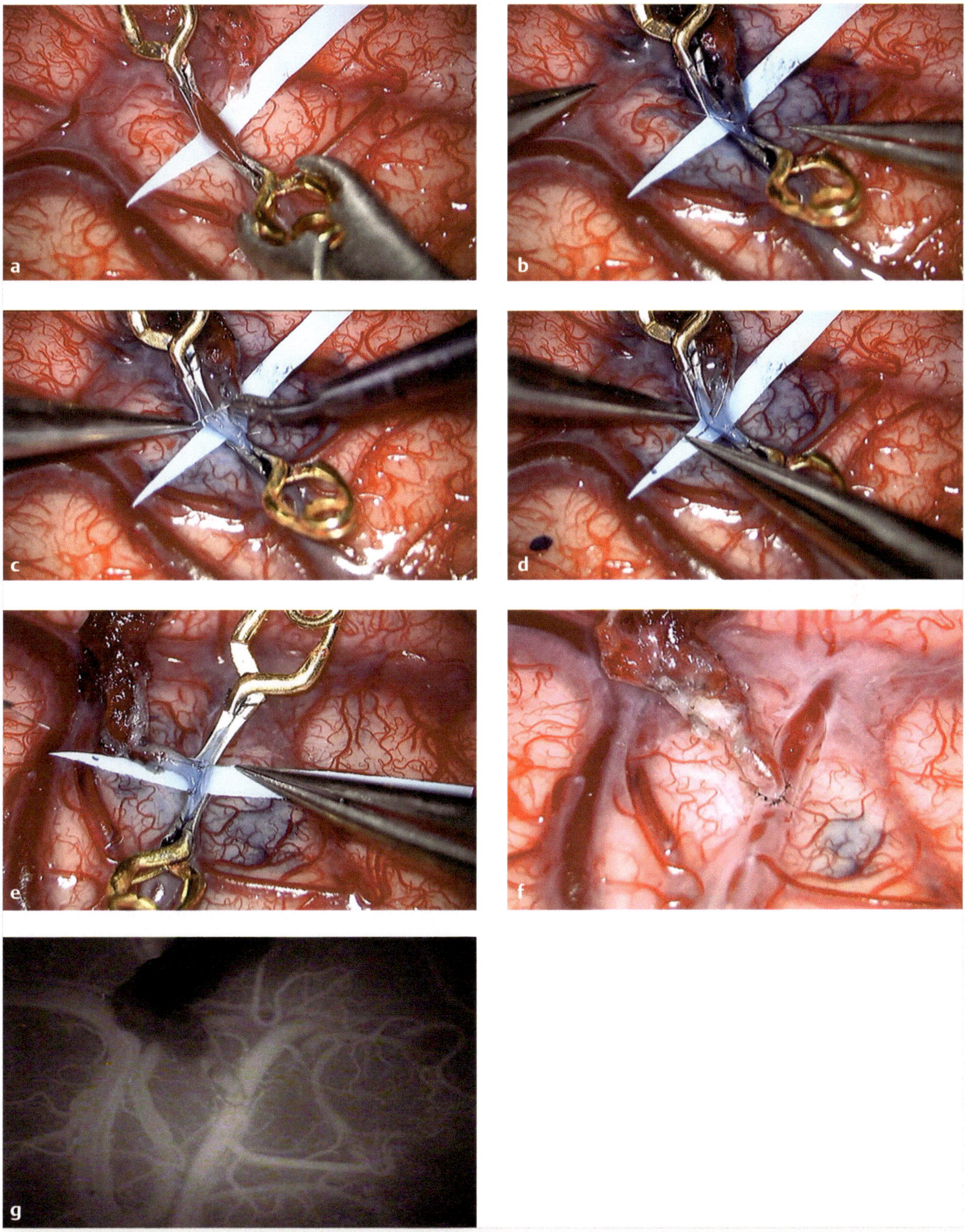

**Fig. 22.4** **(a)** After anesthetic optimization, temporary clips are applied to M4/P4, followed by arteriotomy, and the lumen is flushed with heparinized saline. **(b)** The donor and recipient vessels are tinted with indigo carmine, methylene blue, or a sterile marking pen to better visualize the arteries during microanastomosis. 10/0 Prolene is used for anastomosis, with a toe stitch first. **(c)** A heel stitch follows to anchor the donor vessel to the recipient arteriotomy and provide stability when completing the rest of the suture around the arteriotomy. **(d)** Complete three (sometimes four) interrupted stitches on each side, making sure to not incorporate the opposite vessel wall or stenose the recipient vessel. **(e)** Move the donor graft to expose the back wall prior to completing the anastomosis, followed by three to four stitches. **(f)** Completion of the occipital artery–middle cerebral artery (OA–MCA) or occipital artery–posterior cerebral artery (OA–PCA) direct bypass. **(g)** Use intraoperative indocyanine green angiogram to confirm patency and function of the bypass graft. We also perform flow measurement (Transonics Charbel Flowmeter) of the OA, proximal and distal recipient vessels, and Doppler probe for flow signal transduction.

- Ensure hemostasis prior to closure; use Surgicel for the anastomosis site.

### 22.10.7 Key Procedural Step 7: Closure

- Ensure meticulous hemostasis.
- Dural opposition to not compromise the donor vessel.
- Dural graft overlying the brain: create a plane between brain and bone.
- Bone flap replacement: ensure adequate opening to accommodate the donor graft.
- Perform regular Doppler checks to ensure bypass graft patency.
- Multilayer the scalp closure to muscle, galea, skin.

## 22.11 Tips, Pearls, and Lessons Learned

- Perform meticulous dissection to follow the primary OA.
- Positioning depends on the areas being revascularized.
- Supine with head turned to revascularize posterior MCA, prone for PCA.

## 22.12 Pitfalls

- Inadvertent occlusion or injury to the OA during dissection stage: use careful bipolar coagulation at low power of bleeding points.
- Dissection of the secondary OA branch instead of the primary OA.
- Stenosing recipient artery.

## 22.13 Bailout, Rescue, and Salvage Maneuvers

In case of inadvertent OA occlusion or injury:
- Identify the site of occlusion or injury.
- If the OA graft occluded due to thrombus, pass a 3F pediatric sheath or wire to dislodge the occlusion.
- If the OA graft was coagulated or injured during dissection, excision followed by primary anastomosis of the injured site is warranted.

## 22.14 Postoperative Care

### 22.14.1 Patient Surveillance

- First 24 hours postoperative:
  - Intensive care unit with regular neuro checks.
  - Close monitoring of hemodynamic status (fluid intake, output, and electrolytes).
  - Thresholds for blood pressure MAP goals of 90–110 mm Hg to prevent hypoperfusion, delayed TND, or hyperperfusion and postoperative hematoma.
  - Analgesia, antiemetic.
- Day 2: mobilize, oral intake, transfer to regular ward care.
- Remain in hospital until deemed safe to be discharged by neurosurgical and general surgical team (average hospital stay 2–3 days).
- Post discharge, educate and inform about TND, wound care, and subsequent follow-up plans.

### 22.14.2 Bypass Function Assessment

- Intraoperative OA–PCA or OA–MCA bypass graft assessment using ICG angiogram, Transonic Charbel flow probe, and Doppler probe. Six-month postoperative digital subtraction angiogram (DSA) including a 5-vessel cerebral angiogram, MRI brain including fluid-attenuated inversion recovery (FLAIR)/ DWI sequence, MRI perfusion with/without Diamox (to assess cerebrovascular reserve), and neuropsychological testing.
- Long-term follow-up at 3, 10, 20, and 30 years with clinical and radiological surveillance (investigations as listed at the 6-month check).

## 22.15 Case Illustrations

### 22.15.1 Case 1: OA–PCA Bypass

A 10-year-old girl initially presented at age 7 with mild left arm neglect, and was diagnosed with bilateral MMD. She had bilateral indirect encephaloduroarteriosynangiosis (EDAS) revascularizations at an outside institution that was complicated by a postoperative stroke, requiring a right frontal decompression and lobectomy. After extensive rehabilitation she was left with complete left visual field loss, a spastic left-sided weakness (four out of five weakness), and attended school with a special visual aid due to her poor vision. When seen in our clinic, she was experiencing new episodes of transient blindness, which was worrisome for compromise in the cerebral blood flow in the left occipital region. Cerebral angiogram showed bilateral ICA occlusion with moyamoya vessels (▶ Fig. 22.5**a–d**), and good revascularization of the MCA territories from the bilateral indirect bypass grafts (▶ Fig. 22.5**e–h**). She also had bilateral PCA occlusion with poor filling of both occipital lobes (▶ Fig. 22.5**i, j**). MRI brain showed a large stroke in the right MCA and PCA territory with a smaller left PCA stroke (▶ Fig. 22.5**k–n**). She underwent an uneventful left OA–PCA direct bypass to revascularize her left occipital lobe.

Her 6-month and 3-year angiogram showed a patent left OA–PCA bypass supplying the parietooccipital and

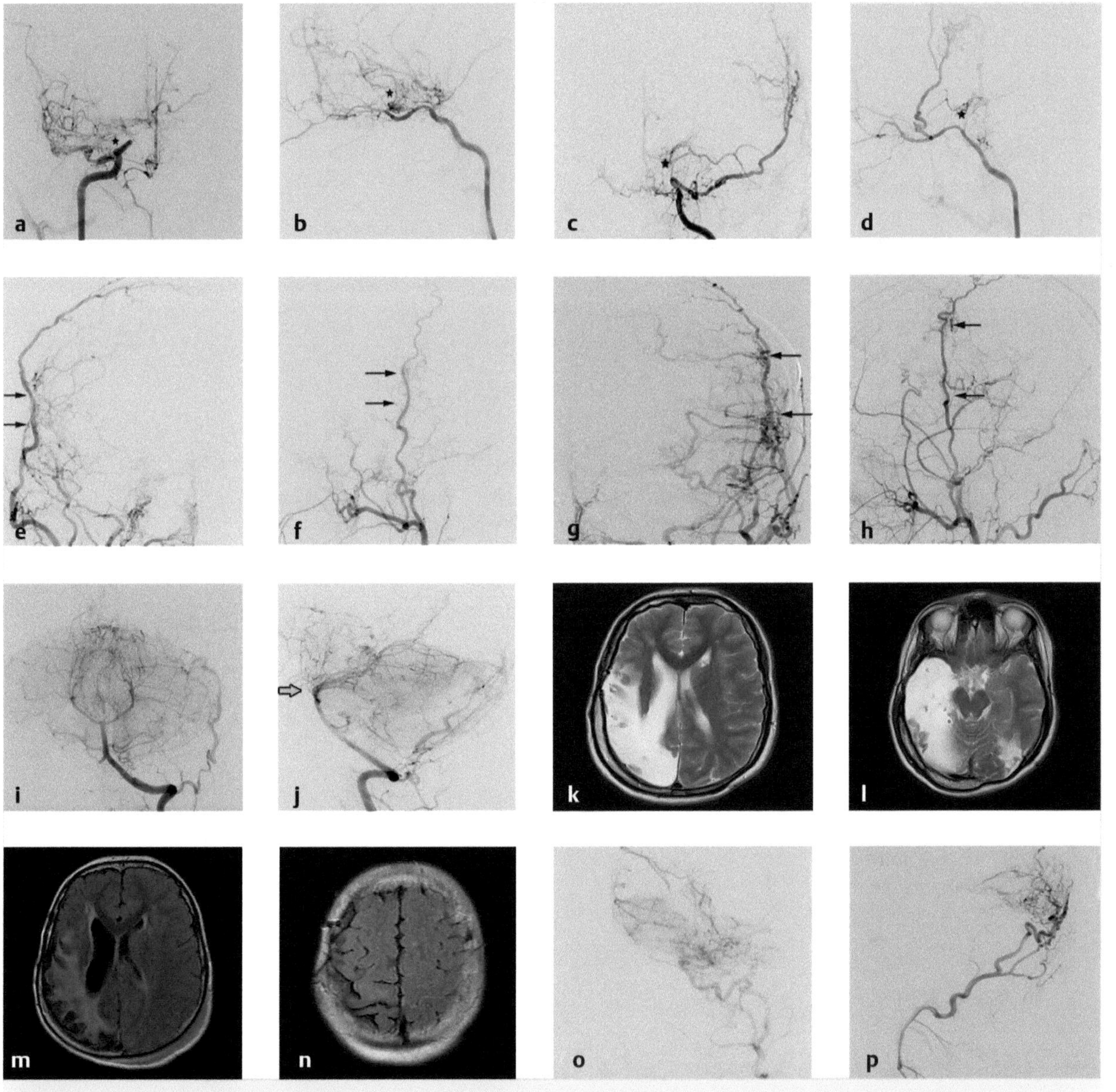

**Fig. 22.5** A 10-year-old girl with bilateral moyamoya disease had bilateral encephaloduroarteriosynangiosis at an outside institution that was complicated by a postoperative stroke 3 years prior. She was left with complete left visual field loss and a spastic left-sided weakness. When seen in our clinic, she was experiencing new episodes of transient blindness. **(a–j)** Cerebral angiogram (**[a]** right interior cerebellar artery [ICA] injection [anteroposterior, AP view], **[b]** right ICA injection [lateral view], **[c]** left ICA injection [AP view], **[d]** left ICA injection [lateral view], **[e]** right ECA injection [AP view], **[f]** right ECA injection [lateral view], **[g]** left ECA injection [AP view], **[h]** left ECA injection [lateral view], **[i]** vertebral artery injection [AP view], **[j]** vertebral artery injection [lateral view]) shows bilateral ICA occlusion with moyamoya vessels (*asterisks*) and good revascularization of the MCA territories from bilateral indirect bypass grafts (*black arrows*). She also had bilateral PCA occlusion with poor filling of both occipital lobes (*block arrow*). **(k–n)** MRI brain (**[k]** T2-weighted axial slice at the level of lateral ventricles, **[l]** T2-weighted axial slice at the level of the orbit, **[m]** FLAIR MRI axial slice at the level of the lateral ventricles, **[n]** FLAIR MRI axial slice at the upper level) showed a large stroke in the right MCA and PCA territory with a smaller left PCA stroke, with evidence of encephalomalacia and ivy signs in the cortical sulci signifying slow cerebral blood flow. She underwent an uneventful left OA–PCA direct bypass to revascularize her left occipital lobe. **(o, p)** 3-year cerebral angiogram (unchanged from 6-month angiogram; **[o]** left OA injection [AP view]; **[p]** left OA injection [lateral view]) shows patent left OA–PCA bypass supplying the parietooccipital and calcarine areas. She remained well and no longer complained of visual disturbance at 8-year follow-up.

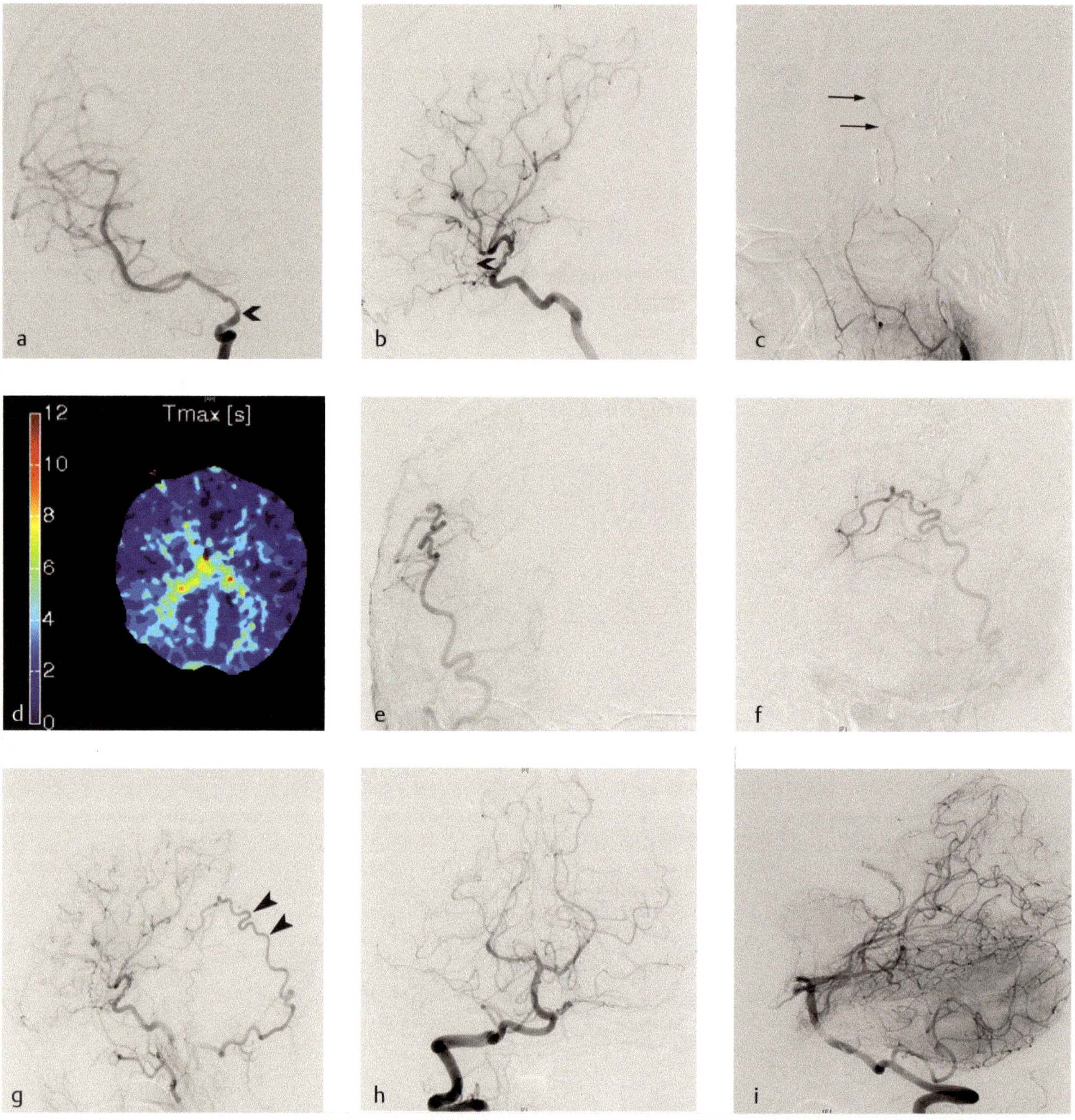


**Fig. 22.6** A 36-year-old patient with transient ischemic attacks affecting her right hemisphere was diagnosed with right unilateral moyamoya disease (MMD). Her cerebral angiogram (right interior cerebellar artery [ICA] injection [anteroposterior, AP view]) **(a, b)** (right ICA injection [lateral view]) showed right-sided high-grade preocclusive stenosis involving the ICA and middle cerebral artery (MCA) with anterior cerebral artery occlusion (*chevron arrows*). After right encephaloduroarteriosynangiosis, her symptoms recurred a year later, with headache, intermittent left-sided weakness and numbness. **(c)** Repeat cerebral angiogram (right ECA injection [lateral view]) showed poor filling of the right indirect bypass graft with little collateralization of the right MCA territory (*black arrows*). **(d)** Magnetic resonance perfusion showed reduced perfusion in the right posterior watershed region. She then underwent right occipital artery (OA) to posterior MCA direct bypass, with symptom reduction postoperatively. Her 6-month cerebral angiogram (**[e]** right OA injection [AP view], **[f]** right OA injection [lateral view]) shows a patent right OA–MCA bypass graft supplying the posterior MCA portion, and stable underlying ICA and MCA high-grade stenoses. At her 3-year follow-up, she was asymptomatic, with cerebral angiogram (**[g]** right CCA injection [lateral view]) still showing a robust and patent OA–MCA bypass graft (*black arrowheads*) supplying the posterior MCA territory. Cerebral angiogram of the posterior circulation (**[h]** vertebral artery injection [AP view], **[i]** vertebral artery injection [lateral view]) shows noninvolvement of the posterior cerebral arteries with MMD and also pericallosal collateralizations.

calcarine areas (▶ Fig. 22.5**o, p**). MRI brain showed no new infarcts, and a nuclear medicine Diamox study showed fixed defects in the known areas of infarct and no Diamox-induced perfusion defect. At her latest follow-up 8 years after left OA–PCA bypass, she remained well and no longer complained of visual disturbance.

### 22.15.2 Case 2: OA–MCA Bypass

A 36-year-old female patient with transient ischemic attacks (TIAs) affecting her right hemisphere was diagnosed with right unilateral MMD (cerebral angiogram [▶ Fig. 22.6**a, b**], showed right-sided high-grade preocclusive stenosis involving the ICA and MCA with ACA occlusion), and underwent right EDAS. Her symptoms recurred 1 year later, with headache, intermittent left-sided weakness and numbness. Repeat cerebral angiogram showed poor filling of the right-sided indirect bypass graft with little collateralization of the right MCA territory (▶ Fig. 22.6**c**). MRI brain showed no new infarcts, but reduced perfusion on the right watershed region (▶ Fig. 22.6**d**). Xenon CT showed suboptimal augmentation of the same region involving the posterior MCA.

She then underwent right OA to posterior MCA direct bypass, with symptom reduction postoperatively. Her 6-month cerebral angiogram showed stable underlying ICA and MCA high-grade stenoses, and a patent right OA-MCA bypass graft supplying the posterior MCA portion (▶ Fig. 22.6**e, f**). MRI brain showed no new infarcts, and MR perfusion showed improved cerebral blood flow to the right posterior watershed area in comparison to preoperative findings. At 3-year follow-up, she was asymptomatic, with cerebral angiogram (▶ Fig. 22.6**g–i**) still showing a patent OA–MCA bypass graft, and MR perfusion showing appropriate augmentation in all vascular territories after Diamox challenge.

## 22.16 Conclusion

OA is a particularly appealing choice for posterior MCA or posterior circulation bypass procedures due to its proximity to the target recipient vessels. Despite the challenges encountered in harvesting the tortuous, highly branched OA, it remains a very good option as a donor graft to achieve the maximal benefit of direct bypass to the posterior MCA or PCA in select patients with MMD vasculopathy.

## Suggested Readings


Ateş O, Ahmed AS, Niemann D, Başkaya MK. The occipital artery for posterior circulation bypass: microsurgical anatomy. Neurosurg Focus. 2008; 24(2):E9

Guzman R, Lee M, Achrol A, et al. Clinical outcome after 450 revascularization procedures for moyamoya disease. Clinical article. J Neurosurg. 2009; 111(5):927–935

Hayashi T, Shirane R, Tominaga T. Additional surgery for postoperative ischemic symptoms in patients with moyamoya disease: the effectiveness of occipital artery-posterior cerebral artery bypass with an indirect procedure: technical case report. Neurosurgery. 2009; 64(1):E195–E196, discussion E196

Khodadad G. Occipital artery-posterior inferior cerebellar artery anastomosis. Surg Neurol. 1976; 5(4):225–227

Yasargil MG, Krayenbuhl HA, Jacobson JH, II. Microneurosurgical arterial reconstruction. Surgery. 1970; 67(1):221–233

# 23 PAA–MCA Bypass

*Menno R. Germans and Luca Regli*

**Abstract**

Sometimes the superficial temporal artery is not available as a donor vessel for extracranial–intracranial (ECIC) bypass surgery. Also, in case of refractory moyamoya disease with an ECIC bypass in situ, there is need for an additional artery that can be used as a donor vessel. The posterior auricular artery (PAA) is a potential donor, if its diameter is large enough. The PAA runs behind the ear and in about half of cases it runs until the temporoparietal region where it can be used as an alternative donor artery for ECIC bypass surgery. The artery runs vertically along the posterior part of a standard craniotomy around the Sylvian point. It can easily be identified on a lateral DSA, where it branches off the ECA and runs behind the external auditory meatus. Note that the DSA needs to be displayed sufficiently caudal to identify the origin of the PAA. The awareness among cerebrovascular surgeons about the presence of a PAA and knowledge about its anatomy may be valuable.

*Keywords:* cerebral revascularization, extracranial–intracranial arterial bypass, posterior auricular artery, middle cerebral artery

## 23.1 History and Initial Description

The posterior auricular artery (PAA) has been used for decades in reconstructive, and ear, nose, and throat surgery, because of its arterial supply to myocutaneous and myofascial flaps.[1,2] It lasted until some years ago, before this artery was used by neurosurgeons for extracranial–intracranial (ECIC) bypass surgery.[3–5]

The PAA supplies a small area behind the ear and the auricle itself. It is usually present as three to five small branches which anastomose with the superficial temporal artery (STA), but sometimes it is suitable as a donor artery for ECIC bypass surgery. In the majority, the PAA branches off the external carotid artery (ECA) just superior to the occipital artery, but in 10 to 15% cases it arises from the occipital artery after an occipitoauricular trunk (see ▶ Fig. 23.1). It continues between the mastoid tip and auricle, and in 33 to 50% cases, it is large enough to extend to the temporoparietal region.[6] In these cases, it runs almost vertically toward the vertex until a mean distance of 7.5 cm from the mastoid tip. Its course at approximately 1.2 cm posterior to the external auditory meatus

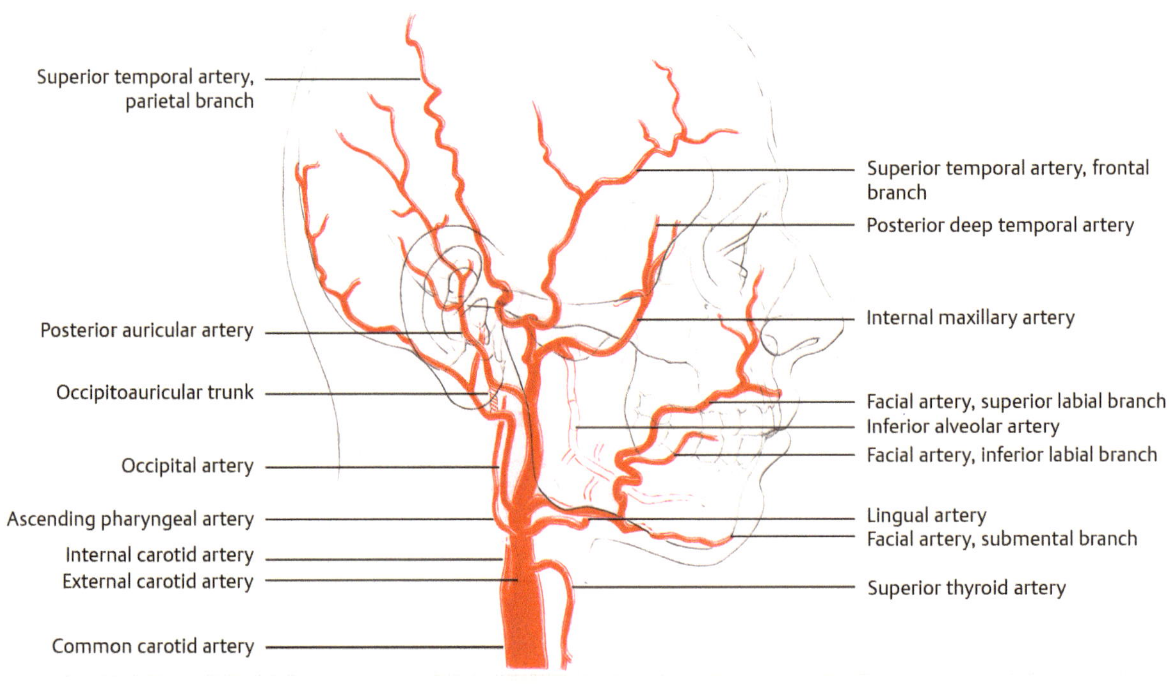


**Fig. 23.1** Simplified anatomy of posterior auricular artery.

is ideal for a bypass, because it is located at the posterior margin of a standard craniotomy around the Sylvian point. In 1.2 to 5.7% of cases, the PAA diameter is large enough to function as a donor artery.[3,6]

## 23.2 Indications

Sometimes the STA is not available as donor vessel for bypass surgery due to hypoplasia of the artery, sacrifice of the artery at previous craniotomy, damage of the artery during dissection, or if it has already been used for a bypass. In such cases, the PAA can be used as an alternative donor artery, if its diameter is large enough. Moreover, in case of refractory moyamoya disease with a standard ECIC bypass in situ, or in case of the need for a double-barrel bypass, the PAA can be used as an additional revascularization technique.[4] Cerebrovascular surgeons must be aware about a PAA when assessing the preoperative angiography of the ECA. When performing a craniotomy for moyamoya disease, knowledge about PAA anatomy may be valuable for planning proper incision and not damaging the PAA.

## 23.3 Key Principles

The PAA is easily identified on a lateral digital subtraction angiography (DSA), where it branches off the ECA and runs behind the EAC (see ▶ Fig. 23.2). In about half the cases, it extends until the temporoparietal region. The diameter must be large enough (> 1 mm) to be used as a donor artery. Its almost vertical course along the temporoparietal region locates the artery at the posterior margin of the standard craniotomy around the Sylvian point. Because only the posterior part of the temporal muscle must be dissected to mobilize to PAA for an ECIC bypass, it causes less injury to the muscle.

## 23.4 SWOT Analysis

### 23.4.1 Strengths

- Procedure comparable to that of STA–MCA bypass, proven to be a successful alternative.[3–5]
- Less injury to temporal muscle.
- Can be used with standard craniotomy around Sylvian point; rescue procedure in case of injury to STA.

### 23.4.2 Weakness

- Low availability of PAA of appropriate size (1.2–5.7%).

### 23.4.3 Opportunity

- To get more acquainted with the presence of an appropriately sized PAA in both neurosurgeons and neuroradiologists minds.

### 23.4.4 Threat

- The use of indirect bypass procedures in (refractory) moyamoya disease offers an alternative to direct bypass procedures such as PAA–MCA.

## 23.5 Contraindications

When the artery is too small (< 1 mm diameter) or not extending to the temporoparietal region, it cannot be used for a bypass. Due to the location of the artery, it is usually too short to revascularize the anterior cerebral artery territory. When a flow of more than 35 mL/min is anticipated, the PAA might not be patent enough to meet this flow rate.

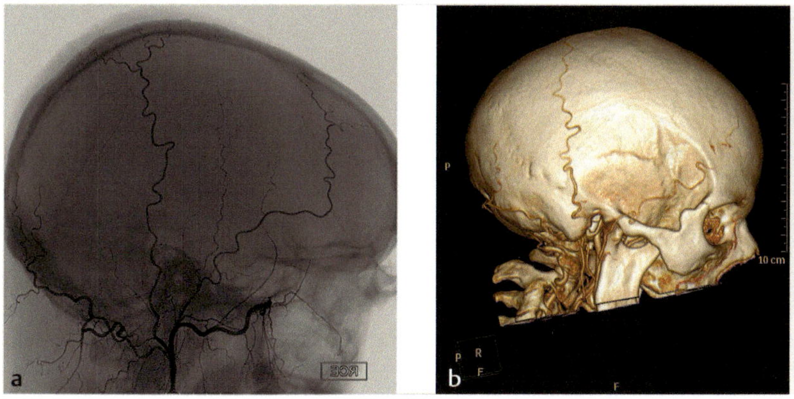

**Fig. 23.2** Digital subtraction angiography **(a)** and 3D reconstruction of CT angiography **(b)** of a right-sided large posterior auricular artery and superficial temporal artery.

## 23.6 Special Considerations

The preoperative DSA of the ECA needs to be displayed sufficiently caudal to identify the origin of the PAA. In addition, radiologists or neurosurgeons reporting the results of the DSA should be aware of the possible presence of a PAA that could be used as a donor artery.

## 23.7 Pitfalls, Risk Assessment, and Complications

The risks for a bypass using the PAA as a donor artery are comparable to that of the STA, and patients can be informed as such.

Although several case reports have described the successful use of the PAA, the long-term patency of this artery is unknown. Nevertheless, the indications, technique, and flow dynamics of the PAA at ECIC bypass surgery are comparable with that of the STA. Therefore, the long-term patency is judged to be comparable with that of an STA–MCA bypass.

## 23.8 Special Instructions, Position, and Anesthesia

Positioning and anesthesiological regimen are comparable to bypass surgery using the STA. It might make it easier to tape the auricle anteriorly to expose the PAA on its complete trajectory. Care should be taken that the auricle is not hypoperfused with this maneuver, because this can lead to ischemia of the auricle.

## 23.9 Patient Position with Skin Incision and Key Surgical Steps

The patient is positioned with a small roll under the ipsilateral shoulder with the head turned to the contralateral side and fixated in the headholder. The trajectory of the PAA and the craniotomy site are then exposed with taping the auricle anteriorly if necessary. The PAA is identified by doppler and/or digital palpation, and a straight incision directly over the artery is planned. As an alternative, one can use the cranial navigation software to draw the location of the PAA as well as the craniotomy. Depending on the area that needs reperfusion and in case of a more posterior location of the PAA, the incision can be made more curvilinear with extension toward anterior to expose the craniotomy site (see ▶ Fig. 23.3). For a double-barrel bypass with both the PAA and STA as donor arteries, a horseshoe or question mark incision can be made, taking care not to interrupt the PAA.

The PAA needs to be exposed and dissected from surrounding tissue at least from the level of the external acustic meatus (EAM) because the artery has to be transposed forward to reach the Sylvian point (see ▶ Fig. 23.4).

For artery dissection, craniotomy around the Sylvian point, and bypass technique, please refer to Chapter 9.

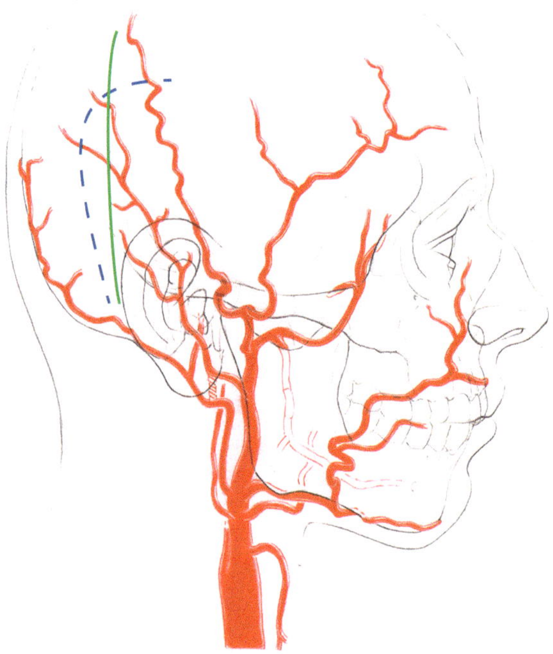

**Fig. 23.3** Incisions that can be used for exposure of the posterior auricular artery (PAA) for PAA–middle cerebral artery bypass (*orange*: straight incision; *blue*: curvilinear incision).

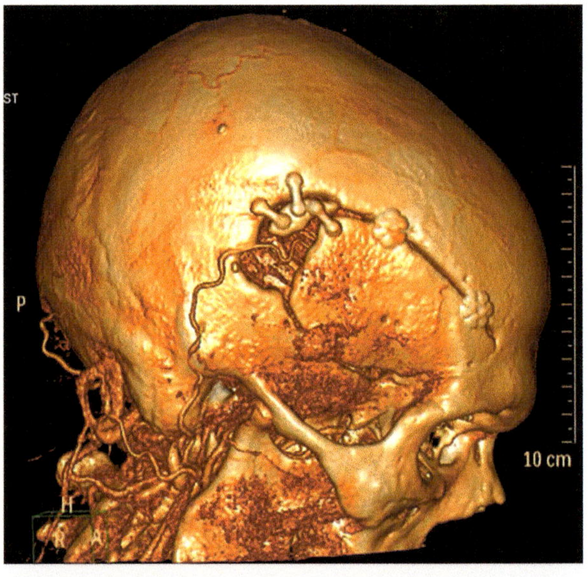


**Fig. 23.4** 3D reconstruction of CT-angiography showing the PAA deflected anteriorly to reach the Sylvian point.

## 23.10 Difficulties Encountered

- When a straight incision over the PAA is used, the craniotomy might be located too posteriorly to expose the Sylvian point.
- Preoperative planning is mandatory to prevent this error, and intraoperative navigation to plan the craniotomy site for localization of the optimal recipient vessel can be considered. Otherwise, a curvilinear incision can be used.
- The PAA only reaches until the posterior border of the craniotomy. Exposure of the artery from at least the level of the EAM makes it easier to transpose it forward.

## 23.11 Bailout, Rescue, and Salvage Maneuvers

The usage of alternative donor vessels, such as the STA or the occipital artery or interposition grafts.

## 23.12 Tips, Pearls, and Lessons Learned

- When the DSA is not showing the origin of the PAA, it might be mistaken for a parietal branch of the STA. In such cases, the incision might be planned too much anterior and the donor artery will not be found.
- Knowledge about the presence of a potential suitable PAA and its relation to the auricle and craniotomy makes preoperative planning easier and safer.

## References

[1] Choung PH. The auriculomastoid fasciocutaneous island flap: a new flap for orofacial reconstruction. J Oral Maxillofac Surg. 1996; 54(5): 559–567, discussion 568

[2] Gibb AG, Tan KK, Sim RS. The Singapore swing. J Laryngol Otol. 1997; 111(6):527–530

[3] Germans MR, Regli L. Posterior auricular artery as an alternative donor vessel for extracranial-intracranial bypass surgery. Acta Neurochir (Wien). 2014; 156(11):2095–2101, discussion 2101

[4] Horiuchi T, Kusano Y, Asanuma M, Hongo K. Posterior auricular artery-middle cerebral artery bypass for additional surgery of moyamoya disease. Acta Neurochir (Wien). 2012; 154(3):455–456

[5] Tokugawa J, Nakao Y, Kudo K, et al. Posterior auricular artery-middle cerebral artery bypass: a rare superficial temporal artery variant with well-developed posterior auricular artery-case report. Neurol Med Chir (Tokyo). 2014; 54(10):841–844

[6] Tokugawa J, Cho N, Suzuki H, et al. Novel classification of the posterior auricular artery based on angiographical appearance. PLoS One. 2015; 10(6):e0128723

# Index

*Note:* Page numbers set **bold** or *italic* indicate headings or figures, respectively.